Law and Ethics for Midwifery

Legal and ethical competence is a cornerstone of professional midwifery practice and an essential part of midwifery training. *Law and Ethics for Midwifery* is a unique and practical resource for student midwives.

Written by an experienced midwifery lecturer, this text draws on a wide variety of real-life case studies and focuses particularly on the core areas of accountability, autonomy and advocacy. Opening with two chapters providing overviews respectively of ethical theories and legislation, the book is then arranged thematically. These chapters have a common structure which includes case studies, relevant legislation, reflective activities and a summary, and they run across areas of concern from negligence through safeguarding to record-keeping.

Grounded in midwifery practice, the text enables student midwives to consider and prepare for ethical and legal dilemmas they may face as midwives in clinical practice.

Elinor J. Clarke is a Senior Lecturer in Midwifery at Coventry University, UK. Elinor trained at Birmingham Women's Hospital and registered as a midwife in 1982. She worked in hospital and community midwifery before undertaking a PG Certificate in Adult Education. Elinor gained a Masters in Child Care Law and Practice at Keele University. The author has many years of teaching on undergraduate and postgraduate courses in midwifery, nursing and allied healthcare professions. Elinor has considerable experience in teaching law and ethics to student midwives. She has served as an elected member of council for the Royal College of Midwives (RCM). Elinor has particular interest in ethical and legal issues around safeguarding babies and female genital mutilation (FGM). Elinor is a member of an FGM national clinical group.

Law and Ethics for Midwifery

Elinor J. Clarke

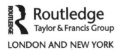
Routledge
Taylor & Francis Group

LONDON AND NEW YORK

First published 2015
by Routledge
2 Park Square, Milton Park, Abingdon, Oxon OX14 4RN

and by Routledge
711 Third Avenue, New York, NY 10017

Routledge is an imprint of the Taylor & Francis Group, an informa business

British Library Cataloguing-in-Publication Data
A catalogue record for this book is available from the British Library

Library of Congress Cataloging in Publication Data
Clarke, Elinor J., author.
Law and ethics for midwifery / written by Elinor J. Clarke.
p. ; cm.
Includes bibliographical references and index.
I. Title.
[DNLM: 1. Midwifery--ethics--England--Case Reports. 2. Midwifery--legislation
& jurisprudence--England--Case Reports. 3. Ethical Theory--England--
Case Reports. 4. Nurse Midwives--ethics--England--Case Reports. 5. Nurse
Midwives--legislation & jurisprudence--England--Case Reports. WQ 160]
RG950
174.2'982–dc23
2014049470

ISBN: 978-0-415-67524-6 (hbk)
ISBN: 978-0-415-67525-3 (pbk)
ISBN: 978-1-315-69105-3 (ebk)

Typeset in Garamond
by Fakenham Prepress Solutions, Fakenham, Norfolk NR21 8NN

This book is dedicated to two amazing women:
Dr Jenny Burton and Baroness Ruth Rendell

Contents

Acknowledgements

I thank my husband, Richard, who enabled me to have time and space to complete the manuscript for this book. I also thank him for the patience and fortitude to encourage me to persevere when publication seemed a long way away. I also thank my children for being patient while I worked long hours in the cabin!

My thanks also go to work colleagues who learned quickly not to ask 'Did you have a relaxing weekend?' and 'How's the book coming on?'. Especial thanks to my parents, who did ask 'How many words?' and 'How's it doing?' and then left it as 'work in progress'.

Thank you to students for asking questions, discussing dilemmas and eventually recognising that midwifery cannot be studied in isolation, and that ethics and law are fundamental to all aspects of midwifery care.

Finally, thank you to all mothers, babies and families that I have been privileged to share childbirth experiences with.

Statutes and statutory instruments

Statutes

Title	Year	Source/comments
Abortion Act	1967	Chapter 12
Abortion Amendment Act	1990	Chapter 12
Abortion Regulations Act	1991	Chapter 12
Abortion (Amendment) Regulations Act	2008	Chapter 12
Access to Health Records Act	1990	Chapter 6
Adoption Act	1976	Chapter 16
Adoption Act	2002	Chapter 16
Adoption and Children Act	1976	Chapter 13
Births and Deaths Registration Act	1953	Section 1 (4) 42 days Section 10 (1) Fathers Section 11 (1) Qualified Informant
Children Act	1989	Section 44–45 Chapter 9
Children Act	2004	Chapter 9
Congenital Disabilities (Civil Liability) Act	1976	Chapter 5, 17
Coroners and Justice Act	2009	Chapter 5, 17
Data Protection Act (DPA)	1998	Chapter 6
Disability Discrimination Act	1995	Chapter 12, 17
Domestic Violence, Crime and Victims Act	2004	Chapter 9
Domestic Violence, Crime and Victims (Amendment) Act	2012	Chapter 9
Family Law Reform Act	1969	Chapter 7
Female Genital Mutilation Act	2003	Chapter 9
Freedom of Information Act (FIA)	2000	Chapter 6, 18

Title	Year	Source/comments
Health Act	2006	Chapter 17
Health Act	2009	Chapter 17
Health Care Professions Act	2002	Chapter 5, 17
Health and Social Care Act	2001	Chapter 6
Health and Social Care Act	2008	Chapter 2, 7
Health and Social Care Act	2012	Chapter 7; Section 1, 3, 4, 5, 10, 11, 12, Chapter 1; Section 61, 62, 68 Chapter 3; 81 Part 8 (NICE) Chapter 2; HSIC Part 10 Abolition NPSA
Health Rights Act	1998	Chapter 6
Hospital Complaints Procedure Act	1985	Chapter 17, 18
Human Fertilisation & Embryology Act	1990	Chapter 12, 15
Human Fertilisation & Embryology (Deceased Fathers) Act	2003	Chapter 6
Human Fertilisation & Embryology Act	2008	Did not change the legislation (remains at 24 weeks)
Human Medicines Regulations Act	2012	Chapter 8
Human Organ Transplant Act	1989	Chapter 7
Human Tissue Act	1961	Chapter 7
Human Tissue Act	2004	Chapter 6
Infant Life Preservation Act	1929	Chapter 13
Infanticide Act	1938	Chapter 13
Medicines Act	1968	Chapter 7; Section 58 (2)
Mental Capacity Act	2005	Chapter 8
Mental Health Act	1983	Chapter 8
Mental Health Act	2007	Chapter 8
Midwives Act	1902	Chapter 4
Midwives Act	1918	Chapter 4
Midwives Act	1926	Chapter 4
Misuse of Drugs Act	1971	Chapter 8
Misuse of Drugs Regulations Act	2001	Chapter 8
National Health Service & Community Care Act	1990	Chapter 2, 11, 17 Health of the Nation (review of the NHS) White paper Working for patients Radical reform of the NHS
National Health Service Act	2006	Chapter 5

Title	Year	Source/comments
Nurses, Midwives and Health Visitors Act	1992	Chapter 3, 4
Nurses, Midwives and Health Visitors Act	1997	Chapter 3, 4
Offences Against the Persons Act	1861	Chapter 17
Prohibition of Female Circumcision Act	1985	Chapter 9
Public Interest Disclosure Act	1998	Chapter 6
Public Records Act	1958	Chapter 6
Safeguarding Vulnerable Groups Act	2006	Chapter 47
Surrogacy Arrangements Act	1985	Chapter 14

Statutory instruments

Title	Year / No.	Focus
SI 1977/1850	1997 No. 1850	Abolished the need for medical supervisors
Prescription Only Medicines (Human Use) Order No. 1997 (SI 1997/1830)	1997	Medicines
The Nurses and Midwives Approval Order SI 1983 No. 873 33/1175	1983	Principle rules Teaching qualifications
The Nursing and Midwifery (Qualifications) Order SI 1983 No. 884	1983	Identification of midwifery qualifications
SI 1986 No. 786	1986	Education
SI 1989 No. 1456	1989	Education
SI 1990 No. 1624	1990	Midwifery training
SI 1991 No. 135 The Nurses, Midwives and Health Visitors (Registration) Modification Rules Approval Order	1991	Changes to principle rules
SI 1993 No. 210 The Nurses, Midwives and Health Visitors (Midwives Amendment) Rules Approval Order	1993	Changes to Midwives Rules
SI 1996 No. 3101	1996	New rules and code
Nursing and Midwifery Order 2001 SI 2002 No. 253	2002 No. 253	Article 5.2.b NMC to prescribe requirements regarding good character
NMC (Education, Registration & Registration Appeals) Rules Order of Council 2004 (SI 2004 No. 1767)	2004 No. 1767 Rule 6	
SI 2013 No. 261 (National Health Service, England, Mental Health, England, Public Health England) Regulations	2012	Updated Midwives Rules

Title	Year / No.	Focus
NHS, England, Mental Health, England, Public Health, England. The National Health service and Public Health (Functions and Miscellaneous Provisions) Regulations 2013	2013 No. 261	Part 3 (9, 10, 11) notification of births and deaths (home birth)
SI 2014 No. 1887 The Healthcare and Associated Professions (Indemnity Arrangements)	2014 No. 1887	Professional indemnity arrangements

Cases

Legal cases

Legal Case	Location	Chapter
P, C & S v *The UK* [2002]	2 FLR 631	9
Pearce v *United Bristol Healthcare Trust*	48 BMLR 118	6, 17
Pretty v *UK* [2002]	2 FCR 97	6
Pretty v *DPP* [2001]	UK HL	
St Georges Heathcare Trust v *S* [1998]	3 All ER 673	6
Sidaway v *Board of Governors of Bethlem Hospital* [1985]	1 All ER 643 HL	6, 17
RCN v *DHSS* (1981)	1 All ER 801, 1 All ER 545	12
Reynolds v *North Tyneside Health Authority* [2002]	Lloyds Rep Med	17
R v *Anderson* (1975)		12
Daniel Pelka	31 July 2013	9
Diane Blood (1999)	2 All ER 687	4
Court of appeal	CA 269–271	
Diane Blood (2003)		
R v *HFEA ex parte Blood*		
R v *Bourne* (1939)	1 KB 687	12
Re *MB* [1997] (adult: medical treatment)	2 FLR 426	6
Re *A* [1987] (adoption, surrogacy)	2 All ER 826	16
Re *B* 1991 (minor, abortion)	*The Independent* 22 May 1991 (Family Division)	12
Re *C* [1985] payments [2002]	1 FLR 909	16
Re *P* [1987] (family)	2 FLR 421	16
Re *S* [1992] (adult, refusal of treatment)	4 All ER 671	6
Re *T* (adult, refusal of treatment)		6
Re *W* [1992]	3 WLR 758	6
R (Axon) v *Secretary of State for Health* [2006]	EWHC 37	4, 12
Potts v *NWRHA* 1983	QB348	6
Jamie Whitaker 2003	HFEA	6
Mr A and Mr B 2002 (IVF mix up)	High Court 2003	6, 17
Justice Butler-Sloss	Lloyds Rep Med	
Leeds Teaching Hospitals NHE Trust v *Mr A*		
Whitehouse v *Jordan* (House of Lords) [1981]	1 All ER 267	17
Wilsher v *Essex Area Health Authority* [1986]	3 All ER 801	17
Natalie Evans 2005	Court of appeal ECHR 2005	6
Beth Williams 2014 (dead husband's frozen sperm)	HFEA	6

Professional misconduct cases

General Dental Council (GDC 2013) Mr Omar Addow (56 years), Birmingham UK. Misconduct hearing: struck off the GDC register for allegedly offering to perform FGM.

General Medical Council (GMC 1993) Doctor Farooque Hayder Siddique, London, UK. Struck off the GMC register for misconduct.

General Medical Council GMC (2004) Doctor struck off the GMC register for misconduct.

Nursing and Midwifery Council (2007) Midwife struck off NMC register for professional misconduct (Paul Beland).

Nursing and Midwifery Council (NMC 2013) Midwife struck off for performing male circumcision without due care (baby died following a haemorrhage) (Grace Adeleye).

Preface

Why should midwives be interested in ethics and ethical theory?

Midwifery is an old and honourable profession, which meets the needs of childbearing women and their families. While the physical act of childbirth itself is fundamentally the same as it ever was, childbirth practices, women's wishes, medical techniques, culture and our understanding of interventions are constantly evolving and changing. Midwifery has also changed and while midwives remain predominantly female, it is unethical to exclude males from joining the profession and the term midwife is not gender-specific. Midwifery practice is changed and shaped by values, beliefs and cultures, which impact upon the relationship between women and midwives. Midwives encounter ethical dilemmas on a daily basis and to ignore or fail to consider the relationship between ethics and midwifery is impossible. Midwifery education is grounded in ethics; from clinical skills through codes of conduct to professional development, NHS Constitution to evidence-based practice, mentorship to preceptorship, birth plans to care pathways, the midwife is immersed in ethical issues. In 1994, a 62-year-old Italian lady became the oldest mother, raising the ethical dilemma: just because something is possible to achieve should it be undertaken? Professor Servino Antinori has subsequently pursued other assisted reproductive techniques which may be morally questionable. Midwives are and will continue to be ethically challenged and a personal midwifery ethic needs to be identified and understood.

Ethical theory is the term given to the explanations of and application of reasoning based upon personal values, morals and behaviours. Midwifery care and maternity services are founded upon an ethical basis regarding childbirth. Attitudes and behaviours may be personal, such as honesty, compassionate and professional. Maternity services can also be ethically based, such as evidence-based, equitable and safe.

Women-focused care is a priority for midwives, and constraints of services, managers' requirements for data (evidence of efficiency and effectiveness) and the need for evidence to support practice challenges midwives to remain focused upon the basics of care. Saving mothers' lives during childbirth necessitates midwives paying attention to five aspects of care (five Cs): continuity, communication, compliance, constraints and complacency (Mander, 2011).

Why should midwives be interested in law?

Midwives should be interested in legislation because it affects all aspects of the role and responsibilities of a midwife. Regardless of where a midwife works or the type of practice the midwife is engaged in, it is necessary to understand the legal framework for practice. Midwives are accountable for their personal and professional conduct and practice. Midwives are required to have an understanding of appropriate ethical, legal and professional frameworks. In the interests of the public, purchasers and providers of services, other healthcare professionals as well as the users of maternity services, it is necessary for midwives to fully understand the implications. The NMC (2008b) identify that 'In order to provide appropriate care for women and their families midwives need to act within the law and help women to make choices, find solutions to care and consent to care.'

If it was not for the tenacity of our forebears, midwifery legislation in the form of the Midwives Act 1902 would not exist, and the right to practise midwifery as we know it today would not be possible. The Midwives Act 1902 gives protection to the name, role and responsibilities of midwives. The system of supervision in midwifery is 'enshrined in legislation'; other professions do not share this requirement. Midwifery supervision serves many purposes, but fundamentally it is intended to protect the public, enable all midwives to continue to develop following registration, and receive support when struggling to fulfil their professional role. The annual notification of intention to practise (NoP) enables the regulating body (Nursing and Midwifery Council – NMC) to fulfil its legal duties, namely protection of the public, by maintaining a live register of all midwifery practitioners (clinical, educational, research and midwifery consultants). Changes to legislation can alter and amend existing statute and midwives need to be proactive in the legislative process.

Control and regulation of midwives

Midwives and midwifery practice are currently regulated and controlled by the NMC. Most midwives, when asked, will say that the NMC is a statutory body, whose function is to protect the public. It is uncertain how many midwives would be able to identify the relevant legislation or the ethical theory and principles which underpin the role and responsibility of either the NMC or midwifery. It is a personal concern of mine as to how many midwives incorrectly think that the Royal College of Midwives (RCM) fulfils the above role. Confusion regarding regulation, professional practice, education and responsibilities need resolving. The RCM and the NMC are very different and distinct organisations: statute defines the NMC, while the RCM attempts to influence statute. A better understanding of English Law may clarify the issue. Midwives and midwifery are controlled by regulations enshrined in legislation. Primary legislation in the form of statute, such as the Midwives Act 1902, identifies how midwives and midwifery practice is controlled. While some controls of midwifery (registration) are in common with other professions, others, such as supervision, are unique. In addition the Health Care Professions Act (2002, §25) identifies the establishment of an overarching regulatory body: the Council for Healthcare Regulatory Excellence (CHRE), whose function is to regulate the regulators.

Change and ethics and law

Keeping up to date with legislation and case law is challenging. However it is important that the law evolves and changes. New legislation may be necessary to meet a developing issue such as the commercialisation of surrogacy, physical abuse or where there is an ethical dilemma (rights of the mother versus the rights of the fetus). Sometimes, court cases do not come to or reach a good outcome, or reach a verdict which if followed would not be considered ethical. An example is the brief venture into forced Caesarean sections, whereby women were subjected to a court order to undergo a Caesarean section delivery due to fetal compromise and likely intrauterine death. A court order requiring a woman to undergo major surgery against her wishes, for the purpose of 'saving' an unborn baby, is removing her basic human right to determine what happens to her (autonomy). Pivotal cases such as *Re S (Adult-refusal of treatment)* [1992] ordered a Caesarean section against the woman's wishes, breached her fundamental human rights, increased her risk of subsequent ill health and provided opportunity for other cases to follow suit. If this case set a precedent, then other similar cases would need to come to the same result. This example illustrates how potentially ethically unsound case law can be. A poor decision should not be applied to another situation. Subsequent case law has not gone down the route of enforced Caesarean section. Even if the facts of the case share some similarity, it is not ethical to set a precedent in such complex cases, each must be considered individually, especially when complicated by other variables such as age, mental health and use of medication.

Another reason for students to be interested in ethics, legislation and case law is the context of maternity services. It is one of the most highly litigious areas (in terms of cost) of healthcare. Of cases held at the National Health Service Litigation Authority (NHSLA), currently 20 per cent concern obstetrics and childbirth cases. The NHSLA identified an expenditure of £729.1 million in 2010–2011. Care should be taken when considering this figure as the amount includes damages paid to claimants (patients, staff and members of the public) as well as legal costs incurred on both sides (claimant and defence lawyers). The NHSLA (2011) also identified a continued rise in the number of claims recorded under the Clinical Negligence Scheme for Trusts (CNST) and Liabilities to Third Parties Scheme (LTPS). While it can be argued that the number of cases for some trusts have not increased, the costs incurred in investigation, preparation for court, fees and payments ensure that NHS trusts cannot afford not to invest in providing high standards of clinical care and effective and efficient services with a good approach to user satisfaction.

Historical aspects of law and midwifery education

Law was introduced into the midwifery curriculum in the late 1980s (Jones and Jenkins, 2004). Students were usually given an overview of the English legal system, including the courts and specific legislation such as the Abortion Act 1967, and focused on professional issues (regulations, rules, codes and supervisors of midwives) as well as legal obligations of a midwife attending a home delivery (Flint, 1986). During the 1980s midwives who were fortunate enough to undertake professional development in the form of an Advanced Diploma in Midwifery (ADM) were provided with the opportunity to critically analyse midwifery regulation and were further educated in other legal aspects, such as independent midwifery and indemnity insurance. Mary Cronk and Caroline Flint captured the specific legal issues relevant to the midwives working in the community in 1989. After a brief overview of the legislation, the authors focus on the Midwives Rules (available from the then United Kingdom Central Council at a cost of £1) and professional conduct. A section of the *British Journal of Midwifery* was dedicated to the national bodies to enable midwives to improve their understanding of the regulation and control of midwifery (Henderson, 1995). The first book dedicated specifically to the legal aspects of midwifery was published in 1994 (Dimond, 1994). The foreword, by Dame Margaret Brain (at the time president of the RCM), identified that 'it is essential that all midwives, regardless of their place of work or type of practice, fully understand the legal framework within which they practice' (Brain, 1994: vi). Since 1994 a succession of legal textbooks for midwives have been produced (Dimond 2002, 2006a, 2013; Jenkins 1995; Jones and Jenkins, 2004), all of which reinforce the message that midwives need to be familiar with the legislative process, have an understanding of litigation and accountability, comply with the statutory provisions associated with childbirth and uphold professional practice. Having an understanding of law and ethics is important, then, but being able to apply this to all aspects of midwifery practice is associated with professional development. Midwives need to develop skills for ethical and legal decision making. Hence the need for *Law and Ethics for Midwifery*!

Why this book, *Law and Ethics for Midwifery*?

The report of the Public Accounts Committee (2014) identifies that

> Having a baby is the most common reason for admission to hospital in England and, in 2012, there were almost 700,000 live births. The number of births has increased by almost a quarter in the last decade, placing increasing demands on the NHS maternity services. Maternity care is thought to have cost the NHS around £2.6 billion in 2012–2013.

Maternity cases account for one-third of total clinical negligence payments and maternity clinical negligence claims have risen by 80 per cent over the last five years. Nearly one-fifth of trusts' spending on maternity services (some £480 million in total, equivalent to £700 per birth) is for clinical negligence cover. The NHS Litigation Authority has recently produced helpful research on the causes of maternity claims, looking at data from the last ten years. The most common reasons for maternity claims have been mistakes in the management of labour, or relating to Caesarean sections and errors resulting in cerebral palsy.

Pre-registration midwifery education currently consists of a combination of theory and clinical practice. Student midwives are unable to graduate if they cannot meet requirements for both theory and practice. While the midwifery curriculum is heavy, ethical thinking and decision making are fundamental to the role and responsibilities of a midwife. *Law and Ethics for Midwifery* defines the subject, considers medical and other ethical theory, and with the use of case studies illustrates the ethical decision-making process. The use of case studies is a practical approach to enabling students to understand theory and practice. For many healthcare practitioners consideration of the law and legal cases is a daunting prospect: 'It does not interest me', 'Its too difficult' or 'If I wanted to be a lawyer I would have done a law degree' are common comments made by students who have yet to recognise that clinical practice does require a good understanding of law and the legal system. Wheeler (2012) considers the English legal system to be the drier notion of law, but recognises that students do require an understanding of the English legal system and how it can affect them and their practice as both students and registered practitioners. Initial student protestations are often followed by a gradual interest when students realise that ethics and law permeates every aspect of their lives (personal and private, as well as professional and within the wider society). Law is a complex subject and requires an appetite and motivation for thought, memory and critique – all higher-level academic skills. Law and legal proceedings are not for the faint-hearted, those lacking stamina or experiencing headaches. The main reasons that midwives may find the law difficult is the use of legal jargon and terminology, hierarchical structure, sections, and finding statutes and cases. Just like labour, English law can be progressive, arrested and complicated. This book is unlike other texts concerning law and ethics for healthcare in that it is specifically intended to focus upon the difficult, different and debatable aspects of midwifery. It has relevance to modern midwifery practice, interests the reader in current issues, and enables midwives to look through a different lens.

Law and Ethics for Midwifery uses the format of identifying the core aspects of ethics and law, and the use of case studies enables students to critically analyse them in relation to specific 'real' dilemmas. The method of using case studies to broaden knowledge and understanding of legal and ethical issues was undertaken by Jones (2000a). She suggests that this approach is useful to both undergraduates and postgraduate students. Case studies also enable the midwife to broaden and develop professional discussion. The case study approach will help midwives and students to ground midwifery practice and use ethical decision making when faced with dilemmas in the changing maternity services. Of particular importance is the emphasis on the legal aspects, which help to focus the midwife regarding statutory requirements. The cases are chosen to enable the linking of theory to practice, and their grounding in real dilemmas will help to bring law and ethics for midwifery to life.

The Legal Aspects of Midwifery (Dimond, 1994) was the first law textbook specifically aimed at midwives (she had previously published *Legal Aspects of Nursing*). Dimond is a prolific writer and has also published law textbooks for physiotherapy, occupational therapy, and radiology and radiography, as well as specifically focusing upon medicines, consent, pain management and mental capacity. In her introduction to *The Legal Aspects of Midwifery* she states that 'the midwife cannot practice her profession in ignorance of the law' (Dimond, 1994: xi). Judging by the content of the first edition, Dimond meant that it was necessary to have an understanding of professional issues as well as statute and accountability. Since 1994 there have been many changes in maternity services: to legislation, clinical practice, and expectations of women, work environments and education. To be a modern midwife, one needs to be able to fulfil the role and responsibilities of a midwife while remaining cognisant of the effects the above changes have on practice. In addition, the modern midwife also has to ensure that whenever he or she delegates any aspect of the responsibilities that he or she supervises, and that standards are maintained.

My experiences of working in midwifery education for the last 25 years suggest that there is a need for midwives to not only have an understanding of law, ethical theory and principles, but to be able to reflect and apply these to midwifery practice. Developing skills of ethical reasoning and the provision of ethical-based care is just as important as providing evidence-based practice.

Abbreviations

ADM	Advanced Diploma in Midwifery
AQP	any qualified provider
ARM	Association of Radical Midwives
ARM	artificial rupture of membranes
ART	assisted reproductive technology
BECG	Birthplace in England Collaborative Group
BFI	baby friendly initiative
BNF	British National Formulary
CAM	complementary and alternative medicine
CCGs	Clinical Commissioning Groups
CHRE	Council for Healthcare Regulatory Excellence
CMB	Central Midwives Board
CNST	Clinical Negligence Scheme for Trusts
COTS	Childlessness Overcome Through Surrogacy
CPD	continuous professional development
CPS	Crown Prosecution Service
CQC	Care Quality Commission (England's healthcare regulator)
CTB	Children's Trust Board
ECHR	European Court of Human Rights
ECJ	European Court of Justice
ECV	external cephalic version
ED	European Directive
EEC	European Economic Community
ELS	Existing Liabilities Scheme
EPR	electronic patient record
EU	European Union
EWO	education welfare officer
FGM	female genital mutilation
FGS	female genital surgery
FFT	Family and Friends Test
GDC	General Dental Council

GMC	General Medical Council
GP	General Practitioner
H&SC	Health and Social Care
HCPAC	House of Commons Public Accounts Committee
HCPC	Health and Care Professions Council
HEE	Health Education England
HPC	Health Professions Council
HRA	Human Rights Act
HSCIC	Health and Social Care Information Centre
ICM	International Confederation of Midwives
INP	independent and supplementary nurse prescribers
LME	Lead Midwife for Education
LSA	Local Supervising Authority
LSAMO	Local Supervising Authority Midwifery Officer
LSB	Local Safeguarding Boards
LSCS	lower segment Caesarean section
LTPS	Liabilities to Third Parties Scheme
MCA	Medicines Control Agency
MDA	Medical Devices Agency
MHRA	Medicines and Healthcare products Regulatory Agency
NAD	no abnormality detected
NHS	National Health Service
NHSLA	National Health Service Litigation Authority
NICE	National Institute for Health and Clinical Excellence
NM&HV	Nurses, Midwives and Health Visitors (Act)
NMC	Nursing and Midwifery Council
NoP	notification of intention to practise
NPSA	National Patient Safety Agency
NRLS	National Reporting Learning Service
PGD	patient group directive
PIL	patient information leaflet
PM	pharmacy medication
POM	prescription only medication
PPP	Personal Professional Profile
PREP	post-registration education and practice
PTSD	post-traumatic stress disorder
QCC	Quality Care Commission
RCA	root cause analysis
RCM	Royal College of Midwives
RCN	Royal College of Nursing
RCOG	Royal College of Obstetricians and Gynaecologists
RMP	registered medical practitioner
RTP	return to practice
SBAR	Situation, Background, Assessment, Recommendation
SCBU	special care baby unit

SI	Statutory Instrument
SI	serious incident
SoM	supervisor of midwives
UKCC	United Kingdom Central Council for Nursing, Midwifery and Health Visiting
UNICEF	United Nations International Children's Emergency Fund
WHO	World Health Organization

Part

1

Theory

1 Introduction to *Law and Ethics for Midwifery*

Knowledge and understanding of ethics and law are paramount to the midwife working in all environments and throughout the world. The purpose of the book is to assist midwives to have an understanding of appropriate ethical, legal and professional frameworks for caring and supporting childbearing women and their families. Of particular importance is the emphasis on the links between theory and practice. It aims to help health and social care practitioners, and specifically pre-registration midwives, understand how ethical dilemmas which occur during clinical practice can be explained by ethical theories and principles and how legislation and litigation has contributed and shaped practitioners' responses and actions.

Law and Ethics for Midwifery is not intended as a traditional textbook. This book is different in that it uses a case study approach (Stake, 1995). The intention is to identify relevant ethical and legal theory and principles, consider through the use of case study analysis an exploration of the ethical dilemmas and the legal implications faced by midwives, and explore the outcomes. The four spheres of accountability (Griffith *et al.*, 2010: 1) are fundamental to the case study chapters. Clinical midwifery practice is a part of an increasingly complex maternity care that is not based solely on routine, guidelines or procedures. Midwifery is an art and a science and as such requires midwifery care to be ethical and lawful, as well as evidenced-based. Relationships between women and midwives are based upon trust and sharing of knowledge, these ethical aspects of the role of the midwife are fundamental to the maternity services. Each case study chapter (6–18) will identify ethical issues and legal aspects, and provide a case study followed by a practice check and useful websites. This case study approach is intended to maximise learning. The book is intended primarily for undergraduate student midwives, but students across health and social care disciplines and other healthcare professionals in clinical practice will be familiar with the specific dilemmas and the experiences identified.

The author has chosen to consider issues which are controversial (abortion and surrogacy); inherently troublesome (assisted reproduction, termination of pregnancy, surrogacy, emergency Caesarean section); and contemporary issues (vulnerable women, birth environment, Caesarean section on demand, criminality of home birth). Ethical and legal aspects (as opposed to clinical care) of midwifery practice are also addressed (medicines, records and confidentiality). Ethical issues will be mainly addressed from a principles-based approach, with the exception of Chapter 17 which will be from a virtues approach. Frequently, textbooks steer away from controversial and complicated issues due to the complexity of the situation or fear of controversy of addressing 'sensitive' issues. Those authors who do tackle controversial or troublesome topics often prefer to address theoretical concepts only. The combining of theory and practice facilitates understanding of ethical concepts and an appreciation of how different people may approach a situation (Jones, 2000a). Midwives have historically been brave and tackled difficult situations, supported women's rights, fought for independence and found themselves to be different from other healthcare professionals. In many situations the midwife has been a lone voice in a variety of settings (social care, education, politics and finance). *Law and Ethics for Midwifery* should help midwives to raise ethical issues and support legislation which addresses the complexity of childbirth. There is a need to debate and discuss difficult or complex issues, to prepare midwives for the variety and complexity of the situations women and midwives experience throughout childbirth.

This book is intended to consider ethical as well as legal issues that are relevant to midwifery practice and to utilise a case study approach to enable the reader to develop understanding of the issues. Traditionally, a case study approach has helped midwives, doctors, midwifery and medical students to explore principles, pathology and skills surrounding childbirth. Clinical skills training has adopted a case study approach to emergency training or skills drills. Rayner *et al.* (2012) used a case study approach to explore maternity emergencies and critical illness. Students may find the case study to be an alternative learning tool, helping them to consider healthcare from different perspectives. The case is instrumental in enabling students to understand how ethical reasoning and different approaches may be adopted. Jones (2000a) suggested that undertaking discussion around constructed cases encourages additional student activity, enables ethical issues to be identified and possible actions to be taken. Case study analysis is a safe approach to explore complex issues. Some students will be familiar with a case study approach and this book adopts such an approach using 'real' incidents from clinical practice. All of the cases are based upon a real incident from clinical practice. The names, location and characters used in the case studies are fictitious to maintain the confidence of individuals, healthcare providers and health services. With regard to legal cases, these are in the public domain and their sources are attributed. The intention is to identify main theory, statute and principles and to then apply these to a clinical case (incident or experience). The author will provide illustrations of possible outcomes and identify relevant legislation and case law. It is recognised that the focus is UK centric; however, midwifery education and practice is informed by European Directives (EDs), which will be identified where relevant. It is not intended to provide an international legal approach at this time, although the author acknowledges the need for such an approach – maybe another book in the future? The learner will have the opportunity to reflect and evaluate their understanding. Throughout this approach professional regulation, conduct and performance will be considered and applied.

The development of law and ethics into the midwifery curriculum has been gradual. Student midwives currently undertake approximately 50 per cent of their programme (NMC, 2008b) in clinical practice and are exposed to and experience situations which challenge their own beliefs and attitudes, cause anxiety and trouble the students (ethical dilemmas). Clinical guidelines (NICE, 2014) increasingly control practice yet they may not be in keeping with a childbearing woman's wishes or expectations. It is understandable that midwives feel caught between providing evidenced-based care (professionally considered to be the goal) and responding to pressures of individualised or personalised care. Traditional education and training does not necessarily address these dilemmas. Midwifery textbooks such as *Mayes' Midwifery* (Sweet, 1982; Henderson and MacDonald, 2004) and *Myles Midwifery* (Fraser and Cooper, 2009) have identified midwifery regulation and rules. In 1994, Brigit Dimond published the first textbook specifically considering the legal aspects of midwifery, and further editions have followed (2002, 2006, 2013). Subsequently, Jones and Jenkins (2004) and Griffith *et al.* (2010) focused on the law and considered legal frameworks, while others (Jones, 2000a; Frith and Draper, 2004) identified ethical theory. In recent years midwifery interest in law and ethics has increased and been evident. Master's courses in medical ethics have been popular with midwives, especially those which encourage multidisciplinary approaches. Midwives (Symon, 1998, 2006a,b,d; Clarke, 1993) have also written about legal issues, published in midwifery journals as well as other publications. The Royal College of Midwives (RCM), in conjunction with Bond Solon (www.bondsolon.com), run annual legal conferences which are well supported and attract midwives who are keen to engage in debate around the legal issues surrounding childbirth. It is timely that a midwife writes *Law and Ethics for Midwifery* using a combination of theory and practice. There is a need for discussion and consideration of ethical and legal issues by midwives. A major conference on Childbirth and the Law (November 2012) at the Royal College of Surgeons in Edinburgh was billed as 'a series of presentations with case studies' which was inspiring and thought-provoking, thus reinforcing the notion that a case study approach is an appropriate way to consider legal and ethical issues.

While this book does not purport to be able to prevent midwives being the subject of legal proceedings, its intention is to discuss the dilemmas and concerns that challenge midwifery practice. It may also serve as an alert to future concerns and dilemmas for midwives. The attempts to criminalise home birth in the Czech Republic and threat to prevent home birth in other countries cannot be ignored. With new processes for commissioning of health services in England, home birth may also be in danger if midwives are unable to maintain skills and promote choice.

Teaching undergraduate students for a large number of years has shown me that for many students legislation does not start off as an interesting aspect of midwifery education. Students may feel that they want a midwifery focus and fewer 'other subjects', and often the relevance of §1.2.32 of a specific statute escapes them. I would suggest that law and ethics is a midwifery focus as ethical principles form fundamental aspects of our relationship with childbearing women. Legislation has an application relevant to midwives, midwifery and the maternity services. As an educator, legal matters are significant; very often students still find legislation and legislative process difficult to learn or apply. Apathy and disinterest in law making is counter-productive. The argument here is that if you do not engage in debate and discussion, and contribute to the legislative process, how could you criticise legislation if it does not then reflect or uphold your views? Gardner (2012c) suggests that midwives should be getting out there and making a difference. Midwives can help change and influence legislation and guidelines, which in turn allows mothers and babies to continue to receive the best possible care. Laws must carry the consensus of the people (Symon, 2011). At the time of writing this chapter, the Health and Social Care Bill is being debated in Parliament. This new legislation will have significant effects upon all health and social care workers (as well as patients). The RCM, along with others, is calling upon the government to scrap the Health and Social Care Bill. The concept of 'any qualified provider' (AQP) is not considered by the RCM to be appropriate for maternity services (Popay, 2012). There is concern that an open market approach does not promote collaboration, may fragment services and destabilise the National Health Service (NHS). In these austere times, savings and efficiencies are important and no one is sure that AQP will be cost-effective or safe, responsive and high quality. Midwives must, and should, contribute to the debate in an attempt to achieve legislation which safeguards maternity services and midwifery care. The right to choose to have a baby at home has been a subject of concern. Symon (2011) suggests that it is necessary to also look to other countries, as an insular attitude will not help and situations (he uses the example of the threat to choices for childbearing women) are not so different from those of the UK. Engagement and participation in the discussion, debates and arguments are vital if midwifery is to ensure that legislation supports the needs of childbearing women. The legal landscape is constantly changing and all healthcare practitioners need to keep up to date with the legislation and engage, contribute and shape it.

It is against this backdrop that *Law and Ethics for Midwifery* is written. Having justified the necessity for a new text, consideration will now be given to the content and layout of the book.

The book is divided into two parts. Here, we consider the structure of each chapter; a background/contextualisation of the themes; and justification of a case study approach. Part I provides: basic theoretical concepts such as ethical theory, principles and values; an introduction to statute and statutory instruments; and the statutory framework for midwifery. The specific formats for the chapters in Part I are: pre-requisites for the chapter, an introduction, theoretical content, conclusion, activities, opportunity for reflection and useful websites or further reading. The format for Part II chapters is similar: pre-requisites, introduction, the focus, during which main ethical and legal aspects are identified, followed by a case study, practice check, reader activity and useful websites.

Chapter 1: introduction to *Law and Ethics for Midwifery*

This chapter consists of an introduction to law and ethics, which is followed by an explanation of the case study approach. Key concepts are identified, namely autonomy, accountability and advocacy. Justification of the need for such a book is provided. **Reflection:** Driscoll's (1994, 2000, 2007) model of reflection.

Chapter 2: ethical theory, an introduction to ethical dilemmas and decision making

Chapter 2 provides an introduction to ethics and ethical theory. This chapter identifies that midwifery practice is complex and requires midwives to understand women's rights regarding care during childbirth. An ethical principle-based approach is considered in relation to decision making. Ethical principles of autonomy and advocacy will be considered. **Reflection:** Gibbs' (1988) model of reflection.

Chapter 3: legal theory, an introduction to English law and the English legal system

Building on legal theory (bills, statutes and breach), consideration is given to differences between criminal and civil law. **Reflection:** a new Midwives Act?

Chapter 4: ethical and legal theory: human, patient and maternity rights

This chapter considers how fundamental human rights are demonstrated and supported in maternity healthcare. It will identify how regulatory bodies support and protect basic human rights. Supervisors of midwives are identified as human rights defenders. Midwives as advocating human rights are explored. **Reflection:** Rolfe *et al.* (2001) reflective writing.

Chapter 5: ethical and legal theory: the legislative framework for midwifery

Ethics and law for midwives demonstrates how midwives are controlled and accountable for care provision. The specific statutory framework for midwifery practice and control of the midwifery profession is discussed. This chapter brings together theory and practice in that registration, regulation and midwives rules are explained. The four pillars of accountability (Griffith, 2012b) will be identified and explored. Midwifery regulation, registration and supervision of the midwife will also be addressed. Midwifery education and the role and responsibilities of the Lead Midwife for Education (LME) are considered. Accountability is reinforced and explained. **Reflection**: Professional portfolios.

Part II: case study chapters – midwifery practice

In Part II there is a change to the chapter structure, and subsequent chapters all have a case study approach. There are a number of chapters addressing ethical and legal issues around accountability and professional practice. Key issues regarding ethical-based midwifery care are considered (medicines, record-keeping and consent), followed by chapters which consider ethical and legal aspects of midwifery and maternity services. Chapters 6–18 all have a case study approach.

Chapter 6: consent and refusal

Consent is an ethical and legal issue. Respect for other human beings is demonstrated in a number of ways. Ensuring that individuals are able to make informed choices regarding their care is fundamental to respectful care. Obtaining consent is a professional requirement and a defence against an allegation of assault or battery. **Case study**: Consent.

Chapter 7: record-keeping

Record-keeping is a fundamental skill of all midwives. Role and responsibilities of a midwife with regard to demonstrating professional practice are considered. Different types of record-keeping and standards are addressed. **Case Study**: Fraud.

Chapter 8: medicines, midwives and the law

The midwife has a clear duty regarding the administration of medicines during childbirth. Ethical aspects are around the human rights, and legal aspects focus upon the relevant legislation and guidelines. The administration of medicines during pregnancy, labour and postnatally can be a dilemma especially when rights may be compromised. The use of drugs and medicines during pregnancy, labour and the postnatal period is a complex issue. Students may find it difficult to understand the responsibilities of the midwife as a prescriber. This chapter enables the reader to consider a variety of aspects of medicines. **Case Study**: Human factors approach.

Chapter 9: safeguarding vulnerable women and babies

Safeguarding is another difficult aspect of the role of the midwife. The health and wellbeing of women and their babies are fundamental to the maternity services. Inequalities, complexities and complicated lives impact upon the provision of midwifery care. Midwifery professional practice often encounters situations whereby the safety of the woman and her baby may be compromised. Women sometimes confide in midwives, offering information which may alert to the possibility of abuse and harm. Midwives themselves may also be at risk or subjected to harm as a result of their occupation. **Case study:** Removal of baby at birth.

Chapter 10: supervision of midwives

Supervision is enshrined in statute, yet midwives may be unsure, confused and suspicious of supervisors of midwives. This chapter explores the ethical and legal basis for supervision and illustrates how supervision promotes the human rights of childbearing women. **Case study:** Emily's waterbirth.

Chapter 11: birth environment

Home or hospital? Dangerous or safe? Clean or dirty? Public or private? Peaceful or noisy? Dull or vibrant? Free or expensive? Freedom to move or restricted movement? There are many birth environments in which women birth babies. This chapter considers the ethical (rights) and legal issues (requirements) regarding the environment of birth in the UK. **Case study:** Scott, Sherrie and the home birth.

Chapter 12: abortion

Many people, owing to religious, moral and personal beliefs, reject abortion. Abortion will always be controversial as personal beliefs, attitudes and values are not universally shared. Ethical principles will be considered. Abortion is illegal in the UK, yet the number of abortions carried out for women resident in the UK in 2011 was 189,931. This chapter explores how and when abortions may legally take place. The case study demonstrates application of ethical reasoning. **Case study:** Sara and termination of pregnancy.

Chapter 13: female circumcision, cutting and genital mutilation

Female genital mutilation (FGM) is illegal in the UK. Women accessing maternity services require holistic and sensitive midwifery care. This chapter explores the ethical dilemmas and legal situation regarding the 'circumcision of females'. **Case study:** Sylvie and her baby daughter.

Chapter 14: episiotomy

Episiotomy is a common intervention during childbirth, which involves a surgical procedure to the female perineum. Episiotomy is controversial but has been performed by midwives for years. Midwives are able to undertake this procedure and consequently need to be clear regarding their duty of care as well as their legal responsibilities. Controversially, this chapter will consider if or when episiotomy is FGM. **Case Study:** Sophie and midwifery skills.

Chapter 15: Caesarean section

This chapter explores both elective and emergency Caesarean sections. Should Caesarean sections be available on demand, and is it ethical to use the court to order a Caesarean section? With rising rates of Caesarean sections it would seem that more women will experience a surgical introduction to motherhood. Perhaps it is time to consider how midwives could be advocates for the woman with complex health needs. The concept of 'best interests' is discussed. Autonomy and advocacy are considered in relation to Caesarean section. **Case Study:** Sienna and elective Caesarean section.

Chapter 16: surrogacy

Surrogacy is not a new concept, yet UK legislation only came to the fore in 1996. Midwives need to be careful to ensure that they fulfil their role and responsibilities and avoid inadvertently breaking the law. Safeguarding and ethical aspects (duty of care) are considered in relation to surrogacy. Concerns are often around the surrogate's ability to 'give up' a baby that she has carried for the last nine months. Disputes are also thought to occur when there are concerns regarding the normality of the baby or specific behaviours of the surrogate mother. Organisations (for example Childlessness Overcome Through Surrogacy (COTS), British Surrogacy Centre and Surrogacy UK) have been established to support the process of surrogate motherhood. These organisations also enable women to contact potential surrogates. Midwives should be careful to ensure that their role and responsibilities in this situation are clear. This chapter considers the many ethical issues as well as considering the legality in the UK of abortion. **Case Study:** Siân, a surrogate mum.

The final chapters of *Law and Ethics for Midwifery* focus upon ethical and legal issues which other healthcare professionals can also find challenging. A quick glance at the national newspapers or listening to television or radio commercials will illustrate the nature and extent of complaints and blame attributed to healthcare professionals. Yet comparatively little time is dedicated in the NHS to training and management of complaints, particularly for midwives.

Chapter 17: professional malpractice, misconduct and negligence

Some may consider that negligence should be earlier in this book. The author, while acknowledging its importance, does not consider that professional malpractice and negligence should be the primary focus of a text on law and ethics for midwifery. Indeed, providing prominence to the topic of negligence would seem to reinforce the notion that midwifery care and maternity services are in a dreadful state and that it is dangerous to birth babies in England today, which is certainly not the case. The placement of this chapter on negligence is deliberate.

Having a baby is the most common reason for admission to hospital in the UK. When things go wrong the financial and emotional costs are high. Ethical and legal frameworks concerning healthcare generally were the focus of Chapters 1–5; this chapter will focus on professional malpractice, misconduct and negligence. Professional regulation, clinical negligence investigations and litigation are used to measure the safety of a service. **Case Study:** Sasha and midwifery competence.

Chapter 18: whistleblowing and complaints

The expectations of women accessing maternity services are high. *Changing Childbirth* (Department of Health, Expert Maternity Group, 1993) identifies choice, continuity and control as being expectations. *Delivering Expectations* (Department of Health, 2010c) outlines how childbirth should be safe but also emotionally satisfying. Maternity services have been stretched and diluted to the point whereby midwives are stressed and women's choices reduced. Blowing the whistle on malpractice and raising concerns are ways in which midwives can safeguard standards: the dilemma for the midwife is how to go about this. **Case study:** Sharon and a busy shift on the labour ward.

Throughout a programme of midwifery education (NMC, 2009b), the care and concern for childbearing women will be the focus of your studies. All activities centre upon the health and wellbeing of the woman and her baby. The NMC make it clear that at all times this is paramount. For some students the acquisition of EU criteria identified by the European Parliament (EEC Midwives Directive 1980) during the programme may be challenging. Without compliance to the EU criteria the student is not considered eligible for registration or working in other EU countries. Students may feel caught between the necessity to achieve EU criteria (e.g. number of deliveries) and the need to provide sensitive and compassionate midwifery care. The dilemmas around vaginal examination are a good illustration of the conflict between women's experiences and the gaining of experience to be confident and competent as a midwife.

Chapter summary

This introductory chapter has set the scene for *Law and Ethics for Midwifery*. Throughout the book the reader will find a series of case studies. These case studies are not fictitious. Some are based upon incidents experienced in clinical practice and clinical cases which have been published; others are cases which have gone to court (legal cases). The case study approach is considered to be useful to enable students to consider a number of perspectives and to support critical thinking. Students may also find the case study provides a trigger for further exploration. For example, Chapter 12 deals with abortion and the case study focuses upon a woman's decision to seek a termination of pregnancy. Students may like to explore termination of pregnancy further and the chapter may trigger an interest in international aspects, women's experiences, inheritance, or a whole host of other aspects. The chapter titles are relevant to modern midwifery and their content considers key ethical midwifery issues of autonomy, advocacy and accountability, and key legal issues such as regulation, registration and supervision. It is important for midwives to be cognisant of the law, but it is equally important for midwives to be participants in law making. Current midwifery education addresses the legal and ethical issues around childbearing, and students are exposed to a variety of situations and complexities which require them to comply with the law. Midwife-led care may save the NHS money (Dabrowski, 2012), but midwives still have to ensure that quality, safety and choice are delivered. The introduction and introductory chapters have not used the case study approach, which will be evident in subsequent chapters; an opportunity to reflect is provided instead.

Reflection

Using Driscoll's (1994, 2000, 2007) model of reflection based around the three stem questions of 'what?', 'so what?' and 'now what?', consider the following:

- **What** opportunities exist for midwives to engage in law and ethics?
- **So what** are the experiences of midwives who have been involved in litigation? Consider the experiences of midwives who have experienced court, attended an NMC professional hearing or been an expert witness.
- **Now what?** Identify any gaps in your knowledge or understanding around legislation. Plan to engage in consultations with the NMC. Consider how you could influence and shape future legislation.

Activities

1. Ask midwives if they have any experiences of going to court. Find out what it feels like to witness the law in action.
2. Keeping up to date with regulations, legislation and current issues can be difficult. Take some development time to access the useful websites found at the end of every chapter.
3. To keep up to date with current ethical and legal issues, check out the Parliamentary reports in each edition of the *RCM Midwives* magazine.

Useful websites

Legislation and Bills: www.legislation.gov.uk
Nursing and Midwifery Council (NMC): www.nmc-uk.org
Royal College of Midwives (RCM): www.rcm.org.uk

To find out more about basic human rights, reproductive rights and children's rights, the following websites are suggested:

Amnesty International: www.amnesty.org.uk
UNICEF: www.unicef.org.uk
White Ribbon Alliance: www.whiteribbonalliance.org
World Health Organization: www.who.int/en

2 Introduction to ethical theory and dilemmas

Pre-requisites for this chapter

It is helpful if you are able to think about ethical dilemmas that you have encountered in clinical environments. While reading this chapter you could apply theory to those situations

Introduction

Ethical theory, ethical behaviour and ethical practice will be the focus of this chapter. Justification for including a chapter on ethical theory is that 'On first hearing the word "ethics" many people believe they know what it means but would have difficulty explaining it' (Jones, 2000a: 4). As identified in the preface, ethical theory and principles have been found in the midwifery curricula since the 1980s. Traditional ethical theory has been used to justify and explain ethical decision making with regard to midwifery care (Jones, 2000a). A midwifery code of ethics (ICM, 1993) was confirmed at the 23rd International Congress in Vancouver. The Midwives' International Code of Ethics covers midwifery relationships, midwifery practice, professional responsibilities and the advancement of midwifery knowledge and practice (ICM, 1993).

So what does ethics in the context of midwifery care mean and can midwives explain it? Ethics may be considered to be about behaviour and doing good or treating people well; so are midwives who undertake artificial rupture of membranes (ARM) behaving unethically? Debating the different approaches to professional practice and the reasons or justification for them is part of the ethos of midwifery practice. This chapter will develop these themes to review the ethical basis for midwifery.

Midwives need to be able to work in partnership with women and have an ability to provide information, identify risks and benefits, and discuss and debate all aspects of care. Midwifery relationships such as partnership, respect of choices, decision making, inter-professional working and collaboration are all-important ethical behaviours. Even the concept of partnership has ethical connotations. Midwives have a very important role in the care of childbearing women and their families. Midwifery practice which meets the cultural needs of a diverse population, working to eliminate harmful practices and promotion of safe birthing practices are all fundamental ethical aspects of midwifery care. The concept of 'best interest' is one of the most misunderstood phrases in maternity care. The 'best interest' of the mother may well be different to that of the fetus. A midwife may feel torn between what would be better for the baby and the 'best interests' of the mother. The professional responsibilities of the midwife and accountability are key to ensuring ethical considerations are upheld. Midwives demonstrate ethical principles when they engage in knowledge transfer, education, development, research and activities that promote the rights of women and children as persons. In summary, ethical-based care is at the core of midwifery, midwifery care and practice! Having a code of ethics provides a statement of midwives' beliefs and values (Thompson, 1994).

The intention of this chapter is to define ethics, identify the three main types of ethics, demonstrate what ethical-based midwifery care is and explain the meaning of ethics. It will also consider how the expansion of medical ethics has also contributed to the increased need for midwives to be able to understand, articulate and demonstrate ethical-based midwifery care. This chapter will also consider the 'ethics of engagement' (FE Thompson, 2004) and the concept of the ethical journey.

This chapter identifies key ethical theories which are relevant for undergraduate heath and social care students. Starting with utilitarianism and deontology, progressing to ethical principles and morals, the author will identify relevance and application to current healthcare. Ethical behaviours that are evident, such as accountability, autonomy, advocacy and confidentiality will be considered. Using the current Codes and Standards (NMC, 2015; HPC, 2010; GMC, 2006) of professional conduct, the author will illustrate how the basic ethical concepts are a fundamental part of a practitioner's practice. Midwifery care that demonstrates that the woman has time to make an informed choice and is empowered to make an autonomous choice is ethically based. Equally, women who are enabled or helped to access services or treatments to which they are entitled is ethically based. Midwives are accountable and to that end those falling short of the standards expected by the regulating body (NMC) are endangering their professional registration and right to practise midwifery.

Ethics and ethical issues are relevant to all midwives, whether you are in clinical practice, research, education or consultancy. Midwives work in a variety of healthcare settings and with a variety of healthcare and social care professions. From prioritising care to screening, developing guidelines to postnatal checks and from supervising students to notification of intention to practise, midwives' work is affected by ethics and ethical decision making. The ethical dimensions (Jones, 2000c) of a midwife's role are numerous: friend, counsellor, educator, researcher, partner, practitioner, advisor, supporter and practitioner. The ethical behaviour of midwives is also apparent, being kind, collaborating, respectful, upholding dignity and professionalism. The main challenge to midwives and midwifery practice is that ethical values change over time.

The table of contents identifies the variety of themes to be confronted throughout the book. As indicated, all of them are 'troublesome' (Meyer and Land, 2004) but they also provoke strong emotions and dilemmas for midwives. Discussions around life and death, carrying a baby that is not genetically related to you, undergoing major surgery to save a compromised or distressed fetus or choosing to terminate a healthy pregnancy are not easily confronted and addressed with confidence. In choosing these topics the author acknowledges the difficult issues encountered by midwives throughout their careers. The types of questions posed are challenging. The answers are not always clear, which in itself presents difficulties for those who like to know exactly what to do or say. However, that is the nature of professional practice, discussion, debate, development and delivery of high-quality care, which is sensitive to individual needs. Fundamentally, midwives also need to know what their own values, beliefs and attitudes towards childbirth and maternity services are before they can consider ethical-based practice.

What is ethics and can midwives explain ethics in the context of midwifery?

Ethics is the application of the processes and theories of moral philosophy to a real situation (Jones, 2000a). An ethical dilemma is identified and arises when there is a choice, decision or action to be taken whereby the alternatives may be unattractive. An ethical dilemma is challenging as there is not a simple decision-making process, and human welfare and wellbeing are affected. FE Thompson (2004) refers to this as mainstream ethics and proposed that in midwifery practice there 'is a "midwifery ethic" or ethics of midwifery which is implicitly available in the lived realities and shared engagement of midwives and mothers'. The argument here is that while it has been traditional to apply bioethics and Western philosophies (Jones, 2000a; NMC codes) to midwifery practice, if midwives look to their practice (care relationships with women and being 'with women') a 'midwifery ethic' is observed. Midwifery ethics is part of midwifery, which concerns relationships with women and the moral commitment that midwives have towards maternity services. Buka (2008: 20) identified that ethics implies a rational and systematic study of moral issues. Logically, then, it is necessary to consider theories of moral philosophy, and apply them to a situation and identify the process of ethical behaviour and conduct. In most textbooks it is customary to start discussing ethics in relation to ethical morals and dilemmas and to distinguish between the two. Morals are about the right or good conduct of a person. Dilemmas are often evident when there is a difference of personal opinion and when guidelines or policy are in conflict. Midwives need to change and adapt when new evidence or interventions and treatments emerge in clinical practice. Keeping pace with developments in healthcare and revisiting ones' own education and training is necessary to ensure that decisions are ethically made. Ethical decision making is a process which requires honesty (knowing your own view, beliefs and attitude), application (consideration of facts, information and understandings) and evaluation (feasibility, success and effectiveness).

What is an ethical issue?

Wilday (1989: 176) suggested that ethics is the study of underlying reasons for deciding what is best when one is faced with conflicting choices. An ethical issue occurs when there is a difference in opinion or understanding of what is right or wrong. A midwifery ethical issue is around differences in opinion regarding a problem or issue, which arise in the context of midwifery practice. For example, where there is a difference in opinion regarding a possible induction of labour or the best way to manage the second stage of labour (this is a deliberate choice of words by the author). Such dilemmas are a daily part of midwifery practice.

In some ways 'ethics' are the decision-making process which go on inside your head when faced with a choice or an option, whereby one thinks 'what if?', 'should I?', 'on the one hand?', 'is this fair?', 'the truth is' or 'does this seem right?' Midwives, like doctors, are autonomous practitioners, and in the provision of maternity care are concerned about and face a number of issues and dilemmas where there are choices, difficult decisions and conflict regarding management and care associated with childbirth.

In 1983 the Royal College of Midwives (RCM) recognised that midwives were concerned about the increasing number of ethical or moral dilemmas they were experiencing in clinical practice: 'Ethical or moral dilemmas are not new, but some have received emphasis in recent years, and others have emerged as a result of scientific advances, changes of attitude in society and the activities of the media' (RCM 1983: 1). At this time some of the main ethical issues were around care of a baby with abnormalities, care of the dying baby, routine screening for abnormality, termination of pregnancy, contraception and sterilisation, artificial insemination by donor, in vitro fertilisation and subsequent implantation, use of surrogate mothers and potential of genetic engineering. The RCM identified that professional responsibility, professional relationships, contractual responsibility and confidentiality were key factors in the midwife's decision making. A checklist (though more like a flowchart) enabled midwives to consider ethical aspects before arriving at a decision. Note that the chart cited that managers, RCM, the supervisor of midwives, colleagues and spiritual advisors should be used to advise and guide the midwife. However, other sources of guidance were not specified. The RCM did not provide definite solutions to problems generally: suggestions and advice would be available to RCM members on an individual basis.

The main ethical issues for midwives have concerned abortion, technology-created dilemmas and research. More recently ethical issues around birth rights, informed consent and the duty of candour (Department of Health, 2014) have challenged midwives in the provision of ethical-based midwifery care.

What is an ethical dilemma?

An ethical dilemma is created when there is a decision to be made or an action taken. Personal beliefs, morals and attitudes will influence an individual's response. In addition, the education and training of midwives will contribute towards the ethical basis or philosophy of a midwife. On the front cover of *Law and Ethics for Midwifery* is a picture of a midwife using technology to listen to the fetal heart rate. Midwives are trained to use a Pinard (mono-auricular) stethoscope to listen to fetal heart rate. Technology has been developed to provide a visual value for fetal heart rate, which is also audible to the mother and midwife. The dilemma for the midwife is: is it better to use a pinard stethoscope or to use Doppler technology to routinely listen to the fetal heart rate? Current guidelines (NICE, 2014) only identify the need to listen and record fetal heart rate. Mothers and midwives may value the audibility of the technology and find it reassuring. The experience of listening to your baby's heart rate early in the pregnancy may enable women to accept and adapt to the pregnancy. Mothers and midwives benefit from sharing the experience and information simultaneously. Some women may wish to use such technology to listen to the fetal heart rate outside of midwifery care. What is the impact of a normal heart rate or altered heart rate on the woman, pregnancy and midwifery care? All these perspectives are important, but what about the fetus? Does the fetus have any rights such as safety, privacy and confidentiality? The picture on the front of this book suggests an ethical dilemma; the discussion and arguments enable midwives to consider the ethical aspects. While English law does not specifically concern listening to fetal heart rates, professional guidelines care pathways and ethical reasoning will provide a solution. The solution to the ethical dilemma regarding routine listening to fetal heart rate will also be based upon the preparation the midwife has received regarding ethical reasoning, research and information, guidelines and the values, beliefs and attitudes of the mother. One of the ways in which midwives can find solutions to ethical dilemmas is to discuss with colleagues. Midwives face ethical dilemmas on a daily basis. It is one of the reasons that midwifery is both an exciting and stressful occupation (vocation). It is not possible to identify every ethical midwifery dilemma or provide solutions so that midwives know the correct way to proceed.

The lack of a clear, specific solution or action is the main reason students find ethical dilemmas difficult. Each dilemma will have moral questions, judgements and values to be considered. At the time of considering an ethical dilemma, the midwife will need to examine moral differences between the woman and him- or herself. Cultural norms at the time, as well as expectations, will also impact upon the process.

Types of ethics

Ethics have been defined according to the focus of the inquiry. In the 1970s bioethics (Mepham, 2005) became topical as ethical issues regarding animal rights, environmental concerns and biological or reproductive technologies were controversial. Biotechnologies have developed and advanced at a rapid rate and for many people have presented solutions, but for others have challenged our beliefs as to what is right or wrong. Medical ethics originated in the issues surrounding end-of-life and life-saving treatments such as dialysis. During the 1980s it became apparent that a broader approach to ethics was required. Healthcare ethics emerged as patients themselves increasingly were aware of their rights and social and political influences impacted upon the nature, extent and type of healthcare received. Midwifery ethics could be considered to be those mores and moral rules which are relevant to midwifery practice and maternity services.

Ethics can be divided for the purposes of discussion into three key elements, namely meta ethics, ethical theory and practical ethics.

Meta ethics are best described as internal or a moral philosophy conducted at an abstract level. Meta ethics are how we work out what we mean by good or bad or if we are happy with our decisions. Ethical theory is the way in which we can explain or solve ethical problems; it is sometimes referred to as a formula for explaining difficult problems. The useful aspect of a formula or structure is that students like to methodically work through. Practical ethics concern daily aspects of life and also include daily aspects of medicine, business and midwifery. Another approach to ethics is described by Buka (2008: 20) as descriptive, normative, meta and applied ethics.

By considering the ethical dimensions of midwifery practice it is clear that, just like with law, a midwife cannot practice in ignorance of the ethical dimension of professional practice. From a practical point of view the NMC provides guidance and standards with reference to and regarding ethical approaches to midwifery care in the form of the Code: Standards of Conduct, Performance and Ethics for Nurses and Midwives (NMC, 2015). An additional consideration is that when inter-professional working such as safeguarding is being used it is necessary to recognise that other professions have their own Codes of Conduct (GMC, HCPC). Conflicts may arise as each profession will be referencing their own code and what is required of them. Most professional codes are based upon ethical principles of confidentiality, accountability and autonomy of the patient, so there should not be any conflict which affects care.

Ethical aspects of healthcare are focused around rights and duties. The rights of the patient are considered paramount (as opposed to the rights of the practitioner). This is an area of current concern in the NHS.

The duties of a healthcare provider are extensive and range from the duty of care to the duty to provide information. Fundamentally, healthcare ethics are based upon the European Convention on Human Rights. The United Nations Convention on Rights of the child (UNCRC) also informs the maternity services and healthcare delivery.

Example of ethical dilemma for midwives

A common dilemma for midwives is with regard to infant feeding. On an international level the World Health Organization (WHO) has a code of conduct/practice regarding the sale of infant formula. On a national level the United Nations International Children's Emergency Fund (UNICEF) (1992) baby friendly initiative (BFI) does not support the promotion of artificial feeding for mothers and families. Any materials produced by infant formula manufacturers being used in the education and training of student midwives, demonstrations to mothers or antenatal education will mean that BFI status is not achieved or is removed. UNICEF (2009) released a statement which identifies that formula milk companies must not mail staff directly with promotional materials or invitations to study days, and any information must be scientific.

The WHO has identified a code of practice for infant formula manufacturers. There has been repeated evidence of infant formula manufacturers breaking the WHO code. One solution to the breaking of the WHO code has been for midwives to boycott the purchase of products by the company breaking the WHO code. The Nestle boycott has been in place for a number of years. Some midwives are choosing not to purchase Nestle products (of which there are many, ranging from cat food to infant formula) in an attempt to draw attention to breaking of the international agreements on advertisement of formula feeds. So, with a Nestle boycott in place it could be argued that midwives are behaving ethically and demonstrating their concern regarding infant formula advertisement. Infant formula companies, however, are increasingly sophisticated in their approaches (UNICEF, 2009). Sponsored study days are an effective mechanism for accessing individual healthcare staff. Individual midwives can be attracted to attend by content that does not arouse suspicion, for example healthy development and growth, allergies, babies with special dietary needs or allergies. On the contrary, others (Jones, 2006) are choosing to work with the companies who subsidise study days. Companies can also engage in subliminal marketing to health professionals on the study day. The dilemma for cash-strapped midwives is whether to attend a 'free' study day sponsored by an infant formula company. Midwives are required to pursue professional development, and not attending could mean failure to maintain the legal requirement to keep up to date. Some infant formula companies have supported midwives in the development of educational materials. If midwives educators wish to receive UNICEF's BFI accreditation they are unable to use the tools developed by midwives, but produced or sponsored by infant formula manufacturers, etc. The issue surrounds the belief (by some midwives) that those who attend study days or use materials by formula manufacturers are a) breaking the WHO code and b) influenced to promote formula feeding. Neither of these arguments are evident.

- A practical situation for the midwife: does she attend a sponsored or subsidised study day or not? (Practical ethics)
- A moral situation for the midwife is that she or he ought to keep up to date with current information and knowledge about babies. By not attending is she or he not improving and meeting NMC PREP requirements?
- Infant formula companies who break the international code are potentially endangering the lives of vulnerable babies. Does the midwife condone this behaviour by attending the study day? Does the midwife demonstrate his/her displeasure by refusing to buy all products made by the parent company? (Ethical dilemma)
- Psychologically, does the midwife believe that breaking a WHO code is important or bad? (Meta ethics)

Defining ethics

Ethics has been defined as the 'application of the processes and theories of moral philosophy to a real situation' (Jones, 2000a: 8) Although the following definition seems easier to apply to midwifery, 'the way people behave based on how their beliefs about what is right and wrong influence behavior' (Ethics Research Center, 2009). Using these definitions the author suggests that midwifery ethics would be the ways in which midwives behave, support and conduct the care of childbearing women.

To a certain extent midwifery education has been dominated by medical approaches to healthcare. Increasingly the midwife professional has become less insular and social and psychological approaches are impacting upon the curricula. A more recent approach has seen student midwives engaging in inter-professional learning around inequalities in health, research and leadership and management. Future directions may include adopting an ethical business approach to the design of healthcare. This is important for all health and social care professionals if they are to reduce the current health inequalities in the UK.

Ethical theories

Ethical theory is the umbrella term given to the overarching aspects dealing with behaviour. Ethical theory is an attempt by scholars to describe and explain how things are or should be. Midwifery ethics are evident in clinical practice and influenced by changes, developments and research, which shape our beliefs about best practice. Ethical theories have been organised into a hierarchy of three levels (Figure 2.1). Ethical theories (for example, deontology and consequentialism), ethical principles and morals. Three ethical theories are frequently cited: deontology; utilitarianism or consequentialism; and virtue. Ethical theory is considered to be the underpinning explanation for a person's focus on decision making. Broadly speaking, deontology is concerned with the duties a practitioner has and how that duty is fulfilled. Consequentialism is concerned with the practitioner considering what the consequences of the action might be. Virtue ethics relate to the moral character of the individual.

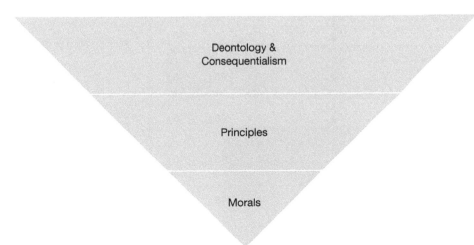

Figure 2.1 Hierarchy of ethical theories.

Deontology (duty-based theory)

Deontology is a duty-based theory. *Deon* comes from the Greek language, meaning *duty*. Immanuel Kant (1724–1804) is considered to be the authority on deontology (Mepham, 2005). Kantian theory is based upon moral agency (Beauchamp and Childress, 2013). Midwives are expected to adopt a deontological approach to their work (law abiding and dutiful) in that they are required to comply with the NMC (2012a) midwives rules. Kant identified seven duties (Table 2.1), all of which are considered equal. Autonomy is thought to be derived from a deontological basis.

Table 2.1 Seven duties

No.	Duty	Meaning
1	Fidelity	To keep promises; be loyal; non-deception
2	Beneficence	To help others
3	Non-maleficence	Not to harm others
4	Justice	Fair play, includes discrimination, distribution of benefits, risks and costs fairly
5	Reparation	Make amends regardless of personal cost
6	Gratitude	Loyalty owed to special people (parents)
7	Self-improvement	To become a 'better' person

Utilitarianism (consequences-based theory)

Utilitarianism is a non-religious ethical theory based upon the end result or outcome. Utilitarianism is forward-looking and has an 'ends justifies the means' approach. In taking a utilitarian approach,

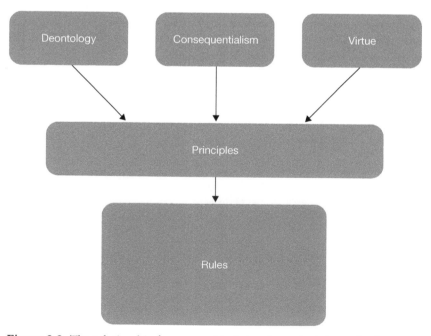

Figure 2.2 The relationship between ethical theories, principles and rules.

midwives would consider if more people would benefit from an action than being harmed by it. Harm to one patient (woman, baby) may be sanctioned (local guidelines) if it is of benefit of a larger group. It is possible to justify immunisations based upon a utilitarian approach, in that babies who are immunised provide protection for the wider community.

Ethical principles

Beauchamp and Childress (1994) identify four biomedical ethical principles which derive from ethical theory. These are

1. Autonomy: determination of what happens to oneself.
2. Beneficence: acts of mercy, kindness and charity. Refers to an action done to benefit someone.
3. Non-maleficence: asserts an obligation not to inflict harm on others.
4. Justice: inequalities in access to healthcare.

Ethical principles are the foundation for all of the professional guidelines regarding healthcare. Ethical principles relevant to midwifery are identified in Table 2.2.

Table 2.2 Ethical principles

Accountability
Advocacy
Autonomy
Beneficence
Confidentiality
Consent
Dignity
Justice
Respect

For healthcare to be ethically based, the ethical principles identified (Table 2.2) should be evident in the design, delivery and the evaluation of maternity services. The ethical principles identified are useful as midwives are able to use them as a framework for resolving ethical dilemmas in all aspects of midwifery. The ethical principles can be applied to our own lives and experiences as well as those of women accepting our care. Professional guidelines are intended to offer guidance for commonly faced dilemmas encountered during the provision of midwifery care. In subsequent chapters the ethical principles are highlighted with regard to the focus of the chapter. An example can be found in Chapter 16 on vulnerable women and the ethical principles of consent and confidentiality.

Autonomy

To be autonomous one has to have maturity (babies and infants are too immature), capacity (incapacity for example due to alcohol) and ability to rationalise. Individuals who are drug-dependent, coerced or exploited are not making autonomous decisions.

Beneficence

This ethical principle provides that midwives should always act in ways which benefit the patient. Beneficence is concerned with balancing the benefits of treatment against the risks and the costs. In application of this ethical principle to maternity services it is easy to understand how a dilemma presents. Antenatal screening clearly presents dilemmas regarding costs, risks and potential benefits. It may benefit an individual as well as communities and public health.

Non maleficence – the principle of doing no harm. Justice – the duty to be fair and not to discriminate.

Paternalism

Paternalism is an attempt to control or regulate 'in the same way a father does those of his children' (Beauchamp and Childress, 1994: 274) Paternalism when applied to maternity services is the concept of making judgements regarding needs and care of women. Paternalism is an illustration of the conflict between beneficence and autonomy (Beauchamp and Childress, 1994: 271). If the intention is to override the woman's choice or preference with a view to avoiding harm, then a paternalistic approach is taken, but it removes the woman's autonomy. A paternalistic approach is sometimes adopted when a woman is thought incompetent to make a decision. Paternalistic approaches can be regarding treatment, information and consultation. Making a decision to withhold or provide healthcare information (for example, regarding screening) is paternalistic. Valid paternalism (Beauchamp and Childress, 1994: 141) is used to justify removal of autonomous decision making.

Morals and virtue

The virtue ethical approach is concerned with the virtues that make for a good life and being a good person. The virtues often associated with midwifery are kindness, caring, compassion and courage. The NMC (2008d) code of professional conduct identifies listening, sharing and collaboration as virtues for nurses and midwives. The Department of Health (2012a) identifies the six Cs associated with healthcare, which provide a framework for high-quality professional healthcare.

Application of ethical theory and principles to healthcare professionals, or practical ethics

The way in which ethical theories are applied to professional practice is through codes of conduct, duties of care and guidelines. Midwives need to be clear of the different status of these documents. In the past midwives have been given specific details as to what is required. Over the years (and different regulatory bodies) the details have been less specific and in the form of principles. An example of this is the Central Midwives Board (CMB) and the NMC.

What could midwifery ethics look like?

In the introduction to this chapter the author suggests the concept of midwifery ethics or ethical midwifery-based care. Midwifery ethics could be considered to be those mores and moral rules which are relevant to midwifery practice and maternity services. The author suggests that midwifery ethics is an emergent concept and is based upon the premise that midwifery is both an art and a science. Moral beliefs and attitudes regarding childbirth stem from the definition of a midwife 'with woman' and justifies our concern with the medicalisation of childbirth. Midwifery ethics are focused regarding rights, duties and changing childbirth principles of choice, continuity and control by women of their birth experiences (maternity autonomy). Other key principles of midwifery ethics are those of dignity, respect and confidentiality. The author also suggests that ethical midwifery care cannot be considered without reference to culture of childbirth and the uniqueness of birth that a midwife is privileged to be a part of. The hospitalisation of childbearing women has (in the opinion of the author) reinforced the notion that care during labour may be provided by carers who have little understanding of ethical-based maternity services.

Forming ethical pathways

Ethical pathways are used to examine a clinical or research situation, analyse the dilemmas and consider the decision-making process. Personal values will impact and influence your views and opinions. Generally when faced with a dilemma, a practitioner may use 'gut feeling' or go through a process of reasoning or following an ethical pathway.

An ethical pathway, then, is used to consider the dilemma following a series of questions to identify the underpinning ethical issues and principles.

An example of an ethical pathway (modified from Johnson and Johnson, 2007) is shown in Figure 2.3.

The ethical pathway shown in Figure 2.3 may be developed for both clinical and research situations and dilemmas. Johnson and Johnson (2007) take ethical decision making further and utilise a series of questions to analyse any ethical dilemma. A key part is deciding if any of the ethical principles are in competition with each other. For example, is the client's autonomy in competition with confidentiality? Further exploration is then necessary to consider if one has a stronger principle than the other. The resolution may be that one takes priority over the other. Long-term consequences may also be considered before a resolution is obtained.

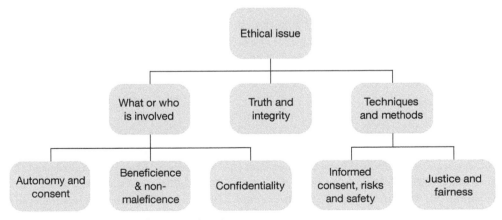

Figure 2.3 An example of an ethical pathway.

Modified from Johnson and Johnson, 2007.

Once the ethical principles have been considered it is then possible to consider issues associated with professional and legal aspects. An example here would be: is there any existing professional guidance (NMC, GMC, other professional bodies or WHO codes or declarations)?

While the above ethical pathway can be used to consider ethical issues and dilemmas, for both clinical and research perspectives to be complete the discussions and debates should include both the client and the multidisciplinary team. Failure to include these demonstrates a lack of understanding of modern healthcare in the UK (client choice and healthcare teams).

Medical ethics

In the past medical ethics have been dominated by two key principles or commandments (Harris, 1985). The commandments were: do not advertise and do not have sexual relations with your patients. When discussing medical ethics with student midwives, most mention the Hippocratic oath that is made by doctors and other healthcare professionals. When asked what the Hippocratic oath is the students relate this to the maxim of 'above all [or first] do no harm (Beauchamp and Childress, 1994: 189). The Hippocratic oath is a sworn statement which outlines the ethical basis for medical care (Beauchamp and Childress, 2009). Changes in society and scientific developments have rendered the Hippocratic oath obsolete as sometimes it is necessary to cause harm to save life. The basic standards of conduct of medical practitioners, like those of other registered practitioners (midwives), need to be modified to reflect the changes in attitudes and beliefs regarding what is ethical, right and equitable. Interestingly, Hippocrates is often referred to as the 'father of modern medicine' for the belief that disease occurs naturally, that is to say a physiological change rather than as a punishment or intervention by the gods. The early Hippocratic oath concerned the relationship between the doctor and patient and the teacher and pupil.

In recent times medical ethics have moved on to consider more fundamental aspects of medicine, such as life (when does it begin?) and death (brain death or cardiac arrest) and the value of life (nature and quality). Medical ethics have been described in terms of moral problems (Gillon, 1985). When does life begin? What value is life? What quality of life? Is it kinder to kill than to allow or maintain suffering? Most definitions of medical ethics identify three concepts: duty, morals and governance (Johnson and Johnson, 2007). Where does this leave midwifery ethics? Where have we placed difficult choices, challenges and dilemmas in terms of problems? If midwifery ethics is all about problems, then this does not take into account the personal beliefs and attitudes that are also part of ethics. Or is this just another attempt by midwives to remain distinct and different.

Midwifery ethics

The concept of midwifery ethics has not to date received great attention in the literature, possibly due to an assumption that medical ethics addresses the dilemmas facing all healthcare professionals. Medical or healthcare ethics also fail to take into account the relationship between the midwife and the childbearing woman. The partnership (or being 'with woman') approach to midwifery care necessitates a midwifery ethic (FE Thompson, 2004). Midwifery ethics is distinct and different from medical ethics as midwives also have the difficult task of providing care for both woman and fetus (baby). When it comes to role and responsibility, many midwives regard their work as including mother and baby, not to mention other responsibilities for partners and families. Midwives (and obstetricians) are the only healthcare professionals who have the delicate task of balancing both the needs and interests of the woman and those of her fetus (Ledward, 2011).

FE Thompson (2004) identifies that in midwifery practice ethics are found to be implicit and explicit.

Ethics in midwifery practice (explicit ethics)

A common feature of all professional regulations is that they are all based upon key ethical theories or principles. A quick comparison of the Nursing and Midwifery Code of Conduct and that of the Health Professions Council Guidance on Conduct and Ethics for Students and General Medical Council reveals commonalities (Tables 2.3 and 2.4).

Table 2.3 Shared principles of good practice

Ethical base	Nursing and Midwifery Council (NMC)	Health and Care Professions Council (HCPC)	General Medical Council (GMC)
Code of conduct, performance	The Code: Standards of conduct, performance and ethics for nurses and midwives (2010)	Standards of conduct, performance and ethics (2013)	Good medical practice (2013)
Confidentiality	The Code: Standards of conduct, performance and ethics for nurses and midwives (2010)	Confidentiality: guidance for registrants (2012)	Good medical practice (2013)
Consent	The Code: Standards of conduct, performance and ethics for nurses and midwives (2010)	Standards of conduct, performance and ethics (2013)	Consent: patients and doctors making decisions together (2009)
Rules and standards	Midwives rules and standards (2010)	Standards of proficiency for Social workers (2012) Operating Department Assistants (2014)	Good medical practice (2013)
Clinical Supervision	Supervision, support and safety: Annual LSA analysis report 2012–2013	N/A	N/A
Professional development	The PREP Handbook (2011)	Your guide to CPD (2011) CPD standards (2012)	Continuing professional development: guidance for all doctors (2012)

Table 2.4 Key ethical behaviours

	Nursing & Midwifery Council
Confidentiality	The Code (2010)
Knowledge and skills up to date	Registration renewal/fee payment
	Annual Intention to Practise Notification
	Midwives Rules and standards (2010)
Effective Communication	The Code (2010)
Informed consent	The Code (2010)
Accurate records	The Code (2010)
Honesty	The Code (2010)
Professional behaviour	The Code (2010)

The RCM has an ethics advisory committee which meets three times per year (Faulkner, 2005). Discussions at the ethics committee focus upon ethical perspectives around concepts of consequences, best interests, harm versus benefits, resource implications, impact on midwifery practice and provision of maternity services.

Ethics in midwifery education

The midwifery curriculum has rightly changed and evolved over the years to provide student midwives with an understanding of the key skills and necessary knowledge to meet the needs of childbearing women and their families. In addition to knowledge and skills, midwives also need to be aware of the need to consider ethical implications of developments and innovations that arise in practice, often on a daily basis. In order to consider the ethical issues the midwife needs to have an opportunity in advance to identify and explore her/his position and gain insight into the reasoning behind decisions made. Ethics have not always been a feature of the midwifery curricula. However, since the late 1990s ethical theory, ethical issues, dilemmas and moral problems have been addressed. Jones (2000a: preface) considers that it is worthwhile to thread ethics throughout the curricula but recognises that the modular structure of undergraduate courses does not always facilitate this. Some universities (Coventry University, 2004) developed law and ethics modules and they feature on undergraduate programmes as well as part of professional development courses. Law and ethics modules can be constrained by University regulations, which control the structure, design and level of activity students are required to engage in. University regulations also require assessment of all intended learning outcomes as well as an amount of essential and recommended reading. These 'controls' over academic modules are intended to ensure equity across courses, assessment parity and transparency for students. Thus, midwifery students can be confident that their law and ethics module is in keeping with those of other undergraduate students and quality mechanisms are in place. Students usually produce individual work for assessment, often in the form of an essay. An alternative model for teaching ethical issues is to consider practice situations and using an inter-professional approach, and to discuss implications and dilemmas to help gain a greater understanding. This approach is advantageous as practitioners can share principles of good practice and recognise how professional codes of conduct are similar (Table 2.3). Increasingly, law and ethics modules are adopting a debated arguments approach, whereby students work individually but come together to debate controversial aspects in a 'safe' environment. Debated arguments can be undertaken in a variety of ways (online, virtual world or 'moot'). The rationale for the diversity of law and ethics modules is to enable students to experience the challenge of professional discussion, acquire presentation skills and demonstrate an ability to listen to alternative points of view.

Ethics in midwifery research

An introductory chapter on ethics would not be complete without considering ethics in midwifery research. Midwives undertaking research – for example Bick and MacArthur (1995), Flint (1991), Kirkham (1989, 1996, 2004), Renfrew (1983), Sleep (1983) and A Thompson (1994) – have been responsible for drawing attention to a variety of ethical issues in midwifery and the maternity services. Models and frameworks for critiquing health research literature (Caldwell *et al.*, 2005) identify questions around ethics for practitioners to consider when evaluating evidence in practice. Ethics committees provide practical experience for midwives wishing to gain insights into ethical aspects of research. For example, opportunities to view preliminary study information sheets, differences between high-, medium- and low-risk studies as well as different timing for gaining consent/types of consent. Anecdotal evidence suggests that seeking advice from Chairs of ethical committees or the ethics committee administrator assists midwives with solving some of the dilemmas around research and maternity services. For example, the appropriateness or not of gaining consent while a woman is in labour. With regard to internet research, Stewart (2006) identifies unique challenges around intellectual property, copyright, online behaviour, anonymity and dissemination of results as well as traditional ethical issues of informed consent and confidentiality. Ethical issues in midwifery research are not uncommon as technological advances, data storage and confidentiality need to be considered. In addition, the basic ethical question regarding rights of women and their babies while undertaking research around childbirth remain.

Human rights and childbirth

Rights are a key concept in healthcare ethics. Basic human rights with regard to healthcare are discussed in detail in Chapter 4. Affording women basic human rights with regard to childbirth is an area of concern for all midwives. The right of confidentiality in particular is fundamental to the relationship between the woman and the midwife. Midwives are in a unique and privileged position to provide care for women during labour. Women have a right to expect that midwives will respect information and observations, and to protect the privacy of family life. Breaches in confidentiality are legally justified when safeguarding is an issue. Rights around childbirth may appear simple, such as the right to birth a baby in a safe environment; they can also be complicated, such as the right to a home birth. Birth rights are those rights or privileges that are often acquired at birth, such as an inheritance or title (Lady). An organisation such as Human Rights in Childbirth provides information around childbirth rights. At their conference in May, 2012 discussion focused upon the fundamental rights of childbearing women. In 2013 discussion focused upon the circumstances in which women give birth.

As has been identified, all aspects of ethics and midwifery are intertwined. This chapter has introduced ethics and provided explanation of ethics, ethical decision making and ethical practice. The role and responsibilities of the midwife mean that for the most part midwives will need to have a good understanding of ethics and ethical practice. There are many challenges to midwifery care and also many demands made upon midwives. Students struggling to explain ethics could start by considering NMC Codes, Standards and Guidelines as they are based upon ethical principles. Other students can use the Health and Care Professions Council. It should be easy to identify the specific theory (principles) upon which they are based.

Duty of care

A duty of care is said to exist when there is a relationship between you and a person who can be directly affected by your acts and omissions. A duty of care exists between the woman and the midwife. What is less clear is whether there is a duty of care between the midwife and the fetus and the woman's partner. A good example of the dilemmas facing midwives is with regard to pain relief in labour. If a midwife has a duty of care to both mother and fetus, should she administer pain relief? Pain relief comes in the form of Pethidine, a drug that is known to affect both mother and baby. Green (2008) questions the use of Pethidine and suggests that ethical judgements will be different in different situations. Using ethical theory to solve the dilemma, she identifies that ethical theory has limited use and that experience, intuition and shared ethical understandings are the cornerstones of good midwifery care. The premise here is that the mother's birth experience (pain relief and comfort) has long-term effects upon her relationship with her baby. Midwives supporting women in labour are morally bound to provide as much of a positive experience as possible. This has to be weighed up against the baby's experience (side-effects from Pethidine) and care at birth to rectify the effects of Pethidine. The midwife has a duty of care to the baby at birth to provide support with breathing, feeding and temperature control.

What are the ethical dimensions of the midwife's role?

The ethical dimensions of the midwife's role are those aspects which challenge, concern and cause dilemmas for midwives. The role (autonomous practitioner, advisor, friend, advocate) and responsibilities of a midwife (educator, counsellor, clinical skills and researcher) necessitate difficult decisions and efficiencies which can cause stress and anxiety. Midwives require emotional resilience to cope with the variety and amount of decisions encountered.

Ethical decision making

Midwives face many ethical dilemmas during their work. The dilemma may be caused by a difference of opinion, employment conflicts or technical innovations and perceptions regarding particular intervention (for example, induction of labour). When faced with an ethical dilemma there are a number of sources of guidance for the midwife. Sources of ethical guidance may be from midwifery tutors, managers, supervisors of midwives, the RCM or spiritual advisors.

Ethical decision making is the process by which midwives can make sense of and understand complex dilemmas that are found in maternity services and midwifery care. Ethical discussions, debate and decisions are usually considered using theoretical concepts of duty and consequences. Ethical dilemmas based upon or raised by technological innovations can be considered using the ethical matrix (Mepham, 2005: 63). Ethical frameworks for decision making are available such as a four quadrant approach (Schneider and Snell, 2000).

The chapters in this book contain case studies which are intended to help midwives develop ethical reasoning skills. The case study acts as a trigger for exploration of the ethical theory, principles and morals around a variety of topics. There are a number of ethical decision-making models (Storch et al., 2004) that are used to consider the options or approaches to a situation or dilemma.

Chapter summary

In this introductory chapter traditional application of ethical theory to midwifery is provided. Following consideration of ethical theory, principles and morals, the concept of midwifery ethics is identified. Justification for this detour is based upon the word *midwife*, meaning 'with woman'; this relationship also impacts upon the care given. Implicit ethics and explicit ethics are thought to be evident in midwifery care and may explain the unique relationship between midwives and women that is distinct and different from other healthcare practitioners and their patients.

Reflection

Using Gibbs' model of reflection (reflective cycle: focus, feelings, evaluation, analysis and action plan) reflect upon a recent episode of midwifery care you have provided. Consider the ethical issues underpinning care provided (Figure 2.4 offers an example).

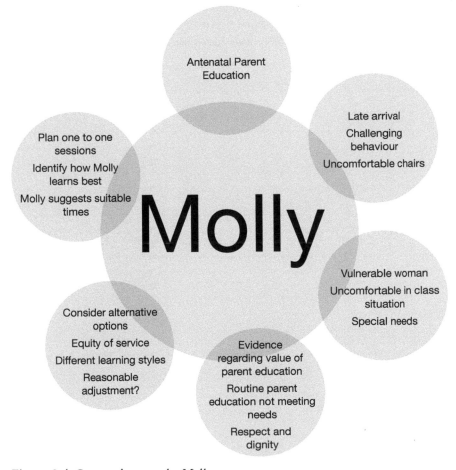

Figure 2.4 Case study example: Molly

Activity

1. Identify four situations in clinical practice and consider which ethical theories and principles are relevant.
2. Have a discussion with another student or midwife and consider how you would uphold basic human rights for childbearing women in a busy labour ward.

Useful websites

Birthrights (UK-based, protecting human rights in childbirth): www.birthrights.org.uk
Ethics Research Center (USA): http://ethics.org
General Dental Council: www.gdc-uk.org
General Medical Council (GMC): www.gmc-uk.org
Health & Care Professions Council (HCPC): www.hpc-uk.org
Human Rights in Childbirth (American-based): www.humanrightsinchildbirth.com
Nursing and Midwifery Council (NMC): www.nmc-uk.org
United Nations International Children's Emergency Fund (UNICEF): www.unicef.org/crc
United Kingdom Clinical Ethics Network (UKCEN): www.ukcen.net/index.php/main
World Health Organization (WHO): www.who.int

3 Introduction to English law and the English legal system

Pre-requisites for this chapter

You may wish to access the government website and identify current Bills going through the legislative process (there is a link to the website at the end of this chapter)

Introduction

This chapter will consider why an understanding of the law is essential for midwives, justify its inclusion in the midwifery curriculum and identify basic theoretical aspects of the English legal framework without which practitioners will not understand the complexity of English law. The English legal framework (see Figure 3.1) is a basic illustration of the English legal system. In this chapter the Health and Social Care Act 2012 will be used to demonstrate legal process. Consideration will be given to legal theory, sources of law and the legislative process. Recourse to the courts to solve disputes is increasingly common (Symon, 2013). Midwives should be mindful of litigious culture and understand the processes. This chapter does not seek to make you into a 'mini' lawyer, but helps you to have a basic understanding of the legal framework in England.

Law is fundamental to the role of all healthcare professionals, regardless of whether you are a support worker, student or registered midwife; legislation affects your daily work. For example, following every delivery the birth of the baby or babies must be notified. This statutory duty is identified in the National

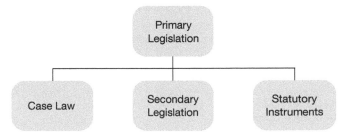

Figure 3.1 Illustration of the English legal framework.

Health Service Act 1977, whereas the requirement on the mother (or other qualified person) to register the birth of a baby is found in the Births and Deaths Registration Act 1953. Like most statute, the legislation was based upon a problem or issue which was so significant it required laws to ensure that something did (or did not) happen. The Births and Deaths Registration Act is necessary to ensure that all babies born are recorded. The information ascribes a status to the baby, after which it is entitled to benefits related to that status. The consequence of not registering a birth is that the person does not exist, and as such is not entitled to anything, including health and social care. If a midwife fails to notify a birth she has not upheld the law, is accountable for that inaction and is failing to provide a satisfactory standard of care.

Most midwives do not find themselves involved in legal proceedings during their career. Many of those who do experience legal proceedings do so as witnesses, expert witnesses or to provide support for a colleague who has the misfortune to be called to account.

Why is law so complex?

Any system that has a hierarchical structure is going to be complicated. Groups, sub-groups and divisions will require identification and distinction. Whole books have been written about the English legal system (Walker, 1980). Most books focus on historical sources of law, legal and literary sources of law, justice administration, procedures and practices (such as evidence). All of the above theoretical aspects are important, but it is sometimes easier to understand when the practicalities are considered. For example, a key source of English law is statute or legislation. The practicalities of legislation are that there is debate and discussion of the need for legislation, purpose of legislation and support for the legislation; having formulated the statute there has to be the granting of Royal Assent by Her Majesty the Queen. Most legislation is expected to last for a long time – after all the above time and trouble it would seem reasonable to expect that the legislation was robust and effective at addressing the original problem or concern. Student midwives have recently had a unique opportunity with the passage of the Health and Social Care Bill 2010 through the respective Houses of Parliament to witness the debate and discussion. The press and media have reported daily on the controversial aspects. Midwives are not the only profession that have concerns about the content of the Bill. Other professions (for example, nurses, medical professions and other allied healthcare professions) were also anxious.

Understanding case law using a practicalities approach is less attractive to student midwives. Attending court and observing legal procedures, giving evidence and writing affidavits and being a witness are all stressful and anxiety-provoking. To enable student midwives to understand the practicalities, a number of teaching approaches may be taken. Students can be encouraged to attend NMC hearings, use role play in a moot or contribute to classroom debates. All of these can help students to practise communication skills, articulate key information and experience the stress of being 'on the spot'. With the increasing use of technology, it is also possible to participate in a virtual court-room situation that has the advantage of being safe.

All professional regulatory bodies have identified frameworks for grading practitioners:

- The NMC, HCP and GMC all have well-established standards of competence and conduct that must be achieved by all practitioners.
- Law influences all aspects of our lives (personal, professional and employment).
- The legal profession has specialist areas (medical negligence).

Judicial review is a mechanism for challenging the law and legislation.

Legal theory

Hamilton and Nash (2008) suggest that there are three sources of English law: statutory law, common law and European law. However, a further consideration is that of judicial review, which serves to challenge the legality of the law and clarify or state a point of law.

Statutory law or primary legislation: how is primary legislation made?

The legal process usually starts with a dilemma, problem or necessity. It is followed by consultation and debate, before finally a solution in the form of legislation is agreed. A statute, which results from this process, is known as primary legislation. Power and control are features of primary legislation. It therefore follows that if you are going to control something or exert power over something, you need to be absolutely sure that it is well thought out, considers a variety of applications and does what you intended it to do. Primary legislation therefore needs to be drafted, redrafted and written in a way that prevents misinterpretation. It also requires many people to consider whether the law is fit for purpose. It may take considerable time to get the structure, wording and content ready before it can be presented to HRH the Queen in order to give Royal Assent. Midwives should be aware of the process so they may contribute and lobby Members of Parliament to ensure the final legislation is comprehensive and clear. Examples of primary and secondary legislation are:

- Primary legislation, e.g. Midwives Act 1902, Surrogacy Arrangements Act 1985
- Secondary legislation (delegated legislation), e.g. statutory instruments (SIs).

In the past midwives have been proactive and involved in the development of legislation. The Midwives Act 1902 could not have been achieved without the dedication and contributions of midwives. During the 1980s there was considerable concern regarding midwifery legislation. Midwives were anxious that the strength of the Midwives Act 1902 was going to be undermined and that midwives would lose key aspects that make midwifery unique and different from nursing. The Nurses, Midwives and Health Visitors Act 1979 was seen by some to be a takeover of midwifery by a larger group of healthcare professionals. In subsequent years the Royal Colleges of Midwives (RCM) and Nursing (RCN) have contributed to the discussions and debates at all stages of the legislative process towards a new statute. Each has staff dedicated to petitioning government and supporting, responding to and critiquing government reports, papers and recommendations. The RCM launched its RCM Parliamentary Panel at the end of 2011, which consists of 24 Members of Parliament, who work with the RCM to raise issues important to midwives and the maternity services. All of this activity does not mean that individual midwives should not be political. It is important that all midwives engage in politics to influence and shape future legislation.

Example of primary legislation

The following statute is used to illustrate how law and ethics are combined. The example of the Human Rights Act 1998 also demonstrates the formation of one English statute.

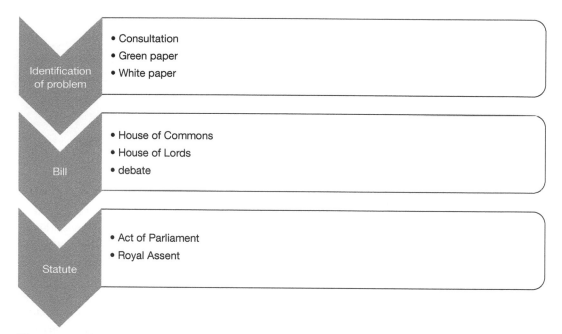

Figure 3.2 The legal process.

Human Rights Act 1998. The Human Rights Act (HRA) is not a midwifery statute *per se*. The HRA has been included to illustrate how primary legislation that does not (on first impression) have relevance to midwives is fundamental to midwifery practice. The HRA 1998 is based upon the European Convention on Human Rights, which emerged after the Second World War to reflect public outrage of the human atrocities experienced. The human rights identified in the convention were considered to be the basic rights associated with a civilised and humanitarian life.

The HRA 1998 has such significance that the author considers it necessary to address this statute early on in the book. One of the key phrases associated with rights is 'responsibility'. As one has rights to do things or to experience things, one also has responsibilities. An example could be that you may have a right to have a child, but that also means you have the responsibility to look after the child.

Students often ask why the date of the legislation is different from the date when the legislation comes into force. With the HRA 1998 it is quite easy to explain as the effect or ramifications of the Act required a lot of changes to large organisations such as the Police Service, who had previously been exempt. Many public authority workers required information, training and skills to avoid falling foul of the new legislation.

The human rights legislation came into force on 2 October 2000. At the time the legislation was needed to address the situation in England whereby public authorities (police, social and healthcare) were not previously required to comply with human rights. Following the introduction of the HRA, all hospitals and health centres were required to demonstrate and maintain basic human rights during the course of their work. The effects of the HRA were threefold:

1. It is unlawful for a public authority to breach the rights set out in the convention.
2. An allegation of a breach of the rights can be brought in the courts of this country.

3. Judges can make a declaration that legislation, which is raised in a case before them, is in breach of the convention. Consequently, cases that had previously been sent to the European Court in Strasburg can be considered in the UK courts.

It may not be immediately apparent as to why the author has chosen to include the following pieces of primary legislation here. The justification is that primary legislation may not have midwifery in the title, but may be relevant to midwifery practice. Midwives need to be able to relate legal aspects to their midwifery practice.

Coroners and the Justice Act 2009. This primary legislation is identified here to illustrate how non-midwifery legislation has an impact upon midwives. The Act has implications for midwives and midwifery when there is a maternal or neonatal death.

Human Tissues Act 1961, 1998; Human Tissue Act 2004. Ignorance of this legislation could cause problems for midwives. The placenta is human tissue and as such it is required by law that it be treated in a respectful and legal manner.

The Health and Social Care Act 2012

This legislation started life as the Health and Social Care Bill 2010. The Bill proposed major changes to the NHS with the aim of improving quality, reducing inequalities, commissioning and reporting of healthcare and reviewing healthcare providers. Re-organisation of the NHS was considered necessary in the context of national debt, austerity measures and the increased demand for healthcare. The Right Honourable Andrew Lansley (Health Secretary) introduced the Bill on 19 January 2010 with the expressed desire to make the NHS more responsive, efficient and accountable. The H&SC Bill spent 14 months going through the legislative process (Figure 3.3), and attracted more than 1,000 amendments before the final vote on 20 March 2012. Royal Assent was given on 27 March 2012.

Progress of the Health & Social Care Bill

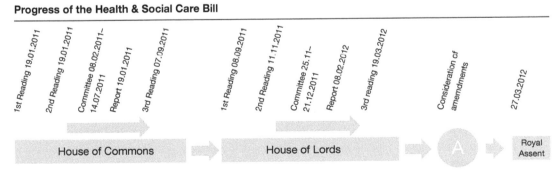

Figure 3.3 The legislative process of the H&SC Act 2012

Secondary legislation

Secondary legislation is a very powerful tool to consider. Secondary legislation may not receive as much publicity as primary but nonetheless has a great impact in that it can spell out details, change details and is generally harder for people to keep track of. Secondary legislation is often used in the regulation and control of professions. An advantage of secondary legislation is the speed in which it can become law as there is no need for Parliamentary time. The proposed legislation or statutory instrument can be drawn up by experts, presented to both the House of Commons and the House of Lords and endorsed. This speedy approach facilitates change and enables professions to regulate and control professional practice. A good example is SI 2001 No. 253, which is discussed in detail in Chapter 5.

Statutory instruments

Statutory instruments (SIs) may be considered as secondary legislation, which fills in the detail of the law without being subject to a full debate in Parliament. SIs are used to enact legislation in a way that can modify, amend or clarify existing statute. Henderson (1995) identifies an article in the *Nursing Times* from 1977 in which the following responses are offered to the question 'If the midwife hands you a statutory instrument would you ...':

(a) Clean it?
(b) Play some stately music on it?
(c) Use it as an essential reference document?
(d) Boil it for 20 minutes
(e) Use it to engrave an inscription on a statue.

While the above illustration is a play on clinical practice and draws our attention to the difficulties practitioners face when confronted with unfamiliar terminology, it is important to recognise that SIs are an important source of law and as such midwives' knowledge regarding them will enable enforcement of English law. SI 1983 No. 1202 is an example of how a change was made to the Nurses Midwives and Health Visitors Act 1979. SI 1983 No. 1202 overturned the original legislation to enable male midwives to provide care. While a statutory instrument is not a clinical tool, it does regulate and control clinical practice through the Midwives Rules (NMC, 2004).

Case law

Case law is also an important source of law influencing healthcare. Legal cases are reported in official law reports as well as local and national press. Keeping up with the latest rulings and outcomes of legal cases is a full-time occupation for many people. The court hierarchical system means that the outcome or ruling of a case will influence the rulings in lesser courts. The rulings in legal cases determined by the judges are used as a basis for subsequent cases. Some cases set what is known as 'precedent', whereby all subsequent cases have to follow the same conventions or outcomes, provided that the circumstances are similar. This is a difficult concept – how do you ascertain similarity between cases? How much similarity does there need to be? Generally it is thought that to share some elements is not sufficient. Certainly similarities regarding age or gender are insufficient. For a case to set precedent it should be of such importance, significance or from a high court.

Case law, then, is a form of law based on decisions made by judges in specific cases. To become 'case law' the case has to have the following characteristics: it should introduce a new principle or develop existing law; the judge may in the summing up clarify terms of existing statute; there may be elements or aspects of the case which are 'distinguished'.

How is law divided/enforced?

Case law can be divided into criminal and civil proceedings. This distinction is important as cases will be directed towards the appropriate court. In addition, the standard and type of evidence will be different for the type of court. The Crown Prosecution Service (CPS) is responsible for deciding which criminal cases go to court. The current director of the CPS is Alison Saunders. The Code for Crown Prosecutors (2013) provides guidance and general principles for Crown prosecutors to follow when making decisions about prosecutions. The Code for Crown Prosecutors is available to download from the CPS website. An important part of the CPS code relates to the treatment of witnesses in court. This is particularly relevant to cases where vulnerable adults and children are involved.

Types of courts

The courts of law in England and Wales are hierarchical in nature. At the top of the legal system are the UK Supreme Court, Court of Appeal and High Court in London. At the bottom of the court system are the magistrates' courts and county courts. Diagrammatic representation of the courts system can be found in Wheeler (2012: 74). The European Court of Justice (ECJ) is arguably the highest court of justice, as decisions made in the ECJ are binding upon English courts.

It is important here to mention the Coroners' Court as all maternal and neonatal deaths are referred here. Midwives who are required to attend a Coroners' Court need support, preparation and training to ensure they can fully participate in the legal process.

Court craft

This is the term given to behaviour, ritual and appearance in court. A fundamental part of law training is the acquisition of courtroom skills. Knowing who sits where in court and how to approach the Bench or present a statement requires preparation and development. Student midwives do not usually gain experience in courtroom skills, although some universities now enable practitioners to experience this in simulations or moots. Mooting is a good way to present, debate and argue in a controlled way. It can enable students to develop presentation, communication and critiquing skills. Mooting also enables the student to gain experience of the court environment and positions held in court. Health and social care practitioners may be intimidated or fearful regarding proceedings and protocol. In addition, health and social care practitioners may feel afraid of anything that could be deemed as 'legal' or become a legal case. Student midwives have positively evaluated opportunities to witness court proceedings or prepare statements or reports. However, it is important to support learners during these opportunities so that they can benefit from the experience.

Expert witness

Expert witnesses are called to court by solicitors to help the legal profession understand and clarify items and issues outside of their expertise. Good expert evidence is thought to be key to good justice. Expert witnesses are often sought by the courts to provide knowledge and experience. They are not required to provide advice, and if they do so they risk becoming the focus of a legal case themselves. Dr Roy Meadows was an expert witness in the Sally Clark case. He suggested that to have 'one cot death is tragic, two is suspicious and three is murder'. It is thought that his statement helped in the conviction of Sally Clark. Summaries of the Sally Clark case and Dr Roy Meadows are provided in the Appendices. In 2014 *Panorama* investigated the conduct of expert witnesses.

Criminal proceedings

While civil proceedings may be more readily associated with healthcare litigation, focus will now be given to criminal proceedings. The rationale is that many students find this aspect of law interesting and most students consider themselves and other healthcare practitioners not to be criminals. The following cases illustrate that crimes against patients not only occur, but also bring the profession into disrepute. A crime is an illegal act and is derived from statute or common law. Examples of potential criminal cases are: murder or manslaughter; theft; fraud; driving offences; and female genital mutilation (female circumcision). Convictions for criminal offences are automatically reported to NMC (no right to confidentiality).

There are a number of criminal cases (Dr Harold Shipman and Nurse Beverly Allitt) that students should be familiar with as they are so serious (and famous) that they provide students with an opportunity to understand how the behaviour of healthcare professionals can be illegal. A short summary of these key cases is included at the end of this book. In the above cases the practitioner committed the crime of murder. The publicity following these cases also focused attention upon healthcare professionals and reinforced the notion that modern healthcare workers do not always behave in an acceptable way.

Criminal proceedings follow an illegal behaviour or act. The key aspect of criminal proceedings is that the accused must be proved guilty 'beyond reasonable doubt'. Beyond reasonable doubt is an important distinction; if there is doubt a lesser charge may be found. For example, with regard to a maternal or neonatal death it must be proved beyond reasonable doubt that murder was intended and that there can be no doubt that the accused directly and deliberately caused the death for a murder charge to be successful. If there is doubt, then a lesser charge of manslaughter will be found. There are two requirements to be met: (1) physical 'actus reus'; (2) mental 'mens rea'.

Civil proceedings

Civil proceedings are the legal mechanism for dealing with civil wrongs or torts. Examples of civil wrongs or torts are negligence, breach of statutory duty, trespass to the person, nuisance and defamation. Civil wrongs are no less significant than criminal actions. Both are subject to legal proceedings. However, the main penalty for a crime is imprisonment or restriction of liberty; the main penalty in civil cases is financial (in the form of compensation). *Law and Ethics for Midwifery* will only focus upon the civil cases of negligence, breach of statutory duty and trespass.

Negligence is a civil wrong. Negligence may affect all aspects of midwifery care in ways that midwives do not always realise. Any wrongdoing that results in injury, stress or death to the woman and/or her baby may result in a negligence claim for compensation. Healthcare is a risky business and obstetrics and childbirth are by their nature associated with risks. An example would be the risk of haemorrhage associated with childbirth. Management of the third stage of labour is normally associated with active management. Does physiological management of the third stage make it more risky for the mother? There are a number of key issues surrounding negligence:

- liability must be proved;
- compensation;
- additional implications for independent midwives;
- breach of statutory duty;
- trespass to the person.

Further explanation of the above torts can be found in Chapter 18, where the focus will be in relation to midwifery. For those of you who are interested in further developing knowledge and understanding of the medical concepts, the author suggests a traditional law text such as Claudia Carr's *Unlocking Medical Law* (2012).

What about other legal frameworks?

Health and social care (including maternity services) are not only influenced by statute, secondary legislation and case law. Healthcare is also controlled and influenced by governance. Governance is the way in which a government can exercise its power and control over its departments or business. Healthcare governance is administered or directed by the Department of Health. Regulation of healthcare professionals is an example of governance. Regulation of healthcare practitioners has been established by statute.

The Department of Health influences all aspects of healthcare (clinical care, research, education) through policy, guidelines and protocols. Clinical governance comes in the form of the National Health Service Litigation Authority (NHSLA) and the Clinical Negligence Scheme for Trusts (CNST). The Jackson reforms concern the relief of sanctions when court directions, rules and orders are not met. These are reforms identified by Lord Justice Jackson on 1 April 2013 to civil litigation in an attempt to boost efficiency and reduce litigation costs. The spiralling costs of court cases associated with healthcare litigation has for some time been a concern.

Statutory regulation of healthcare practitioners

Regulation and control of healthcare practitioners is provided by statute. Primary and secondary legislation identify specific frameworks, processes and standards for all healthcare providers. The General Medical Council (GMC) was initially established by the Medical Act 1858, but significant amendments have been made and are found in the Medical Act 1983. The key functions of regulatory bodies are to ensure that its members are up to date and fit to practise. More recent legislation in the form of the Health Care Professions Act 2002 made provision for a regulator for the regulators. The

Council for Healthcare Regulatory Excellence (CHRE) has the task of ensuring that the regulators fulfil their statutory duties. Professional regulators are required to abide by legal processes while performing their functions. Legal challenges to conduct of proceedings by the NMC have increased (Symon, 2013).

The Health Professions Council (HPC)

The HPC regulates and controls 15 different health professions, including paramedics, operating department professionals, physiotherapists, occupational therapists, dieticians, chiropodists/podiatrists and speech and language therapists. Practitioners who meet the standards (training, professional skills, behaviour and health) set by the HPC are identified on the HPC register (this can be checked by the public at http://hpcheck.org). The HPC has now become the Health and Social Care Professions Council (HSCPC).

The General Medical Council

The GMC regulates and controls all medical practitioners (including GPs). In keeping with other regulatory bodies the GMC publishes guidance for its registrants.

The Nursing and Midwifery Council

The NMC regulates and controls nurses and midwives. It has been functional since 1 April 2002. Nurses and midwives who meet the standards (training, professional skills, behaviour and health) set by the NMC are able to register. An annual registration fee is paid. The annual fee was increased in 2014 and now stands at £100 per annum. Midwives are also required to submit an annual Intention to Practise (ItP) form via the Local Supervising Authority (LSA). Further details and discussion regarding the NMC are provided in Chapter 4. The Constitution of the NMC (schedule 1 part 1 to the orders) covers:

- functions of NMC;
- powers of NMC;
- registration;
- education and training – pre-registration and post-registration (PREP).

The legislative framework for midwifery: an overview

There is not one piece of legislation that covers all aspects of midwifery care and practice and the maternity services. Midwives need to be aware of other statutes which affect their practice. In the table of statutes at the front of this book you will find examples of primary legislation which impact upon midwifery care.

The specific and primary legislative framework for the midwifery profession and practice commenced with the Midwives Act 1902. In 1979 the Nurses, Midwives & Health Visitors Act (NMHV Act) was the first piece of legislation that midwives specifically shared with other professions. At the time midwives were concerned that the legislation would erode the midwifery profession and effectively allow other professions to impact upon midwifery. However, a key aspect of the NMHV Act 1979 was to provide for the Midwifery Council and maintain specific arrangements for midwifery (supervision of midwives). The Statutory Midwifery Framework is important as it regulates and controls midwives and midwifery practice, specifically the role and accountability of the midwife, professional autonomy, regulation of practice, supervision of midwives and the professional register.

Secondary midwifery legislation can be found in the publication of SIs such as Statutory Instrument 2002 No. 253 (Nursing and Midwifery Order). SI 2002 No. 253 came into force in April 2002 and it is unusual in that it amended primary legislation to enable the formation and constitution of the Nursing and Midwifery Council to replace the United Kingdom Central Council (UKCC) for Nursing, Midwifery and Health Visiting. Further and specific attention is given to the legislative framework for midwifery in Chapter 5.

Chapter summary

This chapter has identified the English legal system, introducing key aspects such as primary and secondary legislation. A short introduction to the midwifery legal framework demonstrates that regulation and control of the profession is robust. Further details are provided in the next chapter. Clinical practice is provided within a legal framework and policies and procedures enable midwives to be law abiding. Midwives' private lives are also governed and affected by legislation. Professional standards are regulated and controlled. Midwives who fall short of the regulations recognise that they may be subject to the possibility of criminal, civil and malpractice investigations. Supervision of midwives is an important and historical aspect of midwifery and some argue that midwives enjoy the privilege of controlling their profession. The implications of law for midwives may be summarised as follows:

- Midwives are autonomous practitioners; 'blame' may be attributed to the individual.
- Healthcare (surgery/treatments/standards) is often the focus of legal proceedings.
- Complaints often turn into litigation (no explanation, no apology, lack of support).
- Neurological impairment related to or resulting from birth may be the subject of litigation years after the event.
- Negligence claims are increasing (blame culture).

Activities

1. Find an Act of Parliament. Consider if there is any relevance to midwifery or maternity services.
2. Find a report of a legal case. Using a basic framework for learning (definition, description, detail and discussion) consider relevance to midwifery or maternity services.
3. What is the Cardiff Index and is it of use to student healthcare professionals?

Reflection

This chapter has identified how law is made. If you wanted to make a new Midwives Act how could this be achieved? Consider what a new Midwives Bill might address. Outline the main processes required and consider who could help you to do this.

Useful websites

Crown Prosecution Service: www.cps.gov.uk
Legislation and Bills: www.legislation.gov.uk
NHS Litigation Authority: www.nhsla.gov.uk
UK government: www.dh.gov.uk

4 Ethical and legal frameworks: human rights and midwifery care

Pre-requisites for this chapter

It may be helpful to read some chapters from Paul Buka's (2008) *Patient Rights, Law and Ethics for Nurses: A Practical Guide*. Consider the incidence of home birth throughout the world. Think about the inequalities of healthcare for women and consider mortality rates associated with childbirth. Consider your personal view regarding home birth and how this may impact upon your attitude to hospital births.

Introduction

In Chapter 2, ethical theory, principles and dilemmas were introduced. Attention was drawn to all the professional codes of conduct, guidelines and regulations, which are based upon ethical principles or ethical-based care. Ethics touches every aspect of human life. Theorists may categorise ethics into particular areas, for example medical ethics or professional ethics. These categories are useful when studying a particular topic but effectively ethics is not exclusive to a particular area. In 1998, the medical schools produced a consensus statement around how doctors should treat patients fairly, respect their dignity, autonomy and rights. Usually this is referred to as an ethical basis for care. This author will suggest that midwifery ethics is emerging as a focus for care during childbirth and, like evidence-based care, should form the basis of care during childbirth.

Ethics is fundamentally about how we treat each other, how we behave and manage our lives and how we conduct ourselves. It is important to consider personal behaviour of midwives away from the work setting as professional registration relies upon 'good character' (NMC, 2008d). Healthcare ethics, then, is about the ways in which patients, or in the case of maternity services women, are treated and are able to receive care. The relationship between the woman and the midwife can be described as ethically based if trust, information sharing, confidentiality and partnership are evident. A dilemma for the midwife is that in choosing to have a hospital birth women are more likely to be coerced into routines and interventions which may not be in their best interest.

Confidential enquiries (Flemming Report, 2013) and independent reports (Francis Report, 2010, 2013) have identified that ethical-based care is lacking in the NHS and this has resulted in unacceptable levels of patient suffering and mortality. Specifically, the Francis Report (2013) suggests that compassion in the health service is considered to be at an all-time low. Cummings and Bennett (2012) identified 'six Cs' associated with ethical-based care: care, compassion, competence, communication, courage and commitment. These qualities also apply to midwifery care (Dimond, 2013: 31). Modern healthcare needs to demonstrate the ethical basis of care; also increasingly human rights are enshrined in legislation to potentially force compliance and to secure compensation for those whose care is found to be negligent.

Rights usually have ethical origins in that they are about treatment and experiences, fairness and non-discrimination. Rights are universal and are important for humanity. The right to health is a human right and is supported by the World Health Organization. The United Nations International Covenant on Social, Economic and Cultural Rights (United Nations, 1966) specifies the right of everyone to the enjoyment of the highest attainable standard of mental and physical health.

Prior to the Human Rights Act 1989 (HRA), statutory agencies such as the NHS were not required by law to uphold basic human rights such as dignity. The Kennedy Report (2001), which led to the Human Tissues Act (2004) required hospitals and schools of medicine and museums not to store human tissues (e.g. medical specimens) without consent. Prior to 1998, many midwifery teaching environments used aborted fetuses, unusual placenta (succenturiate lobe) and umbilical cords (true and false knots) for teaching purposes. This is no longer tolerated or supported as it breaches the 2004 Act. Students who wish to view these anatomical specimens can still do so, but need to visit the Gordon museum of pathology at Kings College London. The Gordon museum holds a special licence to store and hold human tissue for educational purposes. This chapter focuses on key ethical bases of care (autonomy, rights and dignity) and how primary legislation (the HRA) has enshrined an ethical approach (rights) in statute.

Ethical principles for care (ethical framework)

Ethical theory is informed by values, beliefs and attitudes. Each ethical theorist has their own beliefs and attitudes which impact upon their philosophy. A good example of the dilemma facing the NHS is that of prescription charges. On the one hand, NHS care should be 'free at the point of delivery'; on the other hand, not all patients take their prescribed medications. The dilemma is that there is insufficient funding to provide medication for all. Patients who do not take their medication may be stopping another patient from getting the medication. Is this fair, right or just? Ethical theory can be used to justify or not prescription charges. The philosophy of the NHS is that healthcare is a comprehensive service available to all, irrespective of the ability to pay. The government are able to, in limited circumstances, require that those who are able to afford it or who request a particular brand pay for their medications.

Ethical theory is supported by rights. The right of human beings to be treated in a way that shows:

- respect for autonomy;
- beneficence;
- non-maleficence;
- justice.

Human rights framework for maternity services

Maternity services that are underpinned by basic human rights such as dignity, autonomy and equality provide a framework for the planning and delivery of ethical-based care. There are numerous examples of inequalities regarding childbirth around the world. Concern in Croatia and Japan has alerted us to the pressure being placed upon women to birth their babies in hospitals (often a distance away from family and friends). Confidential enquiries in maternal deaths reveal inadequacies in the NHS regarding skills and expertise, availability of sufficiently experienced staff and access to services for childbearing women. Justice in the maternity services equates to having the right care, at the right time, in the right way.

Law and healthcare (legal framework)

Human rights and healthcare are modern phenomena. Until recently there has been little consideration given to human rights during childbirth. With the hospitalisation of women for childbirth the medical model of patient and consultant prevailed. Attitudes implied that women were lucky to have their babies in hospital as it was more likely that the baby would be safe. The belief that hospital birth is safer for mother and baby still prevails (Birth Place Study, 2012). The rights of women to be decision makers during childbirth has been strong in the UK since *Changing Childbirth* (Department of Health, Expert Maternity Group, 1993) and the adoption of concepts of choice and control for childbearing women. Prior to this the experiences of childbearing women in the UK was that of a patient and the basis of care was paternalistic. Choices and control were not encouraged as health policy was controlling the birth environment; women were encouraged to birth their babies in hospital. Healthy women should be free to choose where and how they give birth (Inch, 1982). What does the exercising of this birth right mean for the midwife, other women and the baby? The dilemma is that the maternity services cannot support choice when it means that some women cannot be provided with basic care. This dilemma is most frequently found on labour wards. A woman may wish to birth her baby in hospital with pain relief (an epidural); if all the women on the labour ward exercise this right it is likely that the service would not be able to support this care. Midwives are also required to have additional training to support this type of pain relief; medical staff are required to supervise its administration.

The NHS Constitution (2013) identifies that the NHS belongs to all of us (England). The principles and values identified in the constitution set out the rights to which patients are entitled. The rights, pledges, duties and responsibilities identified in the Constitution are legally binding and are to be renewed every three years. Technically this could mean that if the NHS does not fulfil the duties, the public have a right to sue for negligence if all the requirements are met (see below for further information).

Human rights in maternity care

One of the main themes regarding human rights is the inconsistency of human rights throughout the world. Furthermore, the inconsistency regarding women's rights is even more prevalent. During childbirth there is the added complexity when there appears to be conflict between the rights of pregnant and birthing women and those of their unborn babies. When talking about midwives I have heard it said that some midwives are 'for the mother' and others are 'for the baby' when dilemmas occur during childbirth. Personal philosophy of midwives will affect the way in which they behave and present information. If a midwife believes that a woman should endure, experience or suffer a procedure that potentially could 'save' the baby, then the woman should endure it. Sometimes the midwife may find women's agency difficult to protect and that the right to be supported, make one's own decisions and have full information is compromised by the threat of safeguarding procedures for the baby. A good example is with regard to alcohol consumption during pregnancy, smoking during pregnancy and other risky behaviours. A key phrase associated with rights is responsibility. As one has rights to do things or to experience things, then one also has responsibilities. An example could be that you may have a right to have a child, but that also means you have the responsibility to look after the child.

Using a basic human rights framework of dignity and respect, it is possible to construct a human rights approach to childbirth.

Birthrights, a human rights childbirth charity based in the UK, actively campaigns for dignity in childbirth. Following a UK survey of women and a selected group of midwives, Birthrights (2013) identified that 18 per cent of women did not feel that health professionals listened to them, 24 per cent who had an instrumental birth said they had not consented to procedures and 42 per cent of women felt that childbirth had a negative impact. From an ethical perspective this demonstrates a lack of respect for women during childbirth.

Universal rights of childbearing women

According to the White Ribbon Alliance (WRA, 2014), pregnant women seeking maternity care may be subjected to varying degrees of ill treatment. The WRA actively campaign to 'break the silence' regarding abuse ranging from subtle disrespect to physical assault and active discrimination. The universal rights of childbearing women are presented as a charter to emphasise that all countries (those that spend a lot of money on healthcare and those who spend relatively little) should be providing care for childbearing women which is ethically based. It is possible to use the seven rights of respectful maternity care (WRA, 2014) to consider and reflect upon our midwifery practice and maternity services. The application of a basic human rights framework to maternity care (Table 4.1) enables the midwife to consider each episode of care using a rights-based approach.

Healthcare regulators as defenders of human rights

Healthcare regulators such as the Nursing and Midwifery Council (NMC), Health and Care Professions Council (HCPC) and the General Medical Council (GMC) have a pivotal role in the maintenance of human rights and healthcare. This role is achieved in a number of ways.

Professional registration identifies practitioners who have undertaken and successfully completed education and training to become a registrant in the relevant discipline. Registration is completed on an annual basis and the practitioner is required to declare that they are confident and competent to undertake their role. In addition to registration the healthcare regulators also use a process of revalidation or renewal of evidence that the practitioner is fit for purpose and fit for the practice of providing appropriate healthcare. All healthcare regulators have a system for ensuring that they investigate any

Table 4.1 A human rights approach to childbirth

Right	Ethical basis	Example
Justice	Fairness Equity	Informed choice rather than informed coercion Equality Prompt and appropriate referral Works within scope of practice
Reproductive rights Assisted fertility	Equality	Safe environment Place of birth Storage and destruction of human gametes
Care during childbirth	Dignity Respect Confidentiality	Nurturing women during childbirth Continuity of care Continuity of carer Courtesy Privacy in clinical care
Choice	Autonomy	Supports women Shares information Informed consent Evidence-based care
Control	Autonomy	Acceptance or refusal of student midwives present at delivery Who may be in the room during examination and during birth
Compassion	Advocacy Privacy	Protect mother and baby from harm Support a partnership approach to childbirth Embrace diversity and ensure that women's voices are heard
Continuity of care	Duty of care Respect Autonomy	Know your midwife Named midwife
Competent care	Equality Safe childbirth	Evidence-based practice Non-discriminatory practice
Professional midwifery care	Duty 'Do no harm' and de-medicalise childbirth Confidentiality	Informed consent Safe environment Privacy of information

concerns or complaints regarding a registered practitioner. The process for investigation is often referred to a misconduct investigation.

Supervisors of midwives: defenders of human rights?

Supervisors of midwives (SoMs) have a duty to support women's right to health. Supervision ensures that midwives provide a high standard of care to women, support women and act as role models in clinical practice. Jessiman and Stuttaford (2012) identify that SoMs, in their unique role, are able to defend women's right to health, as they are accountable to women for maternity services and maternity care. SoMs lead on initiatives to promote normality, use audit to improve care provided and support women in their choices, and as such defend women's rights during childbirth.

In order for the NMC to fulfil its role in protecting women from poor care or falling standards, supervision is at the front line for the NMC. Raising the profile of supervision to women has been prioritised by the NMC. Midwives are ideally placed to promote the role of the supervisor by referral to and also by engaging with them as part of their annual meeting, and attending updates and study days provided by supervisors. Opportunities to raise the profile and role of supervisors occur throughout pregnancy, labour and during the postnatal periods. Information leaflets may also be provided (NMC, 2012d). Raising the profile of SoMs has been identified as the responsibility of every midwife (Barker, 2012).

Should a midwife support a woman who has made a decision which the midwife feels is inappropriate?

A midwife may be aware that a woman's decision is morally wrong (such as the decision to terminate a pregnancy), but the midwife is required to respect a woman's decision (NMC, 2004).

Childbirth rights?

Childbirth rights can be considered to be the ethical consideration of practices, interventions and procedures undertaken and associated with childbirth. Childbirth rights may also be considered from a maternity service approach. An example is the right to birth a baby at home or in a non-hospital environment. Inch (1982: 15) identifies that a midwife is important for what she or he does not do as well as what she or he does do during normal childbirth. This distinction is important as it acknowledges that midwives are able to promote birthrights as well as erode them. The sort of birthrights which Inch (1982) focuses upon are choices that women make during childbirth. Inch identifies that responsibility for making decisions regarding childbirth is not limited to the healthcare professionals and that women having babies have a right and responsibility to make decisions for themselves. Birthrights are only obtainable if there is effective communication with women to enable them to understand the care proposed and be able to apply it to their own situation. The responsibility of good communication rests with the healthcare provider and is a fundamental part of the role and responsibility of a registered practitioner (NMC, 2009a).

Childbirth rights can be eroded by poor or inadequate communication, values, beliefs and attitudes of caregivers, lack of skill and a lack of respect. High-quality midwifery care impacts upon women's health and reduces health inequalities. A woman's right to choose where, how and with whom to birth her baby is a fundamental human right; the difficulty is that there is always an argument which concerns the safety and wellbeing of the baby. What childbirth rights are afforded to babies?

Legislation

Human Rights Act 1998

The HRA 1998, is based upon the European Convention on Human Rights. The HRA 1998 is primary legislation, which has been enacted to ensure that the ethical aspects identified above are enforced. The HRA 1998 proposed radical changes to large public organisations such as the NHS. The changes affected all aspects of the NHS and all NHS workers require information, training and skills to avoid a breach of the legislation. The legislation came into force on 2 October 2000. At the time the legislation was needed to address the situation in England whereby public authorities (police and social and healthcare) were not required to comply with human rights. The effects were threefold:

1. It is unlawful for a public authority to breach the rights set out in the convention.
2. An allegation of a breach of the rights can be brought in the courts of this country.
3. Judges can make a declaration that legislation which is raised in a case before them is in breach of the convention.

Consequently, cases that had previously been sent to the European Court in Strasburg are now able to be considered in the UK. The HRA 1998 has enabled patients to challenge the NHS regarding all aspects of healthcare, from storage of sperm to assisted suicide.

Human rights case law

While the HRA 1998 is the key primary legislation relevant to women's reproductive and childbirth rights, there are also examples of common law or case law which are relevant. Case law arises from a number of legal cases (not to be confused with the case studies at the end of Chapters 6–18 in this book).

Gillick v West Norfolk & Wisbech Area Health Authority 1986

This common law case is usually referred to as the Gillick Case, and practitioners often refer to 'Gillick competence' to identify when a young person demonstrates maturity and understanding regarding a proposed treatment or intervention. If the young person is able to decide for themselves what is best for them (weigh up the benefits and the dangers, engage in a decision-making process and make an informed decision for themselves) they are said to be 'Gillick competent' (legal basis) and autonomous (ethical basis). This case is significant as it also gave rise to the Fraser guidelines which surround the provision of contraceptive advice and treatment to children under 16 years of age. To prevent a criminal accusation a practitioner may claim a defence of compliance with Fraser guidelines. In 1986 the House of Lords ruled 'that parents do not have the right to be told that their children were being prescribed contraceptives'.

R (Axon) v Secretary of State for Health 2006

A mother (52) of two teenage daughters lost her battle in the High Court in London. Sue felt that as a parent she had a right to know if her girls (under 16) could be advised on abortion (January 2006). If Fraser guidelines were being used in relation to abortion it was possible that practitioners would be able to sue. Axon claimed that 'guidance infringed her rights as a parent under article 8 of European Convention on Human Rights' (safeguards the right to private and family life). Mr Justice Sibler ruled that the parent's rights were overridden by the children's rights to confidentiality, if they were mature enough to understand the implications and therefore competent to take such decisions. The ruling upholds the guidance issued by the Department of Health (2004c) to try to stem the rise in teenage pregnancies. Children should be urged to talk to their parents, but if there is a risk to a child's health or welfare (serious enough to outweigh the duty of confidentiality), the guidance says the doctor cannot insist that their parents are told. Note: confidentiality is not absolute – where a healthcare professional believed a serious risk is posed to a young person's health, safety or welfare the case should be referred through safeguarding children procedures.

R v HFEA (ex parte Blood) 1999

Diane Blood made legal history when she took her case to the European Court. Diane was a widow and wished to use her dead husband's sperm for assisted conception. As he was unable to provide written consent her request was rejected. The European Court ruled in Diane's favour and she subsequently gave birth to two sons (Liam in 1998, Joel in 2002). In February 2003 she claimed a legal victory as her late partner was recognised as the father of her children. This case illustrates the ethical dilemma of becoming a father after death and the rights of a woman to a family.

R v HFEA (ex parte Evans) 2005

Natalie Evans wished to use embryos which had been created (during IVF treatment) using her partner's sperm. Natalie and her partner had started assisted reproductive treatments (ART) and had both consented to the programme. Following a change in their relationship (they separated) her partner withdrew his consent for the embryos to be used. Natalie took her case to the European Court as she felt her human rights (right to family life) had been breached. The European Court ruled in her ex-partner's favour. He had every right to withdraw consent at any time in the process. The HFA Act requires that the embryos are destroyed after a specified time. Natalie's partner was able to exercise his right to withdraw consent to use his sperm.

Warren v HFEA (ex parte Warren) 2014

Beth Warren won a battle with the UK Fertility regulator (HFEA) to prevent them from destroying her late husband's sperm. The HFEA intended to destroy the sperm in 2015 when his consent would not be renewed. Warren's husband died in 2012 following a brain tumour, and had specifically identified that she could use his sperm to fulfil her right to a family following his death. He also consented to his being named as the father of any subsequent children. The High Court ruled that the law allows for sperm and eggs to be stored for up to 55 years if consent is regularly renewed. Beth wanted the freedom to choose if and when she wanted to use the sperm when she was no longer grieving for her husband.

Chapter summary

This chapter has considered basic human rights in relation to childbirth and family life. Following identification of the variety of rights for childbearing women and their families, consideration has been given to the application of ethical principles and the legal situation. Case law has demonstrated the complexity of regulation and control of assisted reproduction and the balance with individual rights to family life.

Reflection: Rights and care in labour

Petra is a non-English-speaking primigravida. She is booked at a large maternity hospital and her birth partner is her mother. Petra's husband also wishes to be at the birth and they are both keen on having a water birth. On the day that Petra goes into labour the labour suite is very busy and a member of staff (with experience of water births) has gone off sick. Petra, with the help of her husband, arrives with her birth plan and is informed that the delivery suite is busy and there are no midwives prepared to support a water birth.

Evaluation

In choosing to use water during labour, Petra is likely to benefit from mobility during labour as freedom of movement is helped by buoyancy in the pool. Water has been used as a method of pain relief for hundreds of years. In addition to its pain-relieving qualities, water has psychological benefits (encourages relaxation, decreases anxiety) during labour. Cluett and Burns (2009) found that immersion in water during the first stage of labour reduces the need for pain relief. NICE (2007) guidelines identify that water temperature should not exceed 37.5°C. Both the RCM and RCOG suggest that there are no known side-effects of women using water during labour. Petra has made a choice regarding her childbirth and should be supported in that choice. Midwives are trained to provide care during labour which promotes normality and choice (RCOG, 2007).

Analysis

Many commentators identify that ethics are a set of principles (Johnson and Johnson, 2007). A dilemma may occur when one is unable to decide which principle should be followed. Petra has made a choice and a decision regarding childbirth; the midwife has a dilemma in that Petra's autonomy is compromised by the lack of carers and skills, and safety issues regarding support for labouring women. The labour ward coordinator is challenged to provide a safe standard of

(continued)

care for all women and the fear that Petra will not experience the birth she was planning. It is likely that, when completing the Patient Satisfaction Survey, Petra will be ticking the 'we are not performing as we should' box.

What can be done?

Government policy identifies that providing choice for childbearing women is supported. While the Department of Health is seeking to obtain cost savings during the next financial year, there is clearly a tension between short-term savings (reducing choice, continuing to have the same number of staff but providing more care (increased birth rates) and long-term health benefits (less intervention, fewer drugs, lower Caesarean section rates).

Implications for practice

Growing demands from a consumer-led service approach challenge midwives and maternity services to meet their customer needs. The current NHS philosophy (Department of Health, 2013) of a business-style approach (efficiency and effectiveness) to healthcare does not sit comfortably with a maternity service philosophy (Department of Health, 2007a, 2012a) (choice, continuity and compassion) or a midwife philosophy (safety, holistic ('with woman'), empowered positive experiences).

The RCM (2013a) identifies what is happening on the front line of maternity services. There are a number of indicators of the pressures on maternity care and limitations of resources available. In 2012, the latest baby boom, there was a 23 per cent increase in the number of births, which puts pressure on an already stretched service.

Conclusion

The contribution of midwife-led care to improving childbirth experiences of women in the UK must be developed. Midwives are trained and educated to a high standard and must demonstrate this throughout their care and in a variety of environments. Government policy may be an ideal, but midwives have to find ways of 'making it happen'.

Practice check

1. How do you empower women with regard to choices in childbirth?
2. How can midwives ensure that the information provided to women and their families is helpful?
3. What rights do women have during labour?

Useful websites

Association of Radical Midwives (ARM): www.midwifery.org.uk
Nursing and Midwifery Council (NMC): www.nmc.org.uk
Royal College of Midwives (RCM): www.rcm.org.uk
Royal College of Nurses (RCN): www.rcn.org.uk

5 The legislative framework for midwifery

Pre-requisites for this chapter

After reading Chapters 1–4 you should already be familiar with primary and secondary legislation, the legal process and the English legal system. It would be helpful to have access to the Nursing and Midwifery Council website at www.nmc-uk.org.

Introduction

So far I have identified that midwives need to have an understanding of law for professional practice. Medical law usually refers to both the statute and case law, which affect health and social care. Medical law is still a developing discipline, which is shaped by the courts (Mason and Laurie, 2006a). This chapter identifies the key midwifery-specific legislation, that is to say the statute that is specific to midwives and midwifery. Consideration of midwifery legislation reveals that regulation and control of midwives and midwifery practice by the medical profession and others (Church, state) is longstanding and has protected the title *midwife* and contributed to the reduction of mortality and morbidity associated with untrained or uneducated midwives. The primary purpose of midwifery legislation has been to protect the public. By regulating and controlling midwives and circumstances in which midwives practice, the law can govern roles, responsibilities and activities of a midwife. In addition, equality and human rights legislation (Chapter 4) places specific obligations on the NHS regarding non-discriminatory practice as well as equality, and these aspects also apply to maternity services and midwifery care. Midwives need to be cognisant of the specific legislation relating to their profession. After all, midwives are required to demonstrate that they are fit for purpose and fit for practice. A midwife cannot provide good-quality woman-centred care if she or he does not understand the standards that need to be maintained. The current midwifery regulating body is the Nursing and Midwifery Council (NMC); part of its role is to protect the public, and to stipulate rules and regulations which midwives are required to abide by and uphold. The NMC holds the largest register of any UK regulator, at approximately 670,000 nurses and midwives (CHRE, 2012). Being familiar with legislation, legislative process and legal requirements enables midwives to fulfil their role and responsibilities. In addition, knowledge and understanding of legislation will enable them to defend their profession and will support arguments around the specific role and responsibilities of the midwife. Increasingly, boundaries of care are being eroded in healthcare and the midwife is able to use statute to defend the right to practise the profession that is midwifery.

The legislative framework for midwifery is based upon the need to protect the public from midwives who do not meet the standards required of professional practice. In other words legislation regulates the midwifery profession through the auspices of the professional body whose purpose is to identify standards, codes of practice and conduct. The legislative framework also originates from the power exerted by the medical profession and the Church over midwives to control their activities and actions. Donnison (1988: 18), in her work on the history of the struggle for the control of childbirth, identifies that in England the 'first formal arrangements for the control of midwives were made under Henry VIII's Act of 1512 for the regulation of physicians and surgeons'. This Act intended to regulate and control physicians and surgeons who were considered to have no understanding or any other kind of learning. Donnison (1988) argues that while the 1512 Act does not mention midwives specifically, by virtue of the fact that midwifery is a 'manual art' and therefore a part of surgery, midwives were also controlled by the 1512 Act. The control Donnison refers to is the licensing by the Church. A licensed midwife equates to a registered midwife today. As part of the gaining of a licence, midwives were required to take a solemn oath to obey the rules of conduct laid down by the Church regarding their practice. Today, student midwives do not swear on oath, but the Lead Midwife for Education (LME) does have to confirm to the NMC that in good faith she or he believes that the student is of good character. In addition, some universities (e.g. Coventry University) request that students repeat a pledge (regarding the standard of care) during the graduation ceremony.

The NMC (2014d) identified that that legislation concerning nurses and midwives needs to be updated and changed to reflect the challenges faced by the largest regulatory body in the world. The NMC urged the government to fulfil its strategy outlined in the command paper *Enabling Excellence* (Department of Health, 2011c). The main issues are regarding the processes and costs of investigation and hearing of professional misconduct cases. The strategic review of the NMC (CHRE, 2012a), in an interim report, 'highlighted weaknesses in governance, leadership, decision making and operational management. In our final report, additionally we identify poor financial stewardship, a passive, hierarchical culture of "resigned resilience" and provide further detail on the problems with the NMC's management and business systems' (CHRE, 2012b: point 1.5, 4). This sad portrait of the regulatory body does little to promote the confidence of the public, profession or practitioners, and hides the significant work that the NMC has undertaken. The NMC has refocused its work, appointed a new Chief Executive and restructured to support delivery regarding investigation of misconduct cases. The NMC proportionally hear more cases involving nurses than midwives per year and have been criticised for increasing fees to fund increasing costs of misconduct investigations (Warwick, 2014a). *Better Legislation for Better Regulation: The Case for Legislative Reform* (NMC, 2014d) argues the case for urgent legislative changes. In April 2014, the Law Commission published a report explaining and setting out recommendations and a draft Bill for a new single legal framework for the regulation of all health and social care professionals. The reforms aim to sweep away the outdated and inflexible decision-making processes associated with the current legislation. The new legal framework would introduce a clear and consistent legal framework which is needed to enable the regulators to uphold their duty to protect the public. The Bill, while aiming to modernise regulation, suggests that the statutory midwifery committee at the NMC could be abolished (Silverton, 2014). It is against this backdrop that the current legal framework for midwifery is considered.

Legal framework for midwifery (legislation and midwifery)

The legislative framework for midwifery is based upon the need to protect the public from midwives who do not meet the standards required of professional practice. In other words, legislation regulates the midwifery profession through the auspices of the professional body whose purpose is to identify standards, codes of practice and conduct. It should be noted that the same legal system also affects the NMC in the execution of their responsibility. Symon (2010, 2013) identifies how the NMC can also face legal challenges over the way in which it executes its role and responsibilities. The legislative framework identifies and controls how the midwifery profession, midwives and their clinical activities are undertaken.

In Chapter 2 I identified that the rationale for legislation is to solve or address a problem. I also identified that the legislative process starts with a Bill. By 1800 midwives were divided into those who were licensed and those who were not, and those who were trained and those who were not. The problem in the 1890s was that the medical profession were concerned by the threat that midwives might pose to their livelihood. The establishment of the Midwives Institute in 1881 had the specific aim of raising the status of midwives, and the only way to do this was to campaign for a Midwives Act. It was not just the medical profession who were worried. Nurses also felt threatened by the proposals for a Midwives Act (Frame and North, 1996). In early 1890, the first of many Midwives Bills was introduced to the House of Commons by Mr Fell Pease (Donnison, 1977). It would seem that the passage of the Midwives Bills (1890s) was not dissimilar to the recent passage of the Heath and Social Care Bill in 2011–2012. Both Bills share opposition, debate, objection and compromise. The press contributed to the difficulties in the passage of the legislation, as news headlines and reports of public demonstrations escalated the debate. Fundamentally, the cost of the reforms and changes that these Bills proposed contributed to the delays and difficulties. At the heart of both legislative processes is the power and control over the medical profession.

The specific legislation that regulates midwifery practice (legislative framework) is found in the following statutes:

- Midwives Act (1902, 1918);
- Midwives Act (1926, 1936);
- Midwives Act (1951);
- Nurses, Midwives & Health Visitors Act (1979);
- Nurses, Midwives & Health Visitors Act (1992);
- Nurses, Midwives & Health Visitors Act (1997);
- Health Act (1999).

The above legislation forms the basis of primary legislation of midwives and midwifery practice. Secondary legislation in the form of statutory instruments and case law further develop and clarify the legal framework for midwifery.

The 1979 Act was the first piece of legislation that midwives specifically shared with other professions. At the time, midwives were concerned that the legislation would erode the midwifery profession and effectively allow other professions to regulate and control midwifery. This is an interesting argument as men and non-midwives dominated the CMB established under the 1902 Act. However, Inch (1982) identified that as late as 1979, midwifery was the only profession governed by a body on which members of the profession were prohibited by law from being anything but a minority on the Board. Putting a positive spin on the involvement of men and non-midwives in the regulation and control of midwifery, it would seem that this high level of service-user involvement should ensure that the profession and its registrants remained focused on the needs and expectations of women and their families. Concern was expressed in the early 1990s that there was a need for strengthening and regaining control of midwifery regulation in the form of new midwifery-specific legislation. Cardale (1990) outlines some of the issues. The Royal College of Midwives (RCM) set up a commission (chaired by Mrs Jane Wyndam Kaye) to identify the strengths and weaknesses of the 1979 Act.

The business of regulating nurses, midwives and health visitors is an enormous task. Self-regulation involves standard-setting, professional conduct, disciplinary procedures, approval of training, validation of courses and maintenance of the professional register. All regulatory bodies are challenged by the enormity of protection of the public. Trust, Assurance and Safety (Department of Health, 2007b) reports upon the regulation of health professionals in the twenty-first century. The report considers how to deal with the small number of professionals who provide poor-quality care, cause concern for patients, families or professional colleagues. Statutory professional regulation is intended to sustain, improve and assure professional standards, as well as identifying and addressing poor practice. The NMC is required to balance these two responsibilities while maintaining strength and integrity of midwifery and demonstrating flexibility to work throughout the UK (Department of Health, 2007b) The Council for Healthcare Regulatory Excellence (CHRE) provides expert advice on professional regulation. The CHRE was a recommendation of the NHS consultation document *Modernising Regulation in the Health Professions* (DH, 2001c). A review of the NMC in 2012 by CHRE identifies that the main problem with the NMC is in fulfilling a statutory role of fitness to practise.

The Midwives Act 1902

This is the first Midwives Act and is cited (Leap and Hunter, 1993) as a milestone in the history of the midwifery profession. The Midwives Act 1902 arose from 'a desire to reduce the high perinatal and maternal morbidity and mortality', and to 'protect the public from untrained midwives' (Mannion, 2008: 384). The Midwives Institute (founded in 1881 and a precursor of the Royal College of Midwives, founded in 1947) sought 'to make midwifery into a profession for well-educated, middle class women' (Leap and Hunter, 1993: 206) and concerned itself with building a professional basis for midwifery. At this time (and as today) there was a national shortage of midwives. The Midwives Act 1902 created the Central Midwives Board (CMB) and established the registration of midwives. The Act allowed midwives who had been in practice for at least one year and who could produce a written testimony of their good character to register under the auspices of this Act to practise midwifery legally. These midwives would be known as 'bona fide' midwives. This interim system of registration as a 'bona fide' midwife was discontinued after 1905. No woman could use the title *midwife* unless registered with the CMB.

The Midwives Act 1902 was passed on 31 July 1902, and nine members were appointed to the CMB. These nine members consisted of four registered medical practitioners, two persons (one of whom was to be a woman) appointed for a period of three years by the Lord President of the Council, and three other persons (one from Queen Victoria's Jubilee Institute for Nurses, one from the Association of County Councils and one from the Royal British Nurses Association) were appointed for a period of three years. The first meeting of the CMB was held on 11 December 1902 and two resolutions were passed:

(i)   a Secretary to the Board should be appointed at a salary of £400 p.a. and

(ii)   the railway fares of the members in attendance from the country should be part of the general expenses of the Board.

(CMB, 1983: 4)

The Midwives Act 1918

This was an important Act as it addressed the financial issues midwives were experiencing in the fulfilment of their role. In addition, the second Midwives Act enabled the CMB to suspend midwives from practice. Provision was made for midwives to be compensated for loss of earnings while suspended from practice. Midwives were required to complete documentation and maintain records while providing care. The cost implications of postage of statutory notification forms would now be removed.

The Midwives Act 1926

This Act was primarily to address the issue of uncertified women attending births. The uncertified woman was required to satisfy a court that 'the attention was given in a case of sudden or urgent necessity'. If unable to satisfy a court, they were liable for a fine of up to £10.

The 1926 Act identified that maternity homes (private services for childbearing women) needed to be registered with the Local Supervising Authority (LSA) and open for inspection.

To provide education for student midwives, there are courses and examinations for registered midwives (Midwives Institute) to obtain a Midwife Teachers Certificate (MTC).

The Midwives Act 1936

The 1936 Act established a return to midwifery practice (RTP) course of instruction. This Act also made provision for the following;

- Statutory refresher courses for midwives, the length to be determined by the CMB.
- The CMB could grant a midwife a midwife teachers diploma (MTD).
- Qualifications/requirements of supervisors of midwives identified.
- LSAs to provide an adequate salaried midwifery service (including uniforms, pay, annual leave, pensions, equipment and scheduled off-duty for midwives). Those midwives who chose not to work for the LSA could continue to work as independent midwives or be compensated if they were rejected by the LSA or chose to no longer practise as a midwife (surrender their certificates).

The Midwives Act 1951

The Midwives Act 1951 consolidates previous legislation. This Act is significant in that it made it a criminal offence for a person other than a registered midwife or registered medical practitioner to attend at childbirth. Subsequent legislation has not changed this provision. However, Article 45 of the Nursing and Midwifery Order 2001 does identify that 'in a case of sudden or urgent necessity' paragraph 1 of the above Act does not apply. Thus, the current situation whereby a paramedic may be the first healthcare professional to arrive would be considered 'urgent necessity', although the paramedic is required to request the support of a midwife. Student midwives and medical students are also exempt from the above, provided they attend as part of a course of practical instruction in midwifery recognised by the regulating body. Dimond (2002) identifies two cases that have demonstrated the need for legislation to protect the role of the midwife, one from a man (partner) and the other from a registered nurse. Both provided care during delivery without involving a midwife. A midwife who is prevented from providing care during labour or birth by a husband, partner or a non-registered medical practitioner should inform the police.

Nurses, Midwives and Health Visitors Act 1979, Chapter 36

Following the Briggs Report (Report on the Committee on Nursing, 1972) recommendation that there should be a single central body for the regulation of Nursing and Midwifery, the government enacted the Nurses, Midwives and Health Visitors Act in 1979. The NM&HV Act 1979 fully repeals the Midwives Act 1951 (schedule 8). Section 10 (1) identifies that the UKCC 'shall prepare and maintain a register of qualified nurses, midwives and health visitors' (NM&HV 1979, ch.36, 10 (1)). Sections 15, 16 and 17 of the NM&HV Act 1979 regulate midwifery practice.

This major piece of legislation was concerning for midwives (Frame and North, 1996). Supporters of the legislation recognised that the government could not afford to fund many individual regulatory bodies, but streamlining and amalgamation of process and functions could be achieved. Opponents, such as the CMB, warned of the dangers of being engulfed by the statutory framework being proposed and the possible contribution to deterioration in the standard of care provided to mothers and babies. As the CMB was the midwifery regulatory body that stood to be most affected by the proposed legislation, any concerns were considered to be reactionary at this time. National pride was also an issue as each nation (Scotland, England and Wales) wished to have its own board. This Act was significant in that it abolished the CMB. Seventy years of regulating midwifery was to be followed by the newly established United Kingdom Central Council for Nursing, Midwifery and Health Visiting (UKCC). The UKCC was to regulate and control all three professions and its constitution was a matter of concern. At the time of abolishing the CMB, there were a record number of serving midwives. With the new UKCC, midwives would not only again be in the minority, but the business of regulation would be shared with the other two professions. The constitution of the board was an issue that some objected to (Bent, 1989). An attempt was made to placate midwives with the provision of a midwifery committee at the UKCC, but the committee was to advise the board – it had to be listened to but not necessarily acted upon (Kirkham, 1995).

Sections 4, 15, 16 and 17 of the NM&HV Act 1979 specifically relate to midwifery. Statutory bodies changed and Sections 1, 2, 3 and 4 identify constitution, functions and membership; the UKCC replaced the CMB. The UKCC was structured as follows: 45 members (17 appointed, 28 nominated). Section 1 of the 1979 Act required each of the four National Boards to nominate seven members. The English National Board (ENB) membership was identified in Section 5 (2) of the 1979 Act and had a maximum of 45 members (30 elected and 15 appointed). Of the 30 elected, four members should be midwives. Schedule 1 of the 1979 Act identified that at least one midwife from each national board must be nominated to the UKCC (thus ensuring that at least four midwives were on the UKCC at any time). In addition to the Central Council and four National Boards (England, Scotland, Wales and Northern Ireland), the 1979 Act identified a statutory Midwifery Committee at the UKCC and each of the National Boards.

The Midwifery Committee at the UKCC was to be responsible for all matters related to midwifery practice. Section 4 (2) identifies that 'The Council shall consult the Committee on all matters relating to midwifery and the Committee shall, on behalf of the Council, discharge such of the Council's functions as are assigned to them by either the Council or Secretary of State by order' (NM&HV Act 1979: Ch 26, 4 (2)).

Under the miscellaneous provisions about midwifery, the NM&HV Act 1979 identified that

the Council shall make rules regulating the practice of midwives and these rules in particular —
(a) determine the circumstances in which, and the procedure by means of which, midwives may be suspended from practice;
(b) require midwives to give notice of their intention to practise to the local supervising authority (LSA) for the area in which they intend to practise; and
(c) require midwives to attend courses of instruction in accordance with the rules.

LSAs were identified in England as Regional Health Authorities (Section 16 (1a)). National Boards have responsibility under Section 16 (4) of the 1997 Act to provide the authorities with advice and guidance in respect of the exercise of their functions.

Nurses, Midwives and Health Visitors Act 1992, Chapter 16

Following the Peat, Marwick, McLintock (PMM, 1989) review of the five statutory bodies, the government identified proposals for amendment of the NM&HV Act 1979. Key changes to the

Table 5.1 The UKCC Register

Part 1 First level nurses trained in general nursing
Part 2 Second level nurses trained in general nursing (England and Wales)
Part 3 First level nurses trained in the nursing of persons suffering from mental illness
Part 4 Second level nurses trained in the nursing of persons suffering from mental illness (England and Wales)
Part 5 First level nurses trained in the nursing of persons suffering from mental handicap
Part 6 Second level nurses trained in the nursing of persons suffering from mental handicap
Part 7 Second level nurses (Scotland and Northern Ireland)
Part 8 Nurses trained in the nursing of sick children
Part 9 Nurses trained in the nursing of persons suffering from fever
Part 10 Midwives
Part 11 Health visitors
Part 12 First level nurses trained in adult nursing (project 2000 courses)
Part 13 First level nurses trained in mental health nursing (project 2000 courses)
Part 14 First level nurses trained in mental handicap nursing (project 2000 courses)
Part 15 First level nurses trained in children's nursing (project 2000 courses)

constitution of the UKCC were the main outcomes. The UKCC was to be 60 members (20 appointed, 40 elected) and professions were to be able to elect council members directly. However, supervision of midwifery practice was specifically addressed. The National Boards (ENB, SNB, NINB and WNB) would continue to be responsible for providing LSA. This remained unchanged, but the Boards' guidance would now have to be consistent with any rules made by the UKCC.

The UKCC (1992) identified 15 parts to the NM&HV Register (Table 5.1).

In having numerous 'parts' to the UKCC Register, individual disciplines appeared to be distinct and different. For midwives it would seem to reinforce the notion that midwifery was a branch or part of nursing. Midwives felt that it was an erosion of their professional status and further evidence that nurses and the public did not recognise midwifery as being a distinct and different profession.

Nurses, Midwives and Health Visitors Act 1997, Chapter 24

The NM&HV Act 1997 was a consolidating Act. The UKCC was to remain as the Central Council but its constitution was to be increased to 60 members (Section 1 (1)). Two-thirds of the members of UKCC were to be 'elected' members. Key elements were to establish and improve standards of training and professional conduct (2). Section 2 (6) identifies that 'In the discharge of its functions the Council shall have proper regard for the interests of all groups within the professions, including those with minority representation.' This clear remit for the Council was significant for midwifery. Section 4 went further and specified that of the members of the Council's Midwifery Committee 'the majority shall be practising midwives'. This legislation enabled practising midwives on the Midwifery Committee to have control regarding all matters of midwifery and to make, amend or revoke rules. In addition, if the Secretary of State was not satisfied that any proposed rules were framed in accordance with the Midwifery Committee, they would not be approved (Section 4 (1)). The Midwifery Committee was also empowered to deal with 'any matter which is assigned to the midwifery committee' and to 'make a report to the Council as to the way in which it has dealt with the matter' (Section 4 (5)). Midwives had regained control over the midwifery profession.

Section 7 of the NM&HV Act 1997 concerns the registration of midwives and identifies that the Council can make rules concerning the documentary evidence, fees to be paid, additional qualifications to be recorded and that a person's registration is to remain effective without limitation (subject to removal from the register for misconduct or otherwise). Other changes were to be made regarding the 'parts' of the register and certificates of registration to be issued. The NM&HV Act 1979 also details registration for nurses and midwives from the European Community (Sections 8–9). Miscellaneous provisions about midwifery (Section 14) concern regulation of midwifery practice (circumstances in which midwives may be suspended, notice of intention to practise to the LSA and attending courses of instruction). The LSA for midwifery was identified as the Health Authorities (in England and Wales) (Section 15 (1)). Each LSA was required to exercise general supervision over all midwives practising within its area, report any prima facie case of misconduct on the part of the midwife and have power in accordance with the Council's rules to suspend a midwife from practice. Attendance by unqualified persons at birth (Section 16) identifies that 'a person other than a registered midwife or registered medical practitioner shall not attend a woman in childbirth' (Section 16 (1)) However, this does not apply in a case of 'sudden or urgent necessity' or 'a person who, while undergoing training with a view to becoming a medical practitioner or to becoming a midwife' attends a woman in childbirth as part of a course of practical instruction.

There are six schedules in the NM&HV Act 1997 which concern constitution, proceedings and adaptations for Northern Ireland. In addition, the 1997 Act repeals all of the 1979 Act with the exception of Sections 23 (4), 24 and Schedule 7. A number of statutory instruments (SIs) are also revoked (SI 1983/884, SI 1984/1975, SI 196/3101).

In 1998 the government commissioned an independent review of the NM&HV Act 1997. JM Consulting published its review in February 1998 (JM Consulting 1998b) and the government accepted the main recommendations. The Health Act 1999 was used to set out provisions for change to the regulation of nurses and midwives. In order to effect change without remaking primary legislation, the government used secondary legislation or Orders to alter the constitution and name of the regulating body.

Health Act 1999

This Act is significant in that Section 62 (9) set out provision for an Order for the establishment of the NMC. Work to identify draft Orders was undertaken and the consultation document *Modernising Regulation: The New Nursing and Midwifery Council* (NHS Executive, 2000) was published. The final result was the Nursing and Midwifery Order 2001 SI 2002 No. 253 (see below), which transferred the regulation of nurses and midwives to the NMC.

European Union and European Midwives Directives

Since 1972 (when the UK signed the Treaty of Rome) the UK has been a member of the European Economic Community (EEC). The effect of this membership is that laws and regulations made in the European Union (EU) are binding upon all member states. Article 11 of the Council Regulation (EEC) No. 1612/68 confers 'the right, entitled to be treated for the purposes of access to the nursing profession, or the profession of midwifery, no less favourably than a national of such a state'.

European Parliament Directive 2005/36/EC provides legislation for midwifery in Europe. These directives are known as the European Union Midwives Directives or EU Directives. The EU Directives identify regulations regarding midwives, midwifery education and training. The NM&HV Act 1979 also identifies that a 'midwifery directive' refers to Council Directive No. 80/154/EEC, which concerns the mutual recognition of diplomas, certificates and other evidence of formal qualifications in midwifery.

The specific EU Directives are: Article 44 of the European Midwives Directive 80/155/EEC identifies the activities of a midwife. Article 40 focuses upon the training of midwives throughout the EU. It requires that all midwives undertaking training must undertake specific experiences (see appendices) such as providing care for at least 40 women during labour. An EU Directive identifies the outcome to be achieved. The EU Directive does not detail or identify how to achieve the outcome, hence the need to include the EU directives in the rules identified by the regulating body. The directives can be located in the NMC (2004) *Midwives Rules and Standards* and NMC (2009b) *Standards for Pre-registration Midwifery Education*. In order to be eligible to register as a midwife with the NMC, all midwifery students must complete the EU directives. Midwives who come from other European countries who wish to register with the NMC must also demonstrate that they have completed the EU directives.

Secondary legislation/statutory instruments

As identified earlier, primary legislation or Acts of Parliament are not the only source of law. Secondary legislation in the form of SIs provides a source of law which impacts upon midwives and other healthcare professionals. A minister may make an Order or Statutory Order (SO) after the original date of the primary legislation. The effect is that the details of existing legislation can be changed. For example, the primary legislation NM&HV Act 1997 identifies a regulatory body which regulates midwives, but the name, nature and constitution of the regulatory body was changed from UKCC to NMC by the SI Nursing and Midwifery Order 2001. Other SIs and changes are identified below. This type of legislation is no less binding than the original legislation; on the contrary, SIs are as powerful as the original statute and are used to change aspects which do not need to go through the full legislative process. Thus, midwives need to be aware of this process such that when consultation documents are circulated they may ensure that their views are known and that they may influence the resultant legislation (SI) and changes. Failure to pay attention to consultations and proposals can result in significant changes, which may not be welcomed. The following SIs are examples of changes that have taken place.

Statutory Instrument 1977 No. 1850

This statutory instrument abolished the need for medical supervisors. Midwifery maintained the concept of supervision and in 1977 all supervisors of midwives (SoMs) were required to be practising midwives (Thomas and Mayes, 1996). Once designated by the LSA the new supervisors of midwives were also required to undertake preparation for the role. The regulatory body at the time was the CMB and they introduced the first induction courses for supervisors. The supervisors' course lasted two days.

Statutory Instrument 1983 No. 873 (33/1175) (The Nurses, Midwives and Health Visitors' Rules Approval Order)

This order concerns the recording of additional professional qualifications on the Register, such as Teachers of Midwifery. The rules approved by this SI are sometimes referred to as 'the principle rules' as they relate to the training of student midwives for entry to part 10 of the UKCC register. The order specifies the length of training, educational requirements for entry to the course and competencies to be achieved by the end of the course. National Boards were given the responsibility of keeping records of the numbers of midwives undertaking courses. The NM&HV Act 1979 and the Rules Approval Order 1983 repealed previous enactments and rules relating to midwifery education and training. This SI was itself repealed by the SI 1990/1624 (below).

Statutory Instrument 1983 No. 884 (The Nursing and Midwifery Qualifications (EEC Recognition) Order)

This concerns the identification of midwifery qualifications. It was repealed by the NM&HV Act 1997.

Statutory Instrument 1984/1975 (The Nursing and Midwifery Qualifications (EEC Recognition) Amendment Order 1984)

This concerns the identification of midwifery qualifications. It was repealed by the NM&HV Act 1997

Statutory Instrument 1989 No. 1456 (The Nurses, Midwives and Health Visitors (Registered Fever Nurses Amendment Rules and Training Amendment Rules) Approval Order 1989)

The UKCC exercised its powers under Sections 2 (3), 4, 11 and 22 (1) of the NM&HV Act 1979, consulted with the professions and made changes to parts of the UKCC Register, rules and training for admission to part 9 of the register. Of key significance for midwives was the requirement to include the General Certificate of Secondary Education among the educational qualifications on the basis of which a person may enter training with a view to registration as a midwife.

Statutory Instrument 1990 No. 1624 (The Nurses, Midwives and Health Visitors (Midwives Training) Amendment Rules Approval Order 1990)

The UKCC exercised its powers under Sections 2 (3), 4, 11 and 22 (1) of the NM&HV Act 1979, and consulted with the Midwifery Committee and made changes to the rules regarding midwifery training. The new rules are cited as the NM&HV (Midwives Training) Amendment Rules 1990. The main changes concerned length of training: three years (45 programmed weeks per year), and 18 months for students already registered on part 1 or part 12 of the UKCC register. Supernumerary status was conferred upon students. The SI also identified the content of programmes of education, substituted the word 'education' for 'training' and specified that student midwives must have one or more periods of practical experience.

Statutory Instrument 1991 No. 135 (The Nurses, Midwives and Health Visitors (Registration) Modification Rules Approval Order 1991)

The UKCC exercised its powers under Sections 2 (3), 4, 11 and 22 (1) of the NM&HV Act 1979, and consulted with the Midwifery Committee and made changes to the principle rules. They were modified to allow a person who has previously been registered in any part of the Register and whose registration had ceased to be effective, to re-register (attain effective registration) to be able to meet the increased need for a nurse, midwife or health visitor 'which had arisen by reason of the hostilities in which Her Majesty is engaged in consequence of the unlawful occupation of Kuwait by Iraq' (Section 2:c). The modified rules only applied if a declaration was provided that the person intended to practise in response to the hostilities in the Gulf region. The effect was to change liability for fee paying from three years to six months so that ineffective registration is again made effective to meet the demand for additional practitioners.

Statutory Instrument 1993 No. 210 (The Nurses, Midwives and Health Visitors (Midwives Amendment) Rules Approval Order 1993)

The UKCC exercised its powers under Sections 2 (3), 4, 11 and 22 (1) of the NM&HV Act 1979, and consulted with the Midwifery Committee and made changes to the midwives rules. The new rules published were the Midwives Rules (UKCC, 1983)

Statutory Instrument 1996 No. 3101 (The Nurses, Midwives and Health Visitors Act 1979 (Amendment) Regulations 1996)

Following consultation (identified in the NM&HV Act 1979), this SI identified new midwives practice rules and a complementary code of practice (UKCC, 1998). Compliance with the rules is the responsibility of all midwives. Failure to comply is likely to result in an allegation of professional misconduct.

A Midwife's Code of Practice (1986) provides a definition of a midwife (Section 2:a) and the activities of a midwife (Section 2:b). Section 3 relates to matters directly related to the Midwives Practice Rules. Section 4: Home confinement. Section 5: Arranging for a substitute. Section 6: Notification of maternal death, stillbirth or neonatal death. Section 7: Equipment to be carried by a midwife in the community. Section 8: Other legislation to the practice of a midwife.

The Midwives Rules (UKCC, 1986; 1998) are divided into Section A, training rules; Section B, midwifery practice rules (27–44). Midwives Rules and Code of Practice (UKCC, 1998) followed further consultation. This SI was revoked in the NM&HV Act 1997.

Statutory Instrument 2002 No. 253 (The Nursing and Midwifery Order 2001)

This SI resulted from an independent review of the NM&HV Act 1997 by JM Consulting (1998a), the publication of the NHS Executive (2000) *Modernising Regulation: The New Nursing and Midwifery Council* and the NHS Plan (2000). Draft orders were published in April 2001 under Section 62 (9) of the Health Act 1989 (see primary legislation, above) and following further consultation with the professions the Nursing and Midwifery Order became law and came into force in April 2002. The two main changes brought about were change of title of the regulatory body from UKCC to NMC and the identification of three parts to the Register (namely nurses, midwives and specialist community public health nurses). The Nursing and Midwifery Order 2001 is unusual in that it amended primary legislation.

Statutory Instrument 2008 No. 1485 (Nursing and Midwifery (amendment) Order)

This statutory instrument allowed the NMC to make necessary amendments to its structural and operational framework in order to be able to carry out its function as a healthcare regulator under the auspices of the Nursing and Midwifery Order 2001.

Statutory Instrument 2008 No. 2553 (Nursing and Midwifery (Constitution) Order 2008)

This SI enables changes to the number and titles of statutory committees.

Statutory Instrument 2012 (The Nursing and Midwifery (Constitution) (Amendment) Order 2012)

This order made it possible to change the constitution of the regulatory body.

Statutory Instrument 2012 No. 3025 (Nursing and Midwifery (Midwives) Rules Order 2012)

This order enabled changes to be made (updating and reprinting) to the Midwives Rules.

Statutory Instrument 2013 No. 261 (National Health Service, England, Mental Health, England, Public Health, England) Regulations 2013

In Part 3 this SI concerns the notification of births and deaths. This legislation was necessary following the Health and Social Care Act 2012 to identify the changes to relevant bodies for notifications of births and deaths. Following the H&SC Act 2012 the following 'bodies' were created: National Health Service Commissioning Board (the Board) and Clinical Commissioning Groups (CCGs). Part 3:10 concerns the manner and time for providing information regarding births and deaths. Part 3:11 identifies the person to whom particulars of birth or death are to be given.

Statutory Instrument 2014 No. 1887 (The Health Care and Associated Professions (Indemnity Arrangements) Order 2014)

This requires that midwives must possess professional indemnity arrangements in order to be registered with the NMC. Midwives will self-declare that professional indemnity arrangements are in place. Failure to have indemnity arrangements results in removal from the NMC Register. Midwives who work in the NHS already have indemnity insurance. The effect of this SI is that midwives working independently of the NHS will have to acquire personal indemnity insurance. The cost of personal indemnity insurance is prohibitive to midwives.

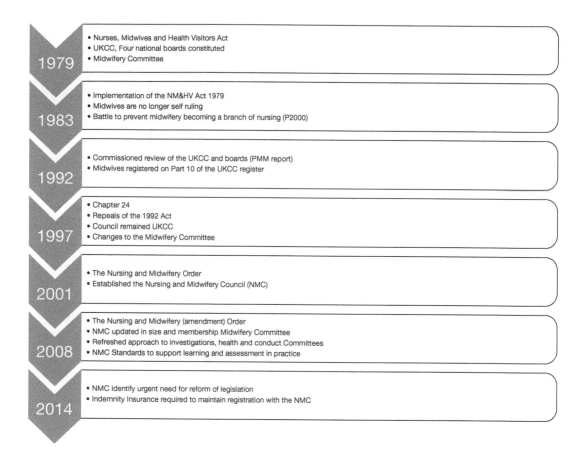

Figure 5.1 The effects of legislation: a recent midwifery timeline

Control and regulation of midwives

Midwives and midwifery practice is currently regulated and controlled by the NMC. Most midwives when asked will say that the NMC is a statutory body, whose function is to protect the public. It is uncertain how many midwives would be able to identify the relevant legislation or the ethical theory and principles which underpin the role and responsibility of the NMC. It is also a personal concern of mine as to how many midwives think that the Royal College of Midwives (RCM) fulfils the above role. Unfortunately, some midwives seem confused by the RCM and the NMC. They are very different organisations: one is defined by statute (NMC) and the other (RCM) attempts to influence it. A better understanding of English law may address the issue. Not all healthcare professionals are regulated. Currently there is debate as to if, when and should support workers/assistant practitioners be registered. Doctors are regulated by the GMC, and others (such as physiotherapists, paramedics and podiatrists) were regulated by the Health Professions Council (HPC), now known as Health and Care Professions Council (www.hpc-uk.org). The healthcare regulators are themselves regulated by the CHRE.

The NMC publish standards and guidelines for healthcare professionals. The midwifery circulars clarify the nature and extent of activities and actions required. A good example is NMC circular

25/2007, which identifies the grading of clinical practice for pre-registration midwifery education programmes. Hence, secondary legislation in the form of SIs identifies statutory regulatory bodies, and statutory regulatory bodies identify rules and regulate and control professional behaviour.

The Midwifery Committee (MC)

The Midwifery Committee is one of two statutory standing committees of the NMC. As identified earlier, the Midwifery Committee can be traced back to the NM&HV Act 1979. The Midwifery Committee 'advises the council on all matters relating to midwifery, including education and training, practice and supervision of midwives' (UKCC, 1994: 4). Each year the Midwifery Committee produces an annual report highlighting its activities. The Midwifery Committee undertakes reviews and consultation regarding the Midwives Rules and Standards as well as education and statutory supervision of midwives. The Statutory Framework for Supervision concerns the establishment of LSAs and the appointment of SoMs. The Midwifery Committee functions and is constituted under the NMC Standing Orders (2009).

Registration as a midwife is a legal requirement and must be maintained to be eligible for clinical practice and the education and assessment of student midwives. Non-payment of the annual retention fee (currently £100) will mean that the midwife is not on the NMC Register and is putting childbearing women at risk if she or he is working as a midwife.

Local Supervising Authority (LSA) (further detail in Chapter 10)

The NMC is required to set rules and standards for midwifery and for the LSA responsible for the statutory supervision of midwives. The LSAs are required to provide annual reports to the NMC. In turn the NMC (2008c, 2009c, 2010e, 2011b) produces an annual report of the quality assurance of the LSAs. The NMC (2012c) identified that all LSAs should continue to promote and publicise opportunities for women to have access to an SoM 24 hours per day, seven days per week and continue to report on initiatives, successes and challenges in this area. Key recommendations are that LSAs must continue to work collaboratively with the NMC to monitor and assure the safety and wellbeing of women using the maternity services through the quarterly quality framework. LSAs should develop guidelines for the annual review of a midwife's practice to ensure that the review undertaken by SoMs is consistent and equitable. The recruitment of SoMs was identified as a challenge in 2011–2012.

Supervision of midwives: an overview (further detail in Chapter 10)

Supervision can be traced back to the Midwives Act 1902. Originally the SoMs were medical practitioners and the role focused around clinical supervision. The intention of supervision at that time was to respond to public concern regarding a falling birth rate and continuing high infant mortality. Supervision is considered to be an effective method of quality measurement and specifically a function to protect the public. It is also thought that supervision of midwives provides professional leadership and a role model. The qualities of an SoM are thought to be ability to be approachable, accessible and accountable. These three As of supervision are underpinned by three other As: advisory, advocacy and accommodating. An SoM is generally described as being a proactive and supporting role. The NMC

(2014c) set new standards for supervision of midwives and for LSAs. The NMC publishes annual reports of the quality assurance of LSAs and they are available from the NMC website.

Supervision of midwives, like clinical supervision, is a formal relationship and forms part of a registered midwife's evidence for notification of intention to practise (ItP). Supervision of midwives is multifunctional in that the relationship may cover managerial, educational and supportive functions. Clinical midwifery supervision is an established, formal relationship in which one professional (SoM) meets regularly with another professional (or sometimes a group of professionals). Clinical midwifery supervision is not part of a performance review, it is not a disciplinary meeting or punishment, but an opportunity to develop and improve the quality of midwifery care.

In 2002, 100 years of statutory supervision of midwives was celebrated. Kirby (2002) identified that the roles, functions and education of the supervisor of midwives had been shaped and defined by changes in social policy, professional development and practice. Jackson (2002) suggested that supervision had moved away from being a punitive and controlling system to a supportive and enabling activity which encourages reflection and peer review. In 2013 the review of the NMC suggested that more should be done to improve supervision of midwives.

In January 2014 the NMC announced that a review of the supervision of midwives system would take place following a report by the Parliamentary and Health Services Ombudsman 'which found that midwifery supervision failed to identify poor midwifery practice following the deaths of three babies and a mother at Furness Hospital' (PHSO, 2013). Supervision of midwives will be addressed in further detail in Chapter 10.

Professional accountability

The NMC is the current regulatory body, governing midwives; the main purpose of the NMC is to protect the public. The way in which the NMC protects the public is by setting standards, producing rules, standards and guidelines for midwives:

- NMC (2004) Midwives Rules and Standards updated in 2008 but were relatively unchanged;
- NMC (2008d) The Code: Standards of Conduct, Performance and Ethics for Nurses and Midwives;
- NMC (2008b) Standards to Support Learning and Assessment in Practice;
- NMC (2009b) Standards for Pre-registration Midwifery Education.

If a midwife does not uphold or comply with the standards, it is misconduct. Investigations into alleged misconduct are reported to the LSA and an action plan is provided. The plan may identify no action or the provision of educational support or a period of supervised practice or both. Case law and professional misconduct cases are identified at the start of this book.

Misconduct and fitness to practise

The NMC currently has responsibility for investigating allegations of professional misconduct. The formal process, while not a criminal or civil court, undertakes proceedings based upon established legal process. The use of the terms 'hearing' and 'striking off order' ensures that the nature of the NMC fitness to practise process is legal. Symon (2013) identifies that it is possible to legally challenge the

NMC regarding conduct of fitness-to-practise decisions. The NMC, like other professional regulators, is required to undertake correct procedures and maintain legal fairness.

Professional misconduct is considered to be any conduct that falls short of the high standards expected of a healthcare professional. Professional conduct cases are scheduled events, which you are able to attend. They take place at a number of venues across the UK and provided you notify the NMC in advance, attendance at hearings is possible. The NMC publishes the names, dates and charge on the website. In addition, the outcomes are also identified. Outcomes may be suspension, removal from the register (striking off the register) or no case to answer. The numbers of midwives referred to the NMC professional conduct committee has remained insignificant (Ackerman, 2012). Employers of midwives (NHS managers) are required to check the registration of all nurses and midwives. Midwives (including those in higher education establishments) are required to inform their employers of any change to their registration.

NMC rules, codes and standards

As part of the statutory responsibilities of a regulatory body the NMC publishes materials to enable practitioners to fulfil their roles and responsibilities and to enable the public to be aware of the standards that are expected of a registered practitioner. It follows that if members of the public are aware of the standards the expectation is that practitioners will uphold them. The NMC publishes guidelines for midwives to enable them to understand the professional requirements of a registered practitioner. In recent years the NMC has been proactive in informing and ensuring that service users are engaging with the regulatory body.

NMC: The Code – Standards of Conduct, Performance and Ethics for Nurses and Midwives

Healthcare professionals have a set of shared values regarding conduct and performance. In the NMC Code the key ethical standard is that of trust. Women must be able to trust their midwife to act lawfully, and this includes both in our personal and professional lives. In reality this means that student midwives are required to be trustworthy both in clinical practice and in their academic work. The NMC Code also stipulates that you must be 'open and honest, act with integrity and uphold the reputation of your profession' (NMC, 2008d: 1).

Different standards are expected from regulatory bodies than those of employers or the legal system. Professional standards are often higher than those of 'a reasonable person'. The NMC requires midwives to make the care of people their primary concern, treating women as individuals and respecting their dignity. Midwives are required to collaborate with those in their care. This includes making arrangements to meet people's language and communication needs. A dilemma occurs when midwives are not able to meet language and communication needs. Finding an interpreter or having funding to make patient information leaflets (PILs) in a variety of formats is not always possible. Midwives may not be multilingual, able to 'sign' or know how to communicate using Makaton. Yet to fulfil the NMC standard she or he must listen to women in their care and respond to their concerns and preferences. The dilemma is: can you continue to provide care when you are unable to meet language needs?

The key elements of the Code are:

- 'Make the care of people your first concern, treating them as individuals and respecting their dignity': 2–3.
- 'Work with others to protect and promote the health and well being of those in your care, their families and carers, and the wider community': 5–6.
- 'Provide a high standard of practice and care at all times': 7–8.
- 'Be open and honest, act with integrity and uphold the reputation of your profession': 9.

The NMC consulted widely regarding revalidation and the content of the proposed structure of the Code. A new NMC Code was published in 2015 and can be obtained at www.nmc-uk.org/Documents/NMC-Publications/revised-new-NMC-Code.pdf.

NMC post-registration education and practice (PREP) and continuous professional development (CPD)

The CMB (1965) reported that between 1 April 1964 and 31 March 1965, 3,281 midwives attended short refresher courses (statutory requirement under the Midwives Act). Short refresher courses were usually residential and midwives were required to attend every five years (rule G1). While refresher courses are no longer stipulated, midwives are now required to demonstrate CPD in order for their registration to be renewed. PREP requirements for midwives were first published in 1994 and have always been a mandatory requirement for maintaining registration as a midwife. PREP (NMC, 2011c) are the standards set by the regulatory body (NMC) with the specific aim of helping midwives provide high standards of care: 'PREP helps you to keep up to date with new developments in practice and encourages you to think and reflect yourself' (NMC, 2008f: 2). The PREP framework is an important component of clinical governance. Key elements of PREP are the need to maintain a Personal Professional Profile (PPP), undertake a return-to-practice programme (if they have been out of practice for five years or more), notify intention to practise and demonstrate every three years that they have attended a number of study days. Early documents (UKCC, 1999, 2000) identified two separate standards – the PREP practice standard (PS) and the PREP CPD standard. The NMC (2008) requires that both standards must be met in order for registration to be renewed.

The PREP PS standard refers to the requirement to undertake a minimum of 450 hours midwifery practice. The PREP CPD standard identifies that midwives must have undertaken and recorded at least 35 hours of learning activity relevant to their practice during the three years prior to renewal of their registration. Midwives are required to maintain a professional portfolio to demonstrate PREP requirements. Portfolios are considered to be the best way for midwives to demonstrate that learning is taking place and that future development will meet the needs of childbearing women. The NMC does not specify nature or type of learning and midwives are considered to be able to make a professional choice regarding their development. Midwives renewing the registration have to provide written and physical evidence to support the PREP declaration. The NMC (2011c) identify that PREP audits may be carried out at any time. In 2013 a sample of PREP audits were undertaken and revealed that not all midwives were compliant. Author's note: PREP supersedes statutory midwifery refresher courses.

NMC midwives rules and standards

Midwives rules and standards (2010) identify standards of proficiency that are necessary for safe and effective practice under Article 5 (1) and 2:a of the Nursing and Midwifery Order 2001. Midwives rules concern education, registration (registration appeals, fees), midwifery and fitness to practise and have been in place in this format since 2004. In the current midwives rules and standards (2010) there are 16 rules starting with citation and commencement through to the publication of an annual report. Key rules (notification, supervision, inspection and responsibility and sphere of practice) are discussed below.

The guidelines often identify standards that are higher than would be expected of a reasonable person. The standard is that of a professional person providing a professional service. Midwives trying to fulfil these standards sometimes have difficulty in clinical practice when time constraints or the application of targets compromise the nature, style and standard of care to be provided. A good example is that of antenatal care. The provision of antenatal care can vary depending upon the environment, caseload and complexity of the pregnancy. Midwives are required to uphold the rules and demonstrate the standards at all times or risk the removal of their name from the Register.

Intention to practise

All midwives registered with the NMC must complete annual notifications of intention to practise (ItP). The completed notification is given to the midwife's named SoM. The SoM will countersign the ItP to confirm that she knows the midwife, and the original is returned to the midwife. If a midwife provides care to a woman or baby in an emergency in an LSA where an ItP has not been submitted, the midwife must complete an additional notification (on the back of the existing notification) and give it to an SoM in the LSA where the emergency took place. All ItPs have to be submitted annually before 1 April. SoMs will not sign ItPs if they are in any doubt that the midwife meets the NMC requirements to practise. The SoM refers to the Local Supervising Authority Midwifery Officer (LSAMO) for advice prior to signing the notification. ItP notifications are one of the ways in which the NMC ensures that midwives have paid their NMC annual fees and have provided confirmation of PREP requirements for maintaining registration.

Revalidation

In January 2014 the NMC commenced consultation regarding revalidation. The NMC identified that revalidation is the process by which registered midwives and nurses will demonstrate to the NMC that they remain fit to practise. The key purpose of validation is to allow the NMC to reassure the public that midwives are fit to practise (in all employment settings) and to discharge the duty of a regulatory body.

Parliamentary and Health Service Ombudsman

While considering primary and secondary legislation it is appropriate to consider the Health Service Ombudsman. Ombudsmen or commissioners were established by the National Health Service Reorganisation Act 1973 to provide an independent person to whom an aggravated, dissatisfied or disgruntled citizen can turn. The Ombudsman is not an alternative to NHS complaints procedures and is concerned with public services. Complaints to an Ombudsman are not considered if the aggrieved person has already appealed to a tribunal or has taken proceedings in a court of law.

Chapter summary

This chapter has identified and considered primary and secondary legislation regulating midwifery and midwifery practice (legal framework for midwifery). The primary purpose of midwifery legislation has been to protect the public. By regulating and controlling midwives and circumstances in which midwives practice, the law can govern roles, responsibilities and activities of a midwife. Consideration of midwifery legislation reveals that regulation and control of midwives and midwifery practice by the medical profession and others (Church, state) is longstanding and has protected the title of midwife and reduced mortality and morbidity associated with untrained or uneducated midwives. Midwives are registered with and regulated by the NMC, which sets the standards for education, training, practice and supervision.

Each of the key statutes have been summarised and each, to an extent represent significant milestones in the development of the midwifery profession. The Midwives Act 1902, in common with the Health and Social Care Act 2012, had a turbulent journey through Parliament. Some legislation, such as the Health Act 1999, does not initially appear to regulate and control midwives, but through the use of 'Orders' or SIs effectively give power and control over the midwifery profession. Attention has also been given to secondary legislation and the way in which SIs have also regulated and controlled midwives and midwifery practice through the identification of rules, standards and guidelines.

Midwifery supervision has been identified as key to the safety and wellbeing of childbearing women. Robust functioning of supervision and effective LSAs are thought to contribute to the safety of women and babies using the maternity services. Midwifery supervision has been fundamental to the profession for over 100 years. Following the publication of CHRE (2012), PHSO (2013), the Professional Standards Authority (2014), Department of Health (2014), the Kings Fund (2015) and the announcement of the NMC (2015), midwifery supervision is no longer publicly supported. Changes to the legislative framework for midwifery are necessary to remove the statutory supervision of midwives. This chapter has raised key areas for discussion and further exploration, such as consent and childbirth rights, as well as concerns regarding the effectiveness and appropriateness of statutory supervision of midwives (PHSO, 2013) (see also Chapter 10).

Midwives need to have an understanding of law for professional practice. While it is thought that a wide range of laws regulates the relationship between a nurse and a patient (Griffith and Tengnah, 2008), midwives also have to consider the specific midwifery legislation which regulates the relationship between a midwife, the regulatory body, childbearing women and the baby.

Activity

Undertake a self-audit of two episodes of care you have provided. Using the following two standards, identify whether you have met the conduct required by the NMC:

- Standard 1: 'You must inform someone in authority if you experience problems that prevent you working within the code' (NMC, 2008d: 6).

- Standard 2: 'You must ensure that any advice you give is evidence based if you are suggesting healthcare products or services' (NMC, 2008d: 7).

Reflection

Using this chapter and NMC publications, have a closer look at the following aspects of midwifery legislation and the ethical basis for midwifery care:

1. Read the background to midwifery supervision. Is the rationale for supervision still valid today?
2. Do you have any questions or concerns in this area that the chapter does not address?
3. Is there anything in the study which makes you want to take some kind of action (further reading, changing the way in which you practise or identification of an action plan)?
4. Access the latest supervision, support and safety report (NMC, 2013). What are the key achievements of supervision evidenced in this report?

Useful websites

Council Healthcare Regulatory Excellence (CHRE): www.chre.org.uk
Makaton Charity (sign language): www.makaton.org
Midwifery legislation: http://legislation.gov.uk
Nursing and Midwifery Council: www.nmc-uk.org
Revalidation: www.nmc-uk.org/Nurses-and-Midwives/revalidation
Royal College of Midwives: www.rcm.org.uk

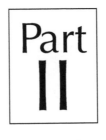

Part II

Practice

6

Consent and refusal

Pre-requisites for this chapter

You should have an understanding of the ethical principles of autonomy and advocacy. It would be helpful if you could access the Mental Health Act 1983 and the Mental Capacity Act 2005.

Introduction

Consent is an ethical and a legal issue and fundamental to demonstrating willingness to receive care, treatments and interventions, as well as reinforcing the basic trust between the woman and her midwife. Women should be at the heart of decision making (*Lancet*, 2014). Theoretical perspectives are around ethical principles, the process of consent and the legality regarding standards and potential for civil or criminal actions. Consent is not an end in itself but a process, which enables childbearing women to have control and make informed choices regarding their childbirths.

From a maternity service point of view there are three main problems or dilemmas surrounding consent and childbirth: the first problem is around a belief that a woman will undergo any treatment or intervention necessary to improve the health of the fetus, save the fetus or reduce the likelihood of trauma to the baby. This belief is flawed as no one individual can be expected to receive treatments, undergo surgery or participate in practices against their wishes. The second problem is regarding the decision-making capacity of the pregnant woman. The capacity is not usually questioned until the woman makes a choice or decision, which does not 'fit' with the maternity service or care providers. The final problem is that decision-making capacity may also fluctuate during childbirth; fear, anxiety, pain and stress can impact upon the decision-making process.

The ethical issues are around the right of an individual to determine what happens to their own body or to be autonomous. This is often referred to as self-determination. The ethical basis for gaining consent is that it demonstrates a respect for the patient/client/woman or individual receiving care. By care I mean any treatment, intervention, investigation or participation. Consent is synonymous with good practice and as such the nursing and midwifery standards of conduct, performance and ethics identify that 'You must ensure that you gain consent before you begin any treatment or care' (NMC, 2008d: 4)

The legal basis for consent is that without it the caregiver or employer may be potentially subject to a negligence claim. Consent is the first defence in a claim for negligence.

Students often ask: what is the law of consent? There is no specific law as in a statute or one specific case law that covers consent. While no single statute covers consent, case law has established the legal mechanisms, and professional requirements have established standards regarding communication and information-giving. It would be difficult for one statute to cover all aspects, instances and circumstances around consent. Some statutes (Children Act 1989; Family Law Reform Act 1969; Human fertilisation and Embryology Act 1990) do not appear to relate to consent but on closer inspection have significant impact.

Professional standards regarding consent (GMC, NMC) identify how and why consent is necessary. Gaining consent requires good communication skills and midwives have to ensure that for consent to be valid it must be given freely (uncoerced), understood (informed) and communicated (verbally, written or participatory). The courts have removed the idea that a signature on a piece of paper amounts to consent.

Dimond (2002) identifies 32 decisions during pregnancy for which the client should provide consent. Taking account of decisions during labour and the postnatal period, it is more likely that most women will be providing consent for upwards of 60 occasions. The ethical dilemma for the midwife is around the woman's capacity to make decisions and her competence in doing so. Key concepts with regard to consent are capacity, competence and special considerations (child and emergency).

Without the consent of patients, activities (care) that involve touching or sharing of patient information may be unethical, illegal and unprofessional (misconduct). The legal issues are around the standards required for consent and the duty of care required to do so. Following a definition of consent, this chapter will consider theoretical perspectives (concept of informed consent), ethical issues (autonomy and rights and professional accountability), legal issues (capacity, competency, duty of care and standards) and provide a case study (Sally) to illustrate consent in practice.

Definitions of consent

Consent may be defined as 'a voluntary, un-coerced decision, made by a sufficiently competent or autonomous person on the basis of adequate information and deliberation, to accept rather than reject some proposed course of action that will affect him or her' (Gillon, 1985: 113). Interestingly, Gillon subsequently suggested that definitions of consent are at best 'ambiguous' (Gillon, 2003: 113) An alternative simplified definition of consent is 'a patient's agreement for a health professional to provide care' (Department of Health, 2001a).

Types of consent

Broadly speaking there are three types of consent: implicit, verbal consent and written consent. Implicit consent is said to be when a patient turns up for healthcare and does not demonstrate any reluctance or verbal disagreement to the process. The woman may expose an arm to receive an injection or abdomen to allow an abdominal examination/palpation. Care has to be taken when a patient arrives in an ambulance, unconscious – is the implication that they would wish to receive all treatment? All healthcare practitioners understand their duty of care in an emergency situation. The dilemmas and difficulty arise when the patient's wishes are not known and a relative or friend presents their views. In the past some healthcare workers may have assumed that because a patient arrives for an appointment that they are consenting to treatments offered. It is necessary to be cautious with the notion that the patient consents to treatment by turning up! Not only does this assumption disrespect the patient, it also undermines the trusting relationship between healthcare providers and their patients. Assumptions like these are dangerous as consent must be specific, understood by the patient and time limited (the patient may change her mind at any time).

Distinctions of consent may be made. Proxy consent, advance consent and unspecific consent all complicate the discourse on consent. Proxy consent is particularly for someone who is unable to consent for herself and has attracted interest from relatives. The next of kin or relative who demonstrates that they know the patient's wishes or what would be in their best interest is challenging during the provision of care. Proxy consent is not usually relevant in the maternity services as childbearing women articulate their own wishes and choices and identify what is in their 'best interest'. There is a caution here: in law the next of kin has no legal right, either to consent or to refuse consent on behalf of another person. A husband or birth partner cannot consent for a Caesarean section on behalf of a pregnant woman. Unspecific consent usually refers to the clause 'and anything else considered necessary'.

Key concepts with regard to consent are that an adult can understand and retain information (competence), has capacity to make an informed choice (can weigh up the pros and cons of a suggested treatment or intervention) and information giving (understands what is being proposed).

Ethical principles applied to consent

Ethical-based care comprises demonstrating the ethical principles of autonomy, beneficence and non-maleficence. Consent is a fundamental part of patient rights, duty of care and professional practice. Consent challenges midwives as the decisions and choices made by childbearing women may not always be in the best interests of the baby or (in the midwife's view) of the woman. In addition, just because something (intervention or treatment) may be available (ultrasound scan) does not mean it should be used. The decision to have an ultrasound scan may identify additional dilemmas that the woman had not anticipated or foreseen. An example of this would be when the ultrasound suggests that the baby is growth-restricted. Consent also challenges midwives when childbearing women make choices that the midwife does not agree with or believe to be in the woman's best interest. An ethical dilemma is also found when the midwife is offering a service, treatment or intervention that is declined. Most midwives are trained to offer choices that are generally considered to be good, healthy options (e.g. routine administration of vitamin K, 'flu vaccination); it is not always comfortable when offers are rejected. Midwives must take into account the personal choice of each woman receiving care.

Autonomy: upholding an ethical principle

Consent is an expression of autonomy. Autonomy is about being in control; the woman is able to express her wishes and act upon information to make an informed choice or decision regarding her care. In other words, a woman has self-determination or the ability to determine or control what happens to her. The midwife should demonstrate respect for self-autonomy in that the woman's decisions should be upheld. Autonomous agents must take responsibility for the course of action chosen. Thus the woman, in choosing to accept or decline a particular course of treatment or intervention, is required to live with the consequences. In applying autonomy to the maternity services this means that one both makes a choice and then is accountable for the choice made (unable to blame others). The reality of the situation relies upon the communication of information and the ability (capacity) of the woman to make a choice. Paternalism is the opposite of autonomy in that a paternalistic practitioner advises or decides what is in a patient's best interest without having concern for their wishes and feelings.

The principle of beneficence

Beneficence is a medical ethical principle of 'acting in the interests of the patient'. It is concerned with the right, wrong, good, bad, ought to do and duty regarding care. The midwife is required to make reasoned judgements in particular situations. An example is the amount of information that it is reasonable for a woman to receive.

Non-maleficence

Primum non nocene – 'first do no harm'. Beauchamp and Childress (2013: 150) consider this principle to be a core value of healthcare ethics. Professional standards of care identify that care providers must provide a high standard of care at all times (NMC, 2008d: 7). The duty of care to 'do no harm' has to be balanced against beneficence or the best interests of the patient. Some philosophers combine non-maleficence with beneficence to form a single principle (Beauchamp and Childress, 2013).

Competency

What, then, is competency in relation to consent? Competency refers to the ability of a person to make decisions. It is not the same as capacity. A competent person is able to understand and retain information.

It is not up to the patient to prove that they are competent to make a decision or choice. The premise is that all adults are competent.

Capacity to consent

The legal premise is that an adult of sound mind will be able to consent or refuse treatment as he or she sees fit. Decision-making capacity is assumed for those persons over 18 years. Children and young persons do not usually have decision-making capacity, but case law has identified that decision-making capacity must take into account a child's age, understanding and ability to retain and make decisions. There are plenty of opportunities during childbearing when a woman's ability to make decisions may be challenged as stress, anxiety and fear may impact upon the process.

Information giving

An action for negligence may be sought by the woman if the midwife has not informed her of the risks and dangers associated with a treatment or intervention. Information must be readily supplied in a way the woman can understand. It is for this reason that during the antenatal period women are encouraged to consider what they feel might be best for them during childbirth. Information giving is a two-way process in the maternity services. Women need to be informed as to what might be possible, choices available, options to consider and decisions to be made. In return, women are required to share medical information, which may impact upon the care pathway or safety during childbirth.

Standard for valid consent

The basic standard for valid consent is that it must be:

- given voluntarily;
- the client has to have capacity;
- the client giving consent must be 'appropriately informed';
- provided by a person with parental responsibility for client under 18 years of age;
- given sufficient information.

Consent: rights and duty of care

The duty of care in gaining consent

The key stages in gaining consent are:

1. information giving;
2. opportunity for questions;
3. agreement.

As part of the process of gaining consent professionals are also required to uphold professional standards regarding consent. Guidelines for consent are provided for healthcare practitioners (Department of Health, 2010b; GMC, 2008; NMC, 2015).

Stage 1: duty of care to inform or information giving

The duty of care to inform women is the first stage in gaining consent and requires midwives to be able to provide up-to-date and relevant information regarding treatments and interventions. In addition, the midwife has to demonstrate that professional standards are met. These standards will include good communication skills and the ability to explain risks associated with the proposed intervention. The midwife needs to be aware that for a successful civil action of trespass, it is not necessary to prove that harm was caused. Breach of duty to inform may also be the subject of a negligence claim.

J Harris (2005) suggested that patients should be able to choose between two different types of giving consent:

> Informed consent is a lost cause, a hopeless ideal. We should now offer a choice between simple and informed consent. Most people would opt for the former and be happy that their doctor to decide whether & how to proceed with treatment – and thereby agree to have no comeback if things went wrong.
>
> (Harris, 2005)

In 2007 a survey of anaesthetists found that there was a great variation in the amount of information given regarding the risks of an epidural analgesia in labour (Middle and Wee, 2009). Consent should be reasonably informed as illustrated in the case of *Hills* v *Potter* (1983).

It is the woman's right to receive information and it is the midwife's duty to provide information that meets the professional standards.

Stage 2: opportunities for questions

If mental capacity is not an issue, having been given relevant information and offered available options, if the patient chooses to refuse treatment that decision must be respected.

Stage 3: agreement

Agreement may be implied, verbal or in writing. A woman has the same right to agree, decline or refuse treatments or interventions.

Standards of professional conduct regarding consent

The standards expected of health professionals by their regulatory bodies may at times be higher than the minimum required by the law (Department of Health, 2010b).

Best interests

The NMC (2008d: 4) identifies that when providing care in an emergency 'you must be able to demonstrate that you have acted in someone's best interests'. The NMC does not stipulate whether it is the woman's best interests or those of the baby. This can present a dilemma for the midwife when an intervention is required to ascertain the wellbeing of the baby but requires participation from the woman. An example of this is undertaking fetal blood sampling during labour.

Legal aspects of consent

So far I have identified that consent is the agreement to treatment or interventions and that obtaining consent is a crucial part of healthcare. Making women our first concern and treating them as individuals is a philosophy that underpins midwifery practice. By treating women as individuals this does not prohibit the use of patient information leaflets (PILs) or generic information regarding a procedure or clinical practice. Providing individualised care means ensuring that the information provided is in a language that is understood, and the woman is able to use the information to make a decision which is appropriate and individual for her. The legal principle is that valid consent must be obtained before starting treatment or physical investigation or providing personal care for a patient. A healthcare professional who does *not* respect this principle may be liable both to legal action by the patient and action by their professional body. Employers may also be liable for the actions of their staff (Department of Health, 2001b).

There is no law of consent as such, and any legal aspects relating to consent are found in case law and guidelines. From a legal perspective, consent is based on legal principles that are laid down in human rights legislation, case law and standards of professional conduct.

Legal principles of consent

The legal framework for consent has been established over the years. The medical profession has explored and debated the types of consent in an attempt to find working solutions. Like other aspects of the law, there are principles and exceptions. The legal frameworks are civil and occasionally criminal. Failure to gain consent may result in an action of trespass, negligence and an allegation of professional malpractice.

Legislation and consent (not in order of significance)

Human Rights Act 1998

Basic healthcare rights are around the right to accept or decline care and to be fully involved in decisions about the care. Consent may be invalid or fraudulent if a midwife uses manipulation, coercion or paternalism in order to gain consent.

The Human Tissue Act 1961, 2004

This requires consent for the removal and use of human tissue. The 2004 Act extends definitions to 'controlled material' which is 'any material which a) consists of or includes human cells and b) is, or is intended to be removed, from the human body ... excepting (a) gametes, (b) embryos' (Section 32 (8), (9)).

Human Organ Transplant Act 1989

This Act requires consent for the removal and use of organs. For the purposes of this Act, gametes and embryos are not considered.

Family Law Reform Act 1969

The Family Law Reform Act amends the law relating to the age of majority, to persons who have not attained that age and to the time when a particular age is attained. It also makes provision for the use of blood tests for the purpose of determining the paternity of any person in civil proceedings. It identifies the evidence required to rebut a presumption of legitimacy and illegitimacy. It makes further provision for entering the name of the father in connection with the registration of the birth of an illegitimate child.

Mental Health Act 1983

This Act is focused on patient rights, while allowing for compulsory detention and treatment of those who are unwilling or unable to consent. Patients' rights regarding controversial treatments such as electroconvulsive therapy are addressed and practitioners are required to consider safeguards regarding consent.

Prohibition of Female Circumcision Act 1985

This makes it an offence to undertake female circumcision in the UK, even with consent.

Female Genital Mutilation Act (2003)

This prohibits anyone from aiding, abetting or procuring a person to excise, infibulate or otherwise mutilate the whole or any part of her own labia majora, labia minora or clitoris.

The Children Act 1989

This Act identifies parental responsibility. A person with parental responsibility is generally entitled to consent to treatment on behalf of an infant or child. There are a small group of important decisions that should not be carried out or arranged by one parent alone (for example, organ donation, sterilisation).

The Human Fertilisation and Embryology Act 1990

The focus here is abortion and embryo research. This legislation relates to assisted fertility and conception. A key concern is that donated gametes (sperm and eggs) must not only be stored and used in specific situations, but that the donor must consent and renew consent over time.

The Children Act 2004

This major piece of legislation extends the rights of children. It establishes a Children's Commissioner as well as new strategy and processes for the safeguarding of children. Children's Trust Boards (CTBs) and Local Safeguarding Boards (LSBs) are established. New targets are introduced for safeguarding and promoting welfare of children. Inspection of Children's Services is to be undertaken.

Mental Capacity Act 2005

A person must be assumed to have capacity unless it is established that she or he lacks it. A person should not be treated as unable to make a decision unless all practical steps have been taken to help them make a decision. The purpose of this Act is to clarify and provide for patients whose mental capacity is compromised. Patients who are mentally incapacitated have difficulty making decisions and the responsibility for decision making (consent) may be legally removed (sectioned under the Mental Health Act 1983).

Table 6.1 Practical steps to enable capacity

- Use simple language and where appropriate pictures and objects rather than words.
- Arrange for a person to have information and explanations in their preferred language.
- Consult someone who knows the person well on the best methods of communication.
- Choose the best time and location where the person feels at ease.
- Take time to make them feel comfortable and not rushed.

Source: adapted from Department of Constitutional Affairs (2007) and the Mental Capacity Act.

Assessment of mental capacity (independent evidence of lack of mental capacity) is not necessary just because someone makes an unwise decision. There are a number of practical steps (Table 6.1) that can be taken to enable a patient to consent.

Legal frameworks (case law) relevant to consent

Case law regarding consent has evolved significantly over the last decade. Case law relates to civil cases brought before the courts. In Re W [1992] Lord Justice Donaldson pointed out that consent plays two quite different functions for the healthcare professional–patient relationship: the first function is a legal function, justification of care without consent means the healthcare professional would commit a crime (battery) and a tort (trespass to person) (civil action). The second function is a clinical function; it secures the patient's trust/cooperation. Counselling on the implications, risks and side-effects of the intervention is necessary to secure a patient's trust. In addition, if the patient subsequently suffers harm as a result of that treatment, it may be a factor in claims of negligence. Case law illustrates the following legal frameworks:

- trespass to person
- negligence
- court orders.

Trespass

When consent is coerced, presumed or provided without information, the consent is invalid and treatments or interventions should not take place. The midwife risks an allegation of trespass (assault or battery) as well as a possible negligence claim. The midwife who does not gain consent is failing in the duty of care and is accountable through investigations into professional malpractice by the NMC as part of their statutory regulatory function.

Trespass to person is a tort. The defence to an action of trespass is that the patient did indeed consent to treatment or that the action was undertaken out of necessity or that there was statutory authorisation (court order under the Mental Health Act, 1983). It may be classed as battery or assault.

Battery: 'an action in battery arises if a patient is touched without her consent'. Assault is considered when a 'claimant is caused to immediately apprehend a contact with this person'. Like other actions for trespass (goods or land), no harm has to be proved. It is worth noting that social touching (holding a hand, arm around a shoulder) would not normally constitute a trespass. If a midwife provides incorrect or misleading information regarding a treatment or intervention the consent obtained will be negative and a liability in trespass can arise. In *Potts* v *NWRHA* [1983] a patient successfully sued for battery when she believed she was having a routine postnatal vaccination, but had actually received a long-acting contraceptive (Depo-Provera).

Case law has established that touching a patient without valid consent may constitute the civil or criminal offence of battery. With regards to determining capacity principles, a key case is that of Re *MB* [1997]. While this case is not maternity-related, it confirms the basic principle that capacity is presumed. However, a relevant maternity case is in the Court of Appeal in the case of *St Georges Healthcare Trust* v *S* [1999].

When providing information to patients regarding risks it is as well to be mindful of *Bolam* v *Friern Hospital Management Committee* [1957], *Sidaway* v *Board of Governors of Bethlem Hospital* [1985] and *Hills* v *Potter* [1989].

Professional misconduct occurs when a midwife does not demonstrate the professional standards when gaining consent. All healthcare practitioners are expected to uphold the standards of their regulatory body. In November 2002 a gynaecologist (Michael Pembrey, 56 years) was struck off the GMC medical register for sterilising patients against their wishes (O Dyer, 2002).

Negligence

Negligence is a civil wrong or tort. Negligence is the term given when either an action or failure to act causes harm to a patient. Negligence is one of the legal mechanisms when a patient perceives that she or he did not provide consent. Harm does have to be proved for a negligence claim to be successful. A key case which illustrates the potential claim of negligence is *Sidaway* v *Board of Governors of the Bethlem Royal Hospital* [1985 2 WLR 480 1985].

The standards of care a woman can expect during pregnancy and childbirth are clearly identified by regulatory bodies (NMC), professional bodies (RCM) and local (NHS trusts) and national guidelines (NICE). The roles and responsibilities of a midwife are identified as duties. Negligence is a civil action, but in the event of the death of mother or baby can become a criminal process as well. Negligence (duty of care, standard of care and breach of duty of care) is considered in further detail in Chapter 17.

Court orders

It is unusual for the law to become involved in healthcare. From time to time there have been occasions when there is a legal case involving a childbearing woman. Court-ordered Caesarean sections were an unnecessary, unhelpful and undesireable development in the 1990s. The Royal College of Obstetricians (RCOG, 1994) considered legal and ethical issues in relation to court-authorised obstetric intervention. Using court orders to force women into treatments and interventions can breach human rights, destroy therapeutic relationships and risk damaging mother–infant relations and potentially increase mental ill health. Forcibly (court-ordered) removing the rights of a competent adult to promote the rights of a unborn child is considered unethical on the grounds of lack of autonomy (on behalf of the woman). See Re *S* (*Adult: refusal of treatment*) [1992] and *St Georges NHS Trust* v *S* [1998].

Doctrine of informed consent

The term 'informed consent' was first introduced into the judicial lexicon in 1957 in the written opinion of an appellate judge in California – DJ Mazur (2003) It relates to the information provided by the practitioner on risks of treatment. Judicial, medical and ethical interpretations of informed consent have created controversy. Two different standards are evident:

1. professional standard of disclosure;
2. new judicial 'reasonable standard'.

Professional standards for consent

Guidelines regarding obtaining of consent are available (Department of Health, 2009; GMC, 2008; NMC, 2008d, 2014; RCOG, 2008). The RCOG (2008: 1) identify that before seeking a woman's consent you should 'ensure that she understands the nature of the condition for which it is being proposed, its prognosis, likely consequences and the risks of receiving no treatment, as well as any reasonable or accepted alternative treatments. Uncertainties should be discussed.' The RCOG also identify that practitioners must be able to discuss 'risk' and if necessary further explain risk with the use of numerical aids. Women need to be able to understand terms such as 'common', 'uncommon', 'rare' and 'very rare'.

Regulatory bodies identify the professional standards for consent (NMC, 2015). The NMC identify that midwives must

- You must ensure that you gain consent before you give any treatment or care
- You must respect and support people's rights to accept or decline treatment and care
- You must uphold people's rights to be fully involved in decisions about their care
- You must be aware of the legislation regarding mental capacity, ensuring that people who lack capacity remain at the centre of decision making and are fully safeguarded
- You must be able to demonstrate that you have acted in someone's best interests if you have provided care in an emergency.

(NMC, 2008d: 4)

The GMC (2008) publish guidelines for medical practitioners regarding gaining consent, and interestingly the guidelines are titled *Patients and Doctors Making Decisions Together*, thus reinforcing the notion that paternalistic care is no longer the bedrock of the medical profession. Guidelines for consent are also published by the Department of Health (2009).

The NMC (2008d: 2) identify that midwives must ensure that they gain consent. This is a basic duty of providing care. The basis for this is the professional ethical standard of making the care of women the primary concern, treating them as individuals and respecting their dignity. In theory, treating women as individuals is not a dilemma for midwives. In reality, treating a woman as an individual while working in an environment which has blanket policies regarding appointments, screening services and routine procedures can prove to be difficult. There is tension between providing an effective, efficient and time-limited service and individualised, supportive and bespoke service. It is not dignified to be herded into clinics or respectful when care is rushed. The midwife standard of care will be judged as well as the waiting times, 'time to treat' and other targets directed by NHS England.

Failure to comply with the professional standards for consent increase the likelihood of complaints, investigations and referral to the NMC. Clinical midwifery supervision is covered in detail in Chapter 10.

Consent: when capacity is compromised

Capacity to consent is compromised if a woman does not understand or is unable to use the information provided to make a decision. Capacity to consent may be temporarily or permanently impaired. Temporary compromised capacity may caused by factors such as panic, shock, fatigue, pain or medication. Capacity may be dependent upon the information the patient is actually given. If the midwife provides a great deal of complex information in a short period of time without giving the opportunity for the woman to think or ask questions, she may be unable to understand. In contrast, the provision of basic information should enable that same patient to possess capacity.

Capacity means that the woman:

- must be able to comprehend and retain information material to the decision;
- must be able to use and consider the information in the decision-making process.

There is no 'test' for capacity in that in order to make a choice or decision the woman is 'assessed or tested' for capacity to consent. Capacity to consent is assumed for a woman over 18 years (Re T (Adult: Refusal of Treatment) 1992). Midwives may find it necessary to communicate complex information to women and need to take care to ensure that a woman understands what is being proposed, how it make affect her and what the outcomes could be. Women are able to make difficult or complex decisions when communications are good. There are many decisions made during maternity care that have risks for the mother and/or fetus; for example, chorionic villus sampling, ultrasound, screening for abnormalities, induction of labour and external cephalic version (ECV). The maternity services recognise that making decisions during labour can be difficult. Women are usually provided with information and encouraged to consider possibilities prior to labour so that their views and preferences are known. If a woman has received pain-relieving drugs or showing signs of severe anxiety or has mental health problems it can be very difficult to gain valid consent. If a woman has been sectioned under the Mental Health Act 2007 it will be clear to practitioners that 'best interests' are the standard required.

Consent in labour

Obtaining consent during labour can be very difficult. Women often have a clear idea of the choices they would like to make during childbirth. Many women identify their wishes on a birth plan or labour care pathway. During labour their needs (or those of the baby) may change and women may need to adjust or change their minds. Coercion is used to describe when someone has been under undue pressure to change their mind.

If consent has to be obtained during labour, the midwife must ensure that information is given between contractions (RCOG, 2008). The woman should have the opportunity to listen and understand what is being suggested and time to make up her mind and consent or refuse as she feels is best for her.

The RCOG (2008) guidelines identify that if possible consent to irreversible procedures should be deferred.

Consent in an emergency

Consent in an emergency situation presents additional problems for the healthcare provider. The targets set regarding time taken between decision and executing healthcare are intended to ensure effectiveness, efficiency and safety of mother and baby. However, these timely targets may also cause difficulty around the ethical and legal aspects of the consent. Women who are unfamiliar with the caregiver, moved to a different environment (birth unit to consultant unit or from a delivery suite to anaesthetic room) may feel pressured into consenting to invasive procedures. If the consent is coerced or uninformed then it is neither ethical nor legal. Failure to gain consent or coercion causing lack of consent for obstetric or gynaecological treatment is associated with post-traumatic stress disorder (PTSD).

One solution to the problem of gaining consent for emergency Caesarean section is to increase women's awareness of the possibility of a lower segment Caesarean section (LSCS) during the antenatal period. By providing information about the current Caesarean rate at a particular NHS trust, women can make informed choices and decisions about where to birth their babies. Information giving during the antenatal period also enables women to identify their choices to midwives, consider the unexpected and use information to make plans, should the unexpected occur.

Consent and under 18 years

Technically, all persons under the age of 18 are considered to be children. A child is defined in the Children Act 1989 as 'a person under the age of 18 years' (Section 105 (1)). The concept of childhood is a socio-legal construct, which is influenced by time and legislation. A good example of this is marriage. History demonstrates that the acceptable age for marriage relates not only to years of age but the specific legislation of a country. In the UK marriage is permitted between young persons over the age of 16 years.

In social environments it may be difficult to ascertain age and people can look much older or much younger than their actual age. In the healthcare environment appearances may be suggestive but most of the time healthcare professionals have access to basic data (date of birth) which indicate a person's age. Discriminatory assumptions based upon age are not acceptable and the Mental Capacity Act 2005 does not allow capacity to consent to be based upon age. Other examples of legislation influencing consent is Section 8 of the Family Law Reform (FLR) Act 1969, which enables a child of 16 or 17 'to give valid consent to any surgical, medical or dental treatment without regard to their parents'. Most parents of teenage children will be familiar with the challenges that are associated with young persons exerting their wishes and feelings. It can be argued that there is a narrow interpretation of the FLR Act 1969 as consent to treatment and examinations for 16–17-year-olds relates only to therapy and diagnosis. Consent for organ transplant or blood transfusion is different, as in Re W [1992] 3 WLR 758.

Common law or case law provides further confusion regarding consent and children and young persons. In *Gillick* v *West Norfolk & Wisbech Area Health Authority* [1986] FLR 224, the issue of providing contraceptive advice to teenagers was the subject of legal debate. The concept of Gillick competence was developed as 'it is not enough that she should understand the nature of the advice which is being given: she must also have a sufficient maturity to understand what is involved'.

Consent for intimate care

Intimate care is difficult to define as perceptions of intimacy vary. Midwives undertake a variety of health assessments, which involve intimate care and may be routine. While it can be argued that abdominal palpation, vaginal examination, perineal care and breast care are fundamental aspects of the role of the midwife, assumptions that women agree to these routines or interventions need to be challenged. If midwives are to respect autonomy, do no harm (including psychological harm) and demonstrate good care, then consent is essential; without consent, control, power and a paternalistic attitude are demonstrated.

A common dilemma for midwives surrounds postnatal care and the promotion of dignity. Intimate care involves the assessment and recording of normal postnatal recovery from childbirth (perineal care, lochia, perineal healing). On the one hand, the midwife could promote dignity, respect the woman's privacy and ask about 'vaginal loss' and perineal comfort. On the other hand, the midwife can observe and check the lochia and perineal healing to assess normality, both of which are undignified. The midwife is acting autonomously in making a clinical decision and upholding the woman's autonomy by the gaining of consent.

Intimate care also concerns supporting women with breast-feeding. It cannot be assumed that because a woman has chosen to breast-feed that she wishes to do so in public or in front of a healthcare worker. Midwives supporting breast-feeding women have a number of tools and techniques that enable them to help women breast-feed successfully without using a hands-on approach. Observation of breast-feeding techniques to confirm positive aspects of infant feeding does not require written consent, but continuity of carer and a compassionate approach increase women's satisfaction and reinforce ethical values.

Consent for intimate examinations

Consent for any intimate examinations, such as vaginal examinations, requires special care. Women's experiences of vaginal examinations are well documented (Clement, 1994; Lewin *et al.*, 2005). Vaginal examinations are used to assess progress during labour and have replaced rectal examination as a more acceptable alternative (Dahlen *et al.*, 2014). It cannot be assumed that during labour a woman automatically consents to vaginal examinations by choosing to birth her baby in a medical environment (hospital). Midwives who follow hospital guidelines regarding routine vaginal examinations during labour need to be confident in the evidence base for the intervention and justify the clinical decision to undertake a vaginal examination. Vaginal examinations are so common in care of women in labour that decisions to undertake them are rarely questioned and are associated with good practice (NICE, 2007). Midwives wishing to undertake a vaginal examination must obtain consent for every examination. Saying to a labouring woman 'just going to check to see if you are progressing' or 'You'll feel me touching you Sweetie' (Bergstrom *et al.*, 1992) is not ethical-based care and does not constitute consent. The dilemma for the midwife is what type of consent should be obtained? Midwives usually ask permission to undertake a vaginal examination and receive verbal consent with minimal explanation. Hospital policy is frequently cited as the rationale, or alternatively to determine progress. Midwives practising defensively might be tempted to request written consent. A signature on a piece of paper does not constitute consent. What should a midwife do? The hospital policy may state that vaginal examinations should be performed four-hourly during labour and professional guidelines state that you should treat people as individuals and respect their dignity. The dilemma is clear – there is a conflict between hospital guidelines, clinical guidelines and the evidence base and women's feelings. In addition, midwives clearly need to know how to protect and maintain dignity while undertaking intimate examinations, and consent is essential to that process. The dilemma is around professional practice versus hospital policy. Ethical-based midwifery care is around supporting women's autonomy in decision making and being able to communicate information effectively to enable the woman to make a choice. The midwife has a professional duty to document the agreement to intervention or examination but does not require a signature from the woman. Verbal consent for vaginal examination is adequate when other aspects of professional care are present. The GMC (2013) identifies guidelines for medical practitioners regarding intimate examinations. Midwives need to be aware of these guidelines to ensure that a woman is not subjected to examination without her consent. This fulfils the role of the midwife in safeguarding women accessing obstetric care.

Frequently asked questions

How long does it take to gain consent?

All communications with patients will take some time and the relationship between the caregiver and the woman will impact upon the process. Women who have continuity of carer and trust their midwives will find it easier to process information provided than those who have just met the midwife and have not established a relationship.

How does a midwife know that a woman has capacity to consent?

It is assumed that all women over 18 years of age have capacity.

How much information should I give?

Sufficient information to enable the woman to identify if the proposal is in her best interests.

The labour ward guidelines state that a midwife should undertake a vaginal examination every four hours while a woman is in labour. Should I undertake this examination?

Only if you have explained the procedure, gained consent and are competent to do so. Examination of a pregnant woman without her permission, with cries of protest and attempts to push you away will result in investigation into professional misconduct, potential civil action, patient complaint and threat of negligence claim.

Chapter summary

Consent is an essential and fundamental part of a quality healthcare service. Any adult, mentally competent person has the right to refuse treatment. It has been demonstrated that consent is a process, not an end result, and consent may be withdrawn at any time. Midwives must gain consent for care provided and need to be especially careful when gaining consent for intimate examinations, due to the risk of unseen psychological effects. There is no authority in English law for a competent patient's refusal of treatment to be overridden, even if the result is certain death. Consent is a complex subject and consent in relation to children is particularly challenging. Case law is constantly modifying and challenging our standards of consent and all healthcare practitioners need to remain up to date with recent changes. If in doubt, seek advice from a supervisor of midwives, the CNST Midwife or the legal department (RCM or NHS trust).

Consent case study: Sally

Sally is in established labour and has stated that she does not want an episiotomy: she would rather sustain a perineal tear. During the second stage of labour the perineum shows signs of 'buttonholing'. Jane (the midwife) recognises that there is a clinical indication for performing an episiotomy. Jane (registered midwife) is qualified to make a clinical decision regarding episiotomy and is legally permitted to undertake the procedure. Jane also understands that to perform an episiotomy does not meet with Sally's wishes.

Evaluation

Sally has exercised her right to be involved in the decision making regarding the management of the second stage of labour. She has exercised her right to determine what happens to her. Sally is acting autonomously in refusing an intervention or treatment (episiotomy). Jane (midwife) considers that performing an episiotomy is for Sally's good (it will prevent a ragged tear), therefore the episiotomy should be undertaken. The dilemma is that if Jane performs an episiotomy she is acting paternalistically and has also disregarded Sally's wishes. Performing the episiotomy without consent will violate a moral (as well as legal) rule. The relationship between a patient and practitioner should be based upon trust. Jane has identified a risk of a perineal tear and should provide appropriate care to meet Sally's best interest. Failure to perform an episiotomy could result in a severe perineal tear which increases the risk of infection, pain and prolonged healing process. In addition, there is a possible negligence claim for failing to uphold a duty of care towards Sally. A further dilemma is whether performing an episiotomy for Sally's good justifies Jane in overruling Sally's wishes.

Analysis

What can be done? Theoretically, ethical decision making is based upon the application of morals, principles and theories to the situation. However, in the second stage of labour there is little time to debate the arguments for performing or not performing an episiotomy. The aim is to achieve a greater balance of benefit over risk. Jane (midwife) may feel that on balance the benefit of an episiotomy in preventing an uncontrollable tear and the possible benefits to the baby outweigh the harm of disregarding Sally's wishes.

Sally believes that she knows what is best for herself and has decided in advance that she would not wish to have an episiotomy during the second stage of labour. The decision was made on the basis of information provided during the antenatal period. It could be argued that during labour (contractions, pain relief and fatigue) that Sally's capacity to make choices has changed. Fluctuating capacity is not unusual during labour but cannot be used to coerce a decision. Sally needs to be able to understand why an episiotomy is necessary at this time.

Performing an episiotomy without consent is a breach of the Human Rights Act 1989 and risks a civil action for trespass and a possible negligence claim. As Sally has been clear that she does not want an episiotomy, if the procedure is undertaken without her consent it is possible that an allegation of professional misconduct will be made. A management and supervisory investigation will need to take place.

Ethical and legal solutions

Jane (midwife), while providing care for Sally, must ensure that she communicates well. Jane must be confident and competent regarding clinical skills and make notes throughout the labour which demonstrate any concerns or clinical issues. Jane cannot undertake an episiotomy without Sally's cooperation or consent. If Jane tries to perform an episiotomy without Sally's agreement it is likely that the procedure will fail, damage may be caused and the relationship will be litigious. Sally's autonomy is paramount and she must be given information to be able to make an informed choice. Jane will need to keep the information simple and specific to Sally's situation. Sally needs to be informed that if Jane does not perform an episiotomy a tear will occur. No one can predict the type of tear or the classification so it is not possible to suggest amount of risks.

Implications for practice (duty of care)

Continuity of care and continuity of carer are fundamental to the relationship between the woman and the midwife. If Sally knows and trusts the midwife providing care she will be able

(continued)

to understand that the midwife would not be suggesting an episiotomy unless it was absolutely necessary.

Communication regarding policies, practices and interventions must be discussed with childbearing women before the onset of labour. Women are entitled to know information relating to delivery rates, intervention rates and health and safety information.

Competence in undertaking an episiotomy is required. Jane (midwife) will be required to be confident and competent if she is going to perform an episiotomy. She will need to uphold professional standards (NMC, 2015) and ensure that her records clearly indicate recognition, responsibilities and sphere of practice.

Conclusion

Episiotomy is a controversial intervention that is primarily undertaken as an emergency procedure. The main justification for episiotomy focuses around expediting the delivery of the baby. The fetus has no legal rights and a woman cannot be made to have an episiotomy against her wishes. However, an episiotomy may be performed if it is in the woman's best interest (risk of severe damage to the perineum). Consent for an episiotomy is usually verbal. The midwife should ensure that the records (including indications) for an episiotomy are clear, so as to uphold professional standards of care and to avoid a potential negligence claim.

Activity

Find and consider standard templates (vaginal examination/abdominal examinations). Identify whether there is a space that reminds you to get consent. Is there a space that reminds you to identify the indication for the assessment?

Practice check

1. What standards of information giving do you demonstrate?
2. How do you ensure that you provide culturally sensitive care?
3. When do you adapt or modify your communication skills to enable a woman to understand? What techniques do you use?

Useful websites

Standards for consent are available at:

- General Medical Council (GMC): www.gmc.org.uk
- Department of Health: www.doh.uk
- Nursing and Midwifery Council (NMC): www.nmc-uk.org

- Royal College of Midwives (RCM): www.rcm.org.uk
- Royal College of Obstetricians and Gynaecologists (RCOG): www.rcog.org.uk

Legislation and Bills are available at:

- Legislation and government: www.legislation.gov.uk

7 Record-keeping

Pre-requisites for this chapter

A good starting point would be to download copies of professional guidelines regarding record-keeping. All regulatory bodies identify guidelines for healthcare professionals (NMC, GMC, HCPC, GDC). Reflect upon the purpose of record-keeping.

Introduction to the issue of record-keeping

Record-keeping is a fundamental skill of all midwives. Dimond (2013) suggests that a midwife does not provide a good service or quality care if she or he does not maintain contemporaneous records, notes and documentation. Keeping records that are comprehensive and clear is part of the duty of care owed to the client (Dimond, 2013). Effective midwifery practice requires midwives to complete records that are accurate, legible and detailed (NMC, 2009a). Professional guidelines (NMC, 2009a) identify that the employer usually sets the way in which midwives should keep and maintain records. While the employer may identify the way in which records should be kept, it is the regulatory body's statutory responsibility to protect the public from practitioners who are unable to maintain records to a satisfactory standard.

Most graduates will be required at some time to write reports and records; this is a common skill which individuals are required to demonstrate from the job application to the letter of terminating employment. The format, presentation and standard of all these records are an indication of the standards maintained. However, the writing of reports and research studies are distinct and different from the writing of professional notes and records associated with care of women and their families. Healthcare graduates must also be proficient in writing professional care records, policies, guidelines, statements and healthcare strategies.

The purpose of record-keeping is to demonstrate care, fulfil a professional duty and provide evidence of the nature and standard of the care provided. The consequences of poor record-keeping may be fatal. Patients who receive the wrong drug, an incorrect dose or a repeated administration (overdose) may do so because the prescription was not clear, recorded or documented correctly. Poor record-keeping may also be identified in legal cases or NMC fitness-to-practise investigations and during the process of supervision of midwives. There is little evidence of research being conducted into record-keeping. Tinsley's audit (2002) of records found practical problems encountered on a daily basis in the maintenance of maternity records. Evidence regarding poor record-keeping is cited in *Confidential Enquiries into Stillbirth and Infant deaths* (CESDI), Confidential Enquiries into Maternal Mortality (CEMACH) and NMC professional conduct investigations. Record-keeping is also perceived as a problem by supervisors of midwives (SoMs) (Tinsley, 2002). Precision with regard to midwifery record-keeping is important as midwives may be required to present evidence of events and actions years after the event. Symon (2009: 395) identifies that midwives are rarely involved in litigation but should be mindful that decision making and events could be subject to scrutiny whereby 'every minute' could be crucial. Student midwives are often anxious regarding records as they experience difficulties with inconsistent advice or conflicting information as to what to record and where to record. From an educationalist's point of view record-keeping skills are something that is firmly embedded in clinical placements. The clinical environment is where students are able to observe, undertake and reflect upon the records made during all aspects of midwifery care. In addition, they have opportunities to see reports, data collection and electronic records unique to the maternity services. Standards observed and demonstrated in clinical practice form the basis for students to gain a number of essential skills. The theoretical basis for record-keeping is reinforced throughout the midwifery curriculum from year one (communication skills, medicines management, antenatal notes, labour records and postnatal assessments), year two (emergency procedures, research, multi-agency working, parent preparation classes) and in year three (governance, medicines management, inter-professional working and complex healthcare).

This chapter will consider the basics of record-keeping followed by specific examples of records, for example, hand-held maternity notes, reports, statements and affidavits. Consideration will be given to the concept of legal documents. This chapter will also address professional portfolios. The NMC (2008d: 8) identifies that 'you must keep clear and accurate records'; this should include discussions that take place, assessments, treatments and interventions, as well as medicines given and their effectiveness.

Finally, this chapter will suggest the urgent need for midwives to self-audit their record-keeping skills and standards as part of their professional development and clinical supervision.

Types of records

Legal documents

Birth certificates, death certificates and marriage certificates are examples of legal documents which are relevant to maternity services. All other records that are kept relating to childbirth are documents which demonstrate care and are evidence of healthcare provision. Every record has the potential to become a legal document or evidence in a court case. It is because of this potential that all records should be made in a professional way and to a professional standard. The labour ward off-duty list has the potential to become evidence that a particular midwife was not on duty, for example.

There has been pressure upon the government to adopt national hand-held maternity notes and standard sheets for recording basic patient observations. The arguments for the adoption are primarily around patient safety, but also about helping practitioners to be compliant. Maternity records have come a long way since the cooperation card utilised in the 1970s and 1980s. The modern hand-held maternity records (Perinatal Institute, 2012) contains sections for professionals and clients to complete which reflect a partnership approach to maternity care, as opposed to a paternalistic approach usually associated with medical care.

Maternity notes

The nature and extent of personal information contained in the hand-held notes is extensive. The woman accepts responsibility for the notes during her pregnancy. While holding pregnancy notes may empower women, some may find it difficult to protect the information contained within them. Midwives also have to ensure that hand-held notes are safe and maintained when they are providing midwifery care.

Partograms and labour notes are important as a record of what happened: the care provided; the standard of care; and the outcomes. Most labour notes contain a partogram and summary sheet which is a copy of the record in the Birth Register. There are specific legal duties associated with childbirth which must be upheld. The labour notes and partogram are particularly significant as they can provide evidence, for example, that a woman was not left alone in labour for long periods of time. The notes may also demonstrate that choices were offered or risks explained. The recording of these professional activities is important for all births as it is difficult to remember at a later date exactly what happened. If the records do not contain information necessary to demonstrate that you have fulfilled your role and responsibility, it is likely that you can lose your registration as a midwife, and this is regardless of a potential negligence claim.

Professional portfolios are used by midwives to demonstrate skills, experiences and professional development. The NMC requires all midwives to maintain a professional portfolio which is also used to audit the professional requirement to keep up-to-date, confident and competent skills as well as professional updating. Professional portfolios provide the evidence that you have fulfilled the PREP (NMC, 2011c) requirements and that your record-keeping is to a professional standard.

Reports are made by midwives for a number of reasons. It may be a report regarding levels of care (maternity dashboards), a report upon a student midwife's progress during clinical placement or a report about proposed change to the maternity service. Midwives are also required to formulate local policy and guidelines.

What are the dilemmas for midwives regarding record-keeping?

Who owns the records made by midwives employed in the NHS? On initial consideration the question regarding ownership of records may seem somewhat irrelevant. However, when it comes to sharing information and use of records as evidence in court, the ownership and safety of those records is important.

The main professional dilemmas for midwives regarding record-keeping are primarily about format, detail or content, style and timing.

Format of records

Most employers stipulate the use of generic documents around patient care which may or may not be appropriate for maternity services. Each NHS trust providing maternity services will also utilise specific documents for maternity care. While there has been a move to provide national maternity records, to date this has not been successful and each NHS trust purchases its own document. In the West Midlands many NHS trusts have utilised the hand-held maternity records developed by the West Midlands Perinatal Institute (WMPI). The advantage of using this document is that it has been developed in conjunction with midwives and utilises evidence from clinical practice to ensure that the documentation meets the needs of the population.

The style of records is sometimes an issue, as too much description may be time consuming and lack of information and detail may imply that care did not happen. The midwife needs to be able to provide care and at the same time ensure that the records contain evidence of care provision. Record-keeping can also be difficult when an emergency arises and priority must be given to the management of the emergency. To some extent, record-keeping during emergencies (such as shoulder dystocia) is facilitated in that there is a proforma or template for standard procedures, include the inclusion of the multidisciplinary team and the allocation of a scribe to specifically record the management.

Good record-keeping

Good record-keeping is an essential midwifery skill. It enables the midwife to demonstrate contact with a client, decision making, provides evidence of care given, identifies information that may impact upon care and facilitates communication and information exchange. Good record-keeping has important functions for clinical practice, administration and logistics, as well as for educational purposes. It is generally acknowledged that good record-keeping improves patient safety, demonstrates care given and is associated with professional practice. Making records that are lengthy, descriptive, illegible or written in a narrative approach are not usually associated with good clinical care, effective or efficient clinical care.

Ethical issues around record-keeping

Ethical principles

Taking into account the basic ethical principle that you should treat others as you would like to be treated, it would seem reasonable that any records that have been made should be shared with the person/persons concerned. Equally, it would seem reasonable that any information recorded should remain confidential and not be available or discussed with anybody. For many years doctors have recognised that confidentiality between the healthcare provider and the receiver of healthcare is paramount. Therapeutic privilege means that the healthcare worker is aware of information and results that are limited to their provision of care and not for sharing with others.

Based on *respect* and taking into account the basic ethical principle that you should treat others as you would like to be treated, it would seem reasonable that any records that have been made should be shared with the person/persons concerned. Equally, it would seem reasonable that any information recorded should remain confidential and not be available or discussed with anybody.

From an ethical perspective the nature and extent of record-keeping can give a good indication of standards and provide evidence of ethical-based practice. What is not written in notes or reports is just as significant as what is written.

Autonomy

Respect for autonomy may be demonstrated in that records clearly show that information was provided, choices made and consent given. Autonomy can also be enhanced if women are able to contribute to the records themselves. An example is the identification of specific care choices in the maternity notes.

Accountability

Fulfilment of the role of a midwife requires a professional approach to record-keeping. The midwife is accountable for the standard of records kept as well as their safety and confidentiality. Legal proceedings in civil or criminal courts, professional misconduct investigations and clinical midwifery supervision all scrutinise the midwife's record-keeping. Failure to meet the required standard or failure of the record to demonstrate that care was given could result in loss of registration, liability and/or a custodial sentence.

Confidentiality

The main dilemmas around record-keeping are to do with confidentiality. Confidentiality challenges midwives and maternity services as personal information is recorded and needs to be kept secure. Sharing of information is also required (safeguarding policy). Midwives, as part of their role and responsibilities, enquire and record information which women provide as part of a professional, therapeutic and trusting relationship with a care provider. Midwives then have a duty to ensure that the trust is maintained and that information which is confidentially obtained does not become common knowledge or shared with others. A phrase that midwives may use is 'need to know basis'.

All midwifery students are required to record clinical experiences.

Consent is an ethical aspect of care, which is demonstrated by the records made by a midwife. While consent is not always in writing, it will be evident from the records that consent for care has been given. The records will indicate the date and time that an observation or treatment was undertaken.

Record-keeping also demonstrates *safeguarding* of vulnerable women as maintaining records ensures that care or medicines are not duplicated. The effectiveness or otherwise of interventions is recorded and evaluated. Records may also provide evidence of occurrence of harm – for example, a documented visit to an accident and emergency department.

Legal aspects of record-keeping

Records are a good way for midwives to protect themselves from litigation in that good, legible records are evidence of the midwife fulfilling their role and responsibilities regarding care and upholding a duty of care. Records, in addition to providing evidence of care given, may also be a formal notification of an event (birth). Midwives have a number of legal duties associated with professional practice. These legal requirements are birth notification, deaths and stillbirths. Failure to maintain professional standards of record-keeping can be used as part of professional misconduct investigations to contribute to sanctions or removal of a midwife from the NMC Register.

Poor recording-keeping can be used in court to suggest poor care and poor standards, and can increase the likelihood of a negligence claim being successful. Record-keeping may be the subject of criminal (fraud) and civil (time limits) litigation. Fraud is a criminal offence and is also considered to be unethical behaviour as trust is a fundamental aspect of the relationship between an employer and employee, patient and caregiver or citizen and community (government).

Births and Deaths Registration Act (1953): birth notification

The law requires all births to be notified. The notification is important for citizenship and the right to healthcare in the UK. Qualified informants notify the authority of the numbers of births and ensure that the government have important data required for planning and provision of services, homes and education.

Data Protection Act (DPA) 1998

The Data Protection Act identifies the law regarding access to records and the right of patients to an explanation of the records made. It is likely that if midwives make notes in the knowledge that women may read them and request information, then records will be accurate and clear.

Public Records Act 1958

This Act states that midwives have a duty to ensure that any records made regarding healthcare are kept safe and secure. In addition, ensuring that any information remains confidential is a professional duty. Midwives are required by this law to ensure that information is secure and locked away when not required. An important aspect is that additions to notes (such as results, electronic monitoring of fetal heart rates or advance directives) must be properly secured and the information cannot be lost or mislaid, and does not fall out of the notes.

Freedom of Information Act (FIA) 2000

Applications can be made under the FIA Act 2000 for information and data from healthcare providers where there is a reasonable and public interest. Patients' personal records are confidential and are not disclosed. Midwives may be asked as part of their management responsibilities to identify numerical data such as numbers of vaginal births following Caesarean sections or number of women who have experienced female genital mutilation who received care in the last six months. The NHS requires that staff maintain records so that compliance with FIA requests is possible.

Affidavit

Most midwives will not be required to provide an affidavit. An affidavit is a written statement that is made in the presence of a solicitor. The statement is taken in front of and signed by witnesses and can be used as evidence in a court case. An example of where an affidavit might be used is in a safeguarding case whereby there is no need for a healthcare professional to be in court. The healthcare professional may have provided a written statement identifying an observed behaviour of a parent while visiting a baby in a special care baby unit (SCBU). The observed behaviour of the parent would be used to demonstrate the behaviour and skills regarding baby care at that time.

Standards of record-keeping

Record-keeping is part of the professional duty of care owed by midwives to the woman. The NMC as regulator of midwifery practice has a duty to ensure that all midwives are familiar with and uphold standards regarding maintenance of professional records. While the NMC does not provide examples of 'good' record-keeping, the regulatory body for midwives provides guidance (NMC, 2009a) and addresses some issues regarding completion and standards.

Basic principles of record-keeping

There are a number of basic principles that are generally applied to professional records:

- Ensure that your writing is legible (practise writing clearly for professional purposes – slanting, small, flourished, enlarged or fancy writing can be saved for personal letters, cards and shopping lists).
- Always use a biro with black ink (so that a photocopy is clear, fading is less likely and smudging/blurring of characters is avoided).
- Record both date and time (do not forget the year ... time flies and it may be difficult to recall at a later date).
- Write facts (avoid excess description and subjectivity).
- Where possible use the correct proforma/tool (for example, when undertaking a vaginal examination use a vaginal examination stencil or sticker; this will ensure that all elements are complete and standards are maintained).
- If you make a mistake or spelling error, do not use white correcting fluid to cover up and write over.
- Students are usually encouraged to acquire skills in electronic record-keeping as well as handwritten notes.

The NMC (2009a) has identified the basic principles of good record-keeping; these can be found in Appendix 3.

What sort of documentation?

In addition to maintaining patient notes, midwives also complete a variety of records that are not directly associated with care. Notifications of intention to practise (ItP), PREP, off duty and meetings with supervisors of midwives professional portfolios are all examples of maintaining professional records. These records should demonstrate the same basic principles of record-keeping.

Electronic patient records (EPRs)

The NHS has the same responsibilities regarding EPRs on healthcare as paper records. There is a professional responsibility for the records to be contemporaneous and accurate. In the same way that paper records may go missing, there is a danger that electronic records can be wiped. The NHS is challenged to develop safe systems for record-keeping that ensure that basic principles are upheld. A number of systems (Lorenzo and BadgerNet) have been developed specifically for the maternity services to provide electronic record-keeping and live patient data management wherever care takes place. This is in addition to the electronic systems for recording fetal heart rates.

Safety and storage

The NMC (2008d: 8) Code identifies that a midwife must ensure that all records are kept securely. Your employer usually identifies the way in which records are kept. The basic principles of format and storage should be similar in each NHS trust. There is currently no national maternity notes system or central repository for maternity notes. The Perinatal Institute in Birmingham has piloted and produced standardised notes for use in the NHS, but not all trusts use these.

Destruction of maternity records

The standard time limits for bringing a civil action of negligence are not relevant in relation to those with a mental disability (neurological impairment). The Limitation Act 1980, Section 33 identifies that a judge has the power to extend the time limit on alleged negligence claims. For this reason, maternity records may be used in court cases a long time after the birth. Case notes, which include the childbirth episode, should therefore not be destroyed.

Professional misconduct

The mechanism for dealing with practitioners regarding record-keeping is professional misconduct. Quality mechanisms surrounding record-keeping are layered. For example, records and record-keeping are part of individual midwives' accountability. The midwife should check and consider whether the records made comply with local guidelines as well as basic principles (readability, clarity and contemporaneity). The clinical negligence scheme for NHS trusts (CNST) undertakes annual inspections of maternity records as part of its review of the level awarded to each trust. Standards of record-keeping and records are reviewed and impact upon the CNST level awarded to each trust. This is a clear indication to midwives that the safety of patients is directly affected by record-keeping. Annual opportunities to check standards of records being made are at the annual performance review with your manager. In addition, the annual meeting with your SoM is useful in identification of standards of record-keeping.

Chapter summary

Good records and record-keeping are synonymous with good care and midwives who are providing good-quality midwifery care will demonstrate high standards in their record-keeping.

While the intention of the NHS is to go paperless, paper-based records are still common in maternity services and care needs to be taken with their writing, storage and access.

Midwives need to know what, how and when to make records relevant to episodes of care. In addition, midwives need to ensure that care pathways are identified in the records and colleagues are clear regarding outcomes of health assessments.

SoMs can do more to support good record-keeping. They can engage with midwives regarding records at their annual supervisor reviews, and can approach the issues of records from a supportive, role model or audit direction. In addition, midwives should enable an SoM, LSA and NMC every 'reasonable facility to inspect' (NMC, 2004b: 24) his/her records.

Managers are accountable for records and record-keeping and should also undertake internal auditing processes, justified as part of clinical governance.

Records are made for the benefit of both the woman and the midwife: carrying one's own maternity notes not only empowers women but enables them to fully participate in the decision-making process and demonstrates respect for the individual. The midwife is able to communicate with colleagues and the woman regarding care choices, care provided and clinical decisions made. Records also benefit the NHS in the identification of care episodes (metrics) and service provision (data).

Case study: Scarlet

Scarlet (an unsupported mother) is a student midwife undertaking a shortened midwifery course; she is on her last placement. She has not achieved 40 deliveries. She is aware that if she cannot demonstrate 40 deliveries she will not be able to register with the NMC as a midwife. Scarlet alters records to enhance her chances of qualifying.

This case demonstrates the amount of pressure experienced by student midwives who undertake the shortened midwifery course (normally between 78 and 88 weeks). All student midwives, regardless of which course (long or short), must achieve specific European Union Criteria in order to register as a midwife. As part of the process of validation of courses, training providers are required to demonstrate that the clinical learning environments have sufficient experiences to enable the student to achieve.

Evaluation

Scarlet has falsified the number of births she has delivered. This is unethical and illegal as Scarlet is trying to qualify as a midwife without having undertaken the number of births required by the regulatory body (NMC). Scarlet has not met the target and this means she cannot register as a midwife. Fraud is defined as a criminal action. Scarlet has deliberately tried to deceive the regulatory body that she has more experience than she has. This behaviour is unethical as it prejudices women's rights to care by a midwife who is competent. Scarlet is likely to be jailed for fraud.

Analysis

The ethical issues in this case are:

- Should Scarlet be able to register as a midwife with less deliveries than other students?
- Are childbearing women in danger? Is there any evidence that less experience of deliveries will put them at risk during labour?
- Should the approved educational institution audit student experiences at regular intervals?

- What lengths are reasonable to support the student gaining opportunities to gain experiences and competencies?

The legal issues are:

- Scarlet's fraud of the care records and the delivery register.
- Scarlet's deception and deliberate attempt to demonstrate that she had more experience and skills than she did.
- Is the clinical environment negligent by not providing the opportunities and time to enable Scarlet to achieve her goal of becoming a midwife?

What can be done?

The argument here is not that Scarlet is uncaring or incompetent, but that she acts in a fraudulent way by changing clients' records. Fraud is punishable with a jail sentence. Persons working in the public arena, however dedicated or caring they are, should not be able to avoid the consequences of their actions.

Midwives have a role in safeguarding the public and in fulfilment of this role midwives who are working with students must ensure that records regarding off duty, experiences and activities are recorded accurately. Approved educational institutions provide documentation, explanations and information regarding the attaining of clinical experiences. Careful auditing and checking of these documents can identify any shortages, discrepancies and deceit.

The role of the NMC is to protect the public. Scarlet is unable to register as a midwife as she has not completed the requirements for professional registration. In addition, she has not demonstrated compassion for childbearing women. Breaking the NMC (2008d) Code prior to registration demonstrates that Scarlet is not able to meet the high standards required of a registered midwife.

Implications for practice

- Loss of job and professional registration.
- The guidance provided by the NMC (2009a) is intended to ensure the provision of safe and effective care.
- Audit of clinical placements and learning environments in practice to ensure that the ratio of staff to students and numbers of experiences is sufficient.
- Is prison the only option for non-violent offenders?

Conclusion

The standard of behaviour expected from a healthcare professional is high. Professionals, by virtue of their public role and responsibility, are expected to know and uphold the law. Ethical issues regarding fairness and equity are principles which professional reputations are built upon. There is a need to consider the role of midwife educationalists regarding the policing of accuracy and detail of record-keeping.

Additional case study

Steve is a newly qualified midwife. He has been providing care during a busy night shift on the labour ward. He has been asked by a colleague to 'look in' on another patient as the named midwife is busy providing care for a woman having a water birth. Steve 'looks in' on patient C, who is obviously upset and requesting pain relief.

Use the following framework to consider the above case study:

- Evaluation
- Analysis
- What can be done?
- Implications for practice
- Conclusion.

Activity

1. Consider how your records demonstrate care, compassion and competence. What or how do the words you have written show a professional approach to standards of records?
2. Practice writing a report, a review or a resume.
3. Identify an action plan to assist in the development of your record-keeping skills.

Practice check

- When was the last time you undertook an audit of your records?
- Are your personal records (delivery register, work diary, client details) maintained correctly, safely stored and legible?
- What level of detail do you normally provide? Date and time, signature and printed name, Personal Identification Number (PIN)?
- At your last meeting with a supervisor of midwives, did you provide examples of and discuss your standard of record-keeping?
- What safety measures are in place with regard to electronic records?

Useful websites

BadgerNet Patient systems: www.clevermed.com/BadgerNet-Platform
Legislation and Bills: www.legislation.gov.uk
Lorenzo medical systems: www.isofthealth.com/en/Solutions/Lorenzo/LorenzoCareManagementUK.aspx
Nursing and Midwifery Council (NMC): www.nmc-uk.org
Royal College of Midwives (RCM): www.rcm.org.uk
Statement-writing guidance: www.lsa.westmidlands.nhs.uk

8 Medicines, midwives and the law

Pre-requisites of this chapter

This chapter is best read after you have read Part I of this book. You should read this chapter with access to the latest copy of the NMC documents regarding standards of medicine administration. You should also be familiar with drugs commonly used in childbirth.

Introduction

Changes to midwives exemptions and the latest legislation, The Human Medicines Regulations 2012, as well as the latest government guidelines regarding whooping cough vaccination will be addressed. The administration of medicines during pregnancy, labour and postnatally can be a dilemma, especially when rights may be compromised. The use of drugs and medicines during pregnancy, labour and the postnatal period is a complex issue. Students may find it difficult to understand the responsibilities of the midwife as a prescriber. This chapter enables the reader to consider a variety of aspects of medicines.

The emphasis on quality care and ever-increasing expectations of childbearing women and their families inevitably puts pressure on the midwife. The numbers of babies being born is increasing but the number of midwives is not increasing proportionately. Midwives can expect to have an antenatal caseload which includes women with different needs, cultural expectations, obstetric risks, fears and anxieties. Complementary and alternative medicine (CAM) is increasingly popular. The midwife will be caring for a number of women during labour, with different requirements and choices regarding pain relief. During the postnatal period the midwife is responsible for the health and wellbeing of the mother and baby, and adaptation to being a family and the acquisition of parenting skills. There is evidence that midwives are stressed, struggling to provide consistently high-quality care while undertaking the safe administration of medicines.

The use of drugs and medicines during pregnancy, labour and the postnatal period is a complex issue. During pregnancy, midwives routinely advise women not to take medicines without first checking that the medicine is safe to use during pregnancy. Midwives are taught that some medicines are contra-indicated during pregnancy because they can cross the placental barrier and affect the fetus. In addition, some drugs may have an abortive effect or induce labour. Midwives are well aware that the timely use of an appropriate therapy and/or method of pain relief can make a difference to the labouring woman and her ability to cope. Midwives are also trained to comply with legislation and standards for the administration of medicines. Some midwives may decide to undertake further training to become an independent and prescriber. The majority of midwives fulfil their role and responsibilities regarding medicine administration through the partnership relationship with medical practitioners (independent prescribers) using supplementary prescribing. During hospital childbirth, competent adults may find restrictions and availability of pain-relieving medicines and therapy unsatisfactory due to staff shortages and lack of competencies. During the post natal period midwives should support women to self medicate where possible to increase autonomy.

This chapter considers medicines, midwives and the law. From an ethical perspective the withholding or delaying of pain relief during childbirth is a breach of human rights and could be considered institutional torture, obstetric abuse and inappropriate use of power and control. It is important that the midwife is equipped with the key legal skills to ensure the safe keeping and administration of a variety of medicines and drugs. Student midwives are instructed upon the safe administration of medicines during clinical placements and theoretical concepts are considered in the curriculum. Sometimes confusion exists as to what a student can or cannot do; this dilemma usually occurs with student midwives on the shortened course/programme as they are already registered adult nurses. Midwifery students need to be given the opportunity to learn about the specific concerns regarding administration of medicines to pregnant women. The midwife needs to understand the duty of care and the specific standards required for all childbirth settings. Key aspects concerning midwives and medicines are: lack of choice and delay in medication; the legal framework for medicines; the midwife as a prescriber; patient group directives; storage of medicines; supply and administration of medicines.

Ethical issues of medicines management

Ethical issues regarding medicines management during pregnancy and childbirth are around rights, autonomy, accountability and pharmacovigilance. Midwives are trained and educated to recognise and respond to the needs of childbearing women. The rights of women to have information and choices regarding all aspects of childbirth are paramount. Details regarding the ethical basis of care around choice and information are provided in Chapters 10, 11 and 14. Midwives provide care for childbearing women in a variety of environments and are expected to promote normality during the childbearing experiences. Complex pregnancies require collaborative care and midwives are familiar with working in a variety of environments, utilising specialist care pathways and administering a variety of medicines and treatments. Against this backdrop, midwives are also aware that relatively minor problems or illnesses can have major health implications for the pregnant woman and her baby. In 2012 the NMC provided advice regarding prescribing in pregnancy to specifically address the complexity of minor illness.

Accountability

Medicines management ensures that every woman and her baby receives the right medicine at the right time and with the right amount of information to be able to accept or reject the treatment. Consent is required and women or their babies should not feel pressured into accepting medicines or treatment because it is a routine. Midwives are accountable practitioners and should promote the rights of the woman to make an informed choice based upon the latest available evidence. A paternalistic attitude towards medicines management could mean that midwives restrict the medicines and drugs available to women.

Pethidine (a common pain-relieving drug), may be restricted at certain times during labour as it has the ability to cross the placenta and effect the fetus. If Pethidine is administered to the mother, the baby may also receive an amount of the drug. Babies born to mothers who have received Pethidine are more likely to be sleepy, lethargic, reluctant to feed and may require respiratory stimulation. If the midwife protects the rights of the fetus by withholding Pethidine for the mother, the midwife is acting paternalistically to the fetus and may also be restricting or failing to uphold maternal rights to appropriate care.

Autonomy

Midwives are the main care provider during pregnancy and childbirth. From an ethical perspective it is 'for the good of the majority' if a midwife is able to prescribe and administer medicines to women during their care. It is not reasonable, just or fair for a women to be subjected to unnecessary delay or limitations regarding the administration of pain relief during labour. As autonomous practitioners, midwives are privileged to identify, provide and demonstrate care for childbearing women. The midwife becoming an independent prescriber can enhance autonomous midwifery practice. All registered midwives can undertake additional training to enable the prescription of any licensed medicine for a medical condition that the midwife is competent to treat. The practicalities of undertaking are often the prohibiting factor as there are cost implications for the course and midwives must be registered with the NMC for at least three years. Independent prescribing is advantageous in midwife-led units, community settings and standalone birth units as it enables prompt and effective medicines management.

Supplementary prescribing is the method whereby midwives are able to administer medicines under the agreement of an independent practitioner for a specific care pathway.

Consent

In order for women to make choices during childbirth, information must be given in such a way that the woman can understand it, retain the information and make a decision as to its suitability for herself. Most medicines are approved for use in a specific way or in certain conditions. An example is vitamin K, which is licensed for intramuscular injection. Vitamin K is not licensed for oral administration. During the antenatal period mothers are given information about the routine administration of vitamin K. Once the baby is born, the midwife gains verbal consent for the drug to be administered. If a medicine is used outside its licensed indications (sometimes referred to as 'off label') midwives must ensure that appropriate consent is obtained. The consent will require explanation of the reasons why the medicine is not licensed for the planned use and information that there is no alternative appropriately licensed medicine available. Record keeping should demonstrate the information given.

Pharmacovigilance

Midwives may be unfamiliar with this terminology. Pharmacovigilance refers to the need to be vigilant and up to date with regard to medicines. Maintaining competency with regard to medicine administration is a requirement of professional registration.

Legal aspects of medicines management

Control regarding the use and administration of drugs during childbirth is required due to the nature and effects of medicines. Patients may be seriously harmed from errors in the medicines management process. Strict controls over drug administration protect the public from harmful effects and drug administration errors. Medicines used during childbirth may be legally controlled due to their nature and addictiveness. Controlled drugs such as Pethidine (Methadone) are frequently used. While drug errors can cause human suffering (and sometimes mortality), they are also a financial burden to the NHS.

The key sources of law relating to medicines are European, public and common law. In addition, professional regulation also identifies and imposes standards regarding midwifery practice. In 2003 the government set up the Medicines and Healthcare products Regulatory Agency (MHRA), which combined the functions of the Medicines Control Agency (MCA) and the Medical Devices Agency (MDA). Like the NMC, the primary function of the MHRA is to protect the public by ensuring that harmful incidents are investigated (and learned from) and the regulation of the usages of medicines and medical devices and equipment. As identified earlier, the use of medicines is not risk-free, and the MHRA acts to safeguard the health of the public in ensuring that risks are minimised. Midwives can report problems about devices to the MHRA direct using an adverse incident reporting scheme, although local policy and procedure should also be followed. Legislation identifies specific control over drug classification. In the UK, regulations (MHRA, NMC) control who, when and how practitioners may manage medicines.

The key legislation

Here consideration will be given to the key legislation regarding medicines that you should be familiar with.

Medicines Act 1968

This Act controls the use of medicines and is the foundation for drug administration in England. The Medicines Act 1968 established the Committee on Safety of Medicines (CSM). Since 2005 the CSM has been known as the Commission on Human Medicines (CHM). The main aim of the Medicines Act 1968 was to require medicines to be licensed before being available for human use. This act identified or classed medicines according to the ways in which control of availability and usage was identified. The classification identified prescription only (POM) and pharmacy medicines (PM). Drugs and medicines which are *Midwives Exemptions* are identified in the 1969 Act Section 58 (2) and have been amended in 2010 and 2011 (statutory instruments). All Midwives Exemptions are reviewed on an annual basis. Further detail on midwives exemptions are given later in this chapter.

The Misuse of Drugs Regulations Act (1971)

This is the main Act concerning the control and administration of drugs. This Act has largely been amended by the Human Medicines Regulations Act 2012.

Medicinal Products: Prescription by Nurses etc. Act 1992

1992 Chapter 28 frequently referred to as Nurses Act 1992 identifies that nurses and midwives who have recorded a prescriber qualification are able to become a nurse or midwife prescriber.

Statutory instruments

From time to time it is necessary for the NMC to use SIs to make changes to the above legislation, such as changes to Midwives Exemptions. The following SIs identify the effect of changes.

Prescription Only Medicines Amendment (Human Use) Order 1997 SI 1997/ 2044

This identifies specific drugs which are POMs, and updates and amends the Act.

Prescription Only Medicines (Human Use) Order 1997 SI 1997/1830

This identifies the classes of medicines in relation to appropriate practitioners. Exemption for certain persons from Section 58 (2) of the Act.

Medicines (Pharmacy and General Sale – Exemption) Order 1980 SI 1980/1924

Exemption from products used by midwives in the course of their professional practice.

Prescription Only Medicines (Human Use) Amendment Order 2004 SI 2004/2

Amends the list of POMs. Identifies specific exemptions. Identifies a number of section changes.

The Medicines for Human Use (Miscellaneous Amendments) Order 2010 SI 2010/1136

This makes changes to the guidance issued to midwives.

The Medicines for Human Use (Miscellaneous Amendments) Order 2011 SI 2011/1327

From 1 July 2011, student midwives are able to administer medicines on the Midwives Exemptions list (except controlled drugs) under the direct supervision of a midwife. This also updates the range of medicines on the Midwives Exemptions list.

Human Medicines Regulations SI 2012/1916

This secondary legislation (SI 2012/1916) identifies the new regulations under the MHRA. The Human Medicines Regulations (HMR) came into force on 14 August 2012. The regulations set out a comprehensive regime for the authorisation of medicinal products for human use; for the manufacture, import, distribution, sale and supply of those products; for their labelling and advertising; and for pharmacovigilance. This legislation is important as it incorporates European legislation. In particular, the HMR SI 2012/1916 regulations implement Directive 2001/83/EC of the European Parliament and of the Council of 6 November 2001 on the community code relating to medicinal products for human use (as amended). HMR Act 2012 also provides for the enforcement in the United Kingdom of Regulation (EC) No. 726/2004 laying down Community procedures for the authorisation and supervision of medicinal products for human and veterinary use and establishing a European Medicines Agency.

Standing Orders (SO) is an old and out-of-date term. It is not a legal term but was used to describe local guidelines that allowed midwives to supply and administer a range of medicines without individual prescription. The purpose of this was to provide seamless care for women (especially in labour).

The midwife and medicines

Midwives prepare for midwifery professional practice by undertaking a long or shortened midwifery course. Student midwives are trained in and required to maintain standards for the administration, dispensing and storage of medicines. Throughout midwifery training consideration is given to the specific and unique issues associated with medicine administration for pregnant and lactating women. Drug calculations are based upon pre-pregnancy size and previous experiences of drug use. Normal considerations regarding administration of medicines (age, physical and psychological aspects) are addressed. In addition, midwives are required to engage in continuous professional development (CPD) following registration (see Chapter 5). Before administering any medication, the midwife will be mindful of the relevant standards and guidelines, which are identified in Box 8.1. Midwives in the course of their professional practice may 'supply and administer on their own initiative any substances specified in medicines legislation under midwives exemptions' (NMC, 07/2011: 1; see Box 8.2). The NMC provide specific guidance for midwives in *The Code: Standards of Conduct, Performance and Ethics for Nurses and Midwives* (NMC, 2008d) *Standards for Medicines Management* (NMC, 2010d) and *Midwives Rules and Standards* (NMC, 2004).

Box 8.1 The key standards for medicines management

NMC (2007) Standards for medicines management
NMC (2006) Standards of proficiency for nurse and midwife prescribers
NMC (2008) The Code: standards of conduct, performance and ethics for nurses and midwives
NMC (2010) Midwives rules and standards

Box 8.2 NMC circulars

NMC Changes to Midwives Exemptions 01/2005
NMC Changes to Midwives Exemptions 06/2010
NMC Changes to Midwives Exemptions 07/2011

The midwife as a prescriber

Independent and supplementary nurse and midwife prescribers are defined as 'nurses and midwives who are competent to make a diagnosis and prescribe the appropriate treatment (independent prescribing) within their sphere of practice' (NMC, 2012b). Midwife prescribers were made possible under the Nurses Act 1992. Where a doctor has made an initial diagnosis, independent and supplementary midwife prescribers may prescribe in accordance with a clinical management plan (supplementary prescribing). Independent and supplementary nurse prescribers (INP) can prescribe all POMs, including some controlled drugs, all medication which can be supplied by a pharmacist or 'bought over the counter'. All independent and supplementary prescribers can only prescribe drugs within their area of expertise and level of competence. It therefore follows that an independent nurse prescriber would not prescribe drugs to pregnant women, whereas an independent midwife prescriber could do so provided she was within her expertise and competence. In addition, an independent and supplementary midwife prescriber would also be expected to share, consult and allow access to the same patient record. For midwives, the sharing of common documentation (hand-held pregnancy records) is normal.

Midwives Exemptions

Midwives are exempt from the general rules of medicines administration for the specific purpose of providing midwifery care. The legislative framework is provided under statutory instruments (identified in Box 8.2). In keeping with other aspects of midwifery care, midwives should be able to identify the evidence base for the administration of medicines, receive appropriate training regarding effects and efficiencies (dosage, side-effects, precautions, contra-indications and methods of administration) and maintain contemporaneous records (date, time, amount and method, signature) using the relevant document (medicines sheet, partogram, ECTG and midwifery notes). The effect of Midwives Exemptions is that midwives are able to supply and administer 'on their own initiative without the need for a prescription or patient-specific direction (PSD) from a medical practitioner' (NMC, Changes to Midwives Exemptions 07/2011: 2). Midwives Exemptions are drugs that are listed under the 1968 Medicines Act. These drug may be administered by a registered midwife without an individual prescription provided they are trained and in the course of professional practice. To find a list of the current midwives exemptions, see the NMC circular 07/2011 Annex 1. The NMC identifies the drug name, use, route and advice for professional practice.

Patient group directives (PGDs)

A patient group directive is defined as 'a written instruction for the supply and administration of a medicine in an identified clinical situation where the person may not be individually identified before presenting for treatment' (Griffith, 2009b: 460). PGDs enable midwives to supply and administer medicines to mothers without an individual prescription. PGDs are mainly used in hospitals in a limited number of situations where it offers an advantage for the care recipient without compromising safety (National Prescribing Centre, 2004). Labour wards are a common place to find a PGD as a medical practitioner may not be readily available to personally prescribe POMs for pain relief. In order to provide appropriate and seamless care, a midwife who is named as competent to supply and administer medicines under the PGD may be exempt from the need to obtain a prescription to supply a POM. Another advantage of PGDs is that they allow for flexibility so that a midwife can use the appropriate dose (taking account of the age and size of the patient).

Non-medical prescribing

The legislation relevant here is the NHS (Miscellaneous Amendments Relating to Independent Prescribing) Regulations 2006. This term refers to independent prescribing. Midwives (who have three years of post-registration experience) can train to become independent prescribers by undertaking an NMC-validated course. Following registration of their prescribing qualification a midwife can start prescribing. Supplementary prescribing is an agreement and a voluntary prescribing partnership between an independent prescriber (doctor or dentist) and the supplementary prescriber (midwife). An advantage of a midwife becoming a non-medical prescriber is that a prescription for any medicine can be made provided it is part of an agreed clinical management plan. Midwife prescribers are particularly valuable while working in the community.

Storage and administration of medicines

The storage and administration of medicines is regulated and controlled by the Medicines Act 1968 and the Misuse of Drugs Act 1971. The legislation has also been amended and updated by the Human Medicines Regulations Act 2012. Controlled drugs are identified under the Misuse of Drugs Regulations Act 2001 and require specific care and control regarding prescription, safe custody and the need to keep registers. Midwives fulfilling their professional role and responsibilities are required to ensure that legal restrictions and controls are upheld. Midwives have extended powers in relation to prescribing and administration of medicines compared to nurses and other healthcare practitioners. The midwife is accountable for the correct storage, administration and records regarding medicines during care provision. Professional accountability (standards and management) is identified by the NMC (2007c, 2010a, 2012a). All midwives also need a copy of the British National Formulary (BNF) to clarify latest requirements and guidance, and provide support for the administration of medicines. A reference guide and information and support regarding storage of controlled drugs is available from the Royal Pharmaceutical Society (you must be a member to download these resources).

Student midwives

Only midwives who are signatories to a PGD are entitled to supply or administer medicines under that directive. Student midwives cannot supply or administer that medicine. However, under the direct supervision of a midwife they can acquire the skills and be supervised in the administration of the medicine. This means that student midwives are allowed to administer medicines on the Midwives Exemptions list (*not* controlled drugs) under the direct supervision of a midwife (The Medicines for Human Use (Miscellaneous Amendments) Order 2011).

Complementary therapies

Pregnant women are just as likely as other women to use complementary therapies to address health issues. Indeed, midwifery and obstetric care positively encourage some supplements such as folic acid. Complementary and alternative therapies are used for a variety of conditions ranging from nausea and vomiting to backache and encouraging a breach presentation to turn into a cephalic presentation with the use of moxibustion. The midwife needs to be aware of the possibility of the woman choosing to use complementary therapies. The NMC (2010a: 37) Code identifies that midwives should 'ensure that the use of complementary or alternative therapies is safe and in the best interests of those in your care'. Midwives who wish to support women with complementary and alternative therapies are required to undertake appropriate recognised training.

Chapter summary

The storage and administration of medicines is a fundamental aspect of a healthcare professional's role and responsibilities. Midwives are autonomous practitioners and are required to assess, administer, record and evaluate medicines throughout the childbearing process. Pain relief in labour is a special skill and concern. The use of drugs during pregnancy and childbirth require specific care as requirements, effectiveness and ability to cross the placenta and affect the fetus should be considered. Drug errors are a concern in the maternity services. CPD is fundamental to ensure that midwives provide and manage medicines appropriately. Midwives are accountable for the medicines they administer and should make every effort to ensure that procedures and practices are safe.

Case Study: Cabrera Case (2008)

Mrs Mayra Cabrera (30 years), a Filipino nurse, was working in theatres at Great Western Hospital in Swindon. In 2003 she became pregnant with her first child. On 11 May 2004 she gave birth to a healthy baby boy (Zac) at 8.14 a.m., with her husband present. Mayra subsequently began fitting, suffered a cardiac arrest and died. During the unsuccessful resuscitation, medical staff noted a 500 ml bag of Bupivacaine had been wrongly connected to a venous cannula inserted into Mayra's right arm. Following a post mortem, the pathologist identified that Mayra had died from Bupivacaine toxicity. Mr Cabrera was present throughout the birth and resuscitation attempts.

(continued)

Mr Cabrera was informed that his wife had died from natural causes. He had no option but to return to the Philippines as his residency status was attached to his wife's work in the UK.

Evaluation

In July 2005 the Hospital Trust confirmed that Mayra's death was caused by an excessive and lethal dose of Bupivacaine. The drug had been wrongly hooked up to Mayra's drip instead of saline solution. A jury inquest took place in 2008. During the inquest it emerged that there had been a least two other fatal accidents (1994 and 2001) in the NHS trust whereby epidural infusions of Bupivacaine had been given intravenously in error.

Analysis

The Cabrera case raises a number of ethical issues. Inequalities in healthcare, safeguarding of vulnerable women, malpractice and human rights in healthcare. Strict control over drug usage is important to protect the public from harm. Mayra birthed her baby in a hospital environment and should reasonably expect that staff would store and use drugs in the correct way. Drugs administration is a careful process involving a checking system to ensure that the correct patient is given the correct drug at the correct time in the correct way. Mayra was a vulnerable patient as she had fitted and entered cardiac arrest, capacity to consent was absent and in an emergency situation she relied upon the healthcare providers to provide good-quality care. Emergency care required the administration of fluids as well as appropriate drugs. Confusion regarding the venous access should not occur when staff comply with drug storage and administration.

What can be done?

- The hospital should have a policy in place which states that Bupivacaine and other epidural drugs should be stored in a locked cupboard away and removed from intravenous fluids.
- Multidisciplinary staff training (using a 'human factors' approach).
- A multidisciplinary review of the storage of drugs.
- Specific equipment for use with epidurals (giving sets, syringes and infusion bags that can only be used with epidurals).

Implications for practice

- Untoward incidents and 'near-miss' incidents should be reported recorded and used for staff training purposes.
- Wrong-route drug errors need to be prevented. Drug administration must follow a specific procedure (even in an emergency); drugs should be checked prior to administration by another professional.

- Mixing drugs (fluid infusions) must be labelled clearly. Storage of local anaesthetic drugs that are combined with a host liquid must not be stored in the same place as normal saline or electrolyte solutions.

Conclusion

Midwives need to demonstrate excellent medicines management at all times. A human factors approach to education, training and skills of drug administration could reduce wrong-route drug errors. All women, including NHS staff, should expect and receive high-quality maternity care. Medicines management is a multidisciplinary responsibility and managers need to ensure that midwives are supported in the correct storage, checking and administration of all drugs.

Practice check

1. What are the rules for students administering medicines?
2. If you have administered Pethidine to a woman during labour, what duty of care do you have to (a) the woman and (b) the baby?

Activity

While working on a postnatal ward, consider the culture of medicines management. Ask yourself the following questions:

1. What is the philosophy underpinning the administration of medicines? (You may wish to consider the following aspects – self-administration, drugs rounds, patient focused and alternative therapy.)
2. What role models are demonstrated (control, procedural or casual)?
3. What principles are demonstrated? (For example, the five 'rights' – 'right dose, right drug, right patient, right time and right route'.)
4. What influences the therapy? In addition to availability, other influences upon therapies and medicines could be knowledge of the patient, maternal age, method of infant feeding, patient abilities and attributes (ability to swallow tablets, fear of injections, preferences).

Useful websites

Legislation and Bills: www.legislation.gov.uk
Medicines and Healthcare Regulatory Agency: www.mhra.gov.uk
Nursing and Midwifery Council (NMC): www.nmc-uk.org
Royal College of Anaesthetists: www.rcoa.ac.uk
Royal College of Midwives (RCM): www.rcm.org.uk
Royal Pharmaceutical Society of Great Britain (legal and ethical issues): www.rpharms.com/support-resources/pharmacy-law-and-ethics.asp

9 Safeguarding vulnerable women and babies

Pre-requisites of this chapter

It is assumed that you have a good anatomical knowledge of normal female genitalia and perineum. You should also be utilising the latest professional regulatory standards (NMC, 2010a): *The Code: Standards of Conduct, Performance and Ethics for Nurses and Midwives*.

The terms 'child protection' and 'safeguarding' are both used and explained in this chapter.

Introduction

This chapter focuses upon safeguarding vulnerable women and babies. Increasingly, midwives are being asked to provide care and support for women and babies with complex health and social care needs. While academics and practitioners frequently consider obstetrical, medical and physical needs, social aspects of childbearing usually receive less attention. However, vulnerable women and babies require special attention as they are unable to experience positive aspects of childbirth that other women are afforded. Gender-based violence is thought to increase during pregnancy (JB Thompson, 2004), alongside morbidity and mortality. Midwives have a duty to reduce inequalities in health. The maternity services are also challenged to ensure that vulnerable women are not further disadvantaged by the lack of care, treatment or insensitivity of the staff or services. Access to midwifery care, evidence-based care and empathetic midwives and culturally sensitive services are important for the health and wellbeing of all women.

The government is anxious to ensure that maternity services are cost-effective, efficient and provide excellent care for childbirth. An experienced midwife once told me that 'a healthy mum is needed for a healthy family'. As a student midwife I was encouraged to 'help and support' new mothers to enable them to get rest, relaxation and to focus on their new baby. This was often a challenge as postnatal exercises were not necessarily high on mum's agenda. Changes in the maternity services have meant that postnatal care has changed radically during the last 20 years. Postnatal visits that once were routine and prescribed are now targeted around newborn blood spot screening and infant weight. Postnatal drop-in centres and clinics have reduced the number of home visits, especially at weekends. Women are encouraged to access information via Sure Start centres, the internet and peer support groups.

These changes enable midwives to focus primarily upon antenatal care and labour and leave women vulnerable and lacking support postnatally. Perinatal mental health is a great concern and yet there are few resources to address this.

A key aspect of caring for vulnerable women and babies is a multi-professional and inter-professional approach to maternity services. Midwives are clear that they are the experts in normal childbirth and that as autonomous practitioners they have a specific role and responsibility regarding childbirth. However, midwives are no longer trained to work in isolation and they are required to 'work with others to protect and promote the health and wellbeing of those in your care, their families and carers, and the wider community' (NMC, 2010: 4). The ability of midwives to work inter-professionally may vary for a variety of reasons. Inter-professional working is difficult as it requires collaboration rather than working alongside. To be able to safeguard women and their families I believe that collaboration is necessary at a strategic as well as at individual level. Accountability of organisations as well as professionals is necessary to ensure that the duty to safeguard women and their families is focused and effective.

There are numerous examples of midwives working inter-professionally, but one aspect of the maternity services that further challenges them is vulnerable women and babies. Midwives historically have recognised the needs for these women and babies but are often constrained or frustrated by the systems and strategies in which they function. An example of this is during the 1960s when community midwives found it necessary to write letters of support for vulnerable women to enable them to have suitable housing. Historically, maternity services were first to recognise the need for relatives to stay with the patient (baby) in special care, and 'family rooms', self-contained flats and facilities were provided close to the baby. Case conferences with medical staff, social workers, nursery nurses, health visitors, midwives, nurses and relatives were often held in these environments. During the 1970s hospital midwives needed to act promptly with referrals when babies were born with congenital abnormalities to enable them to be transferred to centres with specialist care.

What is safeguarding?

Safeguarding is the policy, process and practice of safeguarding individuals from harm or abuse. Safeguarding is a collective term for professionals to use and replaces the term 'child protection'. The term safeguarding is considered to be politically correct as it is recognised that children are not the only age group to suffer abuse. There are three Rs that help practitioners to fulfil their role regarding safeguarding: Recognition, Responding and Reporting of abuse. This chapter considers both vulnerable women and babies and children. Child protection is the term given to the process and mechanism by which babies and children are protected from harm and abuse.

Safeguarding babies and children

Child protection (safeguarding) is a complex, emotive, stressful and undervalued role of the midwife. Much has been written about the prediction of child abuse, e.g. Pringle (1978). Theoretical perspectives have focused upon early warning systems (Kempe and Kempe, 1978), checklists (Browne and Stevenson, 1983) and tools used to identify children at 'high risk' of child abuse. However, screening procedures need to be considered with caution as the universal application of lists fail to consider cultural and social circumstances – the screening technique is not similar to rubella, where screening is based on the premise of immunity being present or not; screening for child abuse is based around risk and probability. Parents cannot be easily identified as potential abusers as factors which lead to abuse are multifactorial. Many adults who have been abused themselves do not go on to abuse their children and many abusers may not have been abused themselves. Abuse is not restricted to physical, neglect and sexual abuse. In modern times psychological abuse is subtle and may go undetected.

During the 1990s, child protection work focused attention away from prediction of abuse and crisis intervention towards preventing the abuse in the first place. The National Commission of Inquiry into the Prevention of Abuse (1996) is an example of the altered approach. In the UK the strategy for safeguarding children is an inter-agency approach and there is a shared responsibility. *Working Together to Safeguard Children* (HM Government, 2010) provides guidelines for safeguarding and promoting the welfare of children. Safeguarding is the term applied to the escalation of concerns regarding the health and wellbeing of babies, children and vulnerable adults.

Safeguarding women

Ethically it is every individual's right to live in safety and to be free from fear and abuse. Abuse is a violation of human and civil rights by another person or persons. Thus the ethical and legal issues regarding abuse (which may be a single act or repeated acts) are important for midwives to understand as midwives have a role and responsibility regarding safeguarding adults. Following the Francis Report (2013), professionals are reminded that safeguarding also applies to patients in both health and community care settings. Domestic violence is unseen and unheard as it takes place in the privacy of home (behind closed doors). New considerations for safeguarding women are around obstetric or childbirth abuse, physical abuse (FGM) and emotional abuse (fear, anxiety associated with pregnancy).

Ethical issues

The birth of a baby is a unique, precious and emotional time for all women. For some women they may have reached this point in a less than ideal way (rape, failed contraception, unable to terminate pregnancy, unwanted pregnancy). All women need midwives to treat them as individuals, provide respectful care and be open and honest with them. In addition to providing midwifery care, the midwife also has a safeguarding duty. The woman's right to confidentially is not absolute, if a midwife has concerns regarding safeguarding she is required to follow procedures to protect the vulnerable. Sharing information about the woman and her family with other agencies is part of the safeguarding process. The Department of Health (HM Government, 2010) make it clear that if a midwife has reasonable cause to believe that a child in a family of a client is being abused the midwife must take appropriate action. The reality is that this means breaching the confidence of the pregnant woman. Making a clinical decision to escalate concerns and share information or observations made as part of a therapeutic relationship is a dilemma for the midwife. The midwife's own values, beliefs and attitudes are called into question. The midwife needs to be able to justify the decision and demonstrate care, compassion and courage in involving other agencies. In an emergency it may be that the decision is easier. During routine care the midwife should involve a supervisor of midwives (SoM) at the earliest opportunity to enable support with the decision-making process.

The right of all individuals to not be subjected to abuse is a challenge. People may become vulnerable for numerous reasons, as a result of birth, illness, age. Also, location (hospital) increases the vulnerability and the ability to address it. Discriminatory, sexual and institutional abuse have been experienced by women. There is increasing understanding that any adult receiving any form of healthcare is vulnerable. Vulnerability in a healthcare context is around a greater risk from harm than others. The Safeguarding Vulnerable Groups Act 2006 identifies the vulnerability of people receiving healthcare.

Children's rights

Children's rights are a relatively new concept. In the past adults have believed it was their right to treat children as they wished. Poland first proposed the rights of children and the United Nations adopted children's rights on 20 November 1989; the UK ratified those rights in 1991. The United Nations Committee on the Rights of the Child identified that all children should have rights regarding health and safety.

Following the Children Act 2004 the British government appointed Children's Commissioners for England, Ireland, Wales and Scotland.

A key right for children is the protection from physical assault (chastisement). Some countries legislate for children to have equal protection from assault as adults – Austria, Cyprus, Denmark, Finland, Germany and Italy.

Strategies for addressing children's rights have been based around:

- identification of vulnerable families, e.g. domestic violence, mental health issues and substance abuse;
- parent education for helping adults understand the needs of young persons (nutrition);
- parental support to be able to meet basic needs of babies and young persons (learning disabilities);
- communication with others (support groups for those with shared medical conditions).
- specific health strategies regarding sudden infant death, shaken babies, pre-term babies, crying babies and smoking;
- providing targeted support for vulnerable groups (Sure Start).

Patient's rights

Patient's rights have also been an under-reported ethical issue. The WHO identify that basic human rights must be met for patients while receiving healthcare. Basic rights for women accessing maternity services are identified by the White Ribbon Alliance (2014). Women accessing healthcare during pregnancy and childbirth are vulnerable. Empowering women during pregnancy and childbirth enables them to make choices that are appropriate for them and provides opportunities for them to gain information; respectful care increases confidence and enables women to be strong to birth their babies in a way that is comfortable for them. Midwives need to be self-aware to understand how they can influence the woman's ability to be strong and confident to reduce the likelihood of power and control over the woman.

The patient's right to *confidentiality* is not absolute. When it comes to the duties of a midwife, the duty to safeguard overrides the duty of confidentiality. If a midwife is worried about abuse it is necessary to share that information (using safeguarding procedures).

Role of the lead midwife for child protection

NHS trusts have a named midwife or lead midwife for child protection. The role of the lead midwife for child protection may be summarised as:

- training;
- knowledge – information provision, procedural accountability;
- support;
- consultation;
- representation at the Local Safeguarding Children Board (LSCB);
- review of records and evidence.

The role of the lead midwife for safeguarding is challenging, not least because of the difficulties surrounding the nature of the work, unsocial hours and high standards of record-keeping required. Colleagues may fail to recognise the upsetting nature of safeguarding and the need to provide support for those involved. Difficult questions have to be asked of all staff involved in caring for vulnerable clients; this includes criminal records checking, de-baring services and consideration of motivation (think about the Jimmy Savile situation).

The report into the death of Victoria Climbié published in 2000 identified that Victoria died in February 2000 despite having had contact with four social services departments, three housing departments, two specialist child protection teams (Metropolitan Police), two hospitals and a family centre managed by the NSPCC. The Laming Report made 108 recommendations:

- general recommendations (1–17)
- social care recommendations (18–63)
- healthcare recommendations (64–90)
- police recommendations (91–108).

The recommendations regarding healthcare are significant as health providers have key responsibilities regarding protecting from abuse and working inter-professionally.

Supervisors of midwives

SoMs are specifically identified by the NMC (2009c) to protect women and babies. This is achieved by promoting and demonstrating safe standards of midwifery practice. In addition, SoMs are challenged with ensuring that maternity services respond to the needs of women. It is no surprise, then, that SoMs have been identified as defenders of human rights (Jessiman and Stuttaford, 2012). Part of the SoM's responsibilities includes ensuring midwives provide a high standard of care and through their practice and interaction with women can demonstrate accessible, high-quality care in a culturally sensitive manner, thus promoting the rights of women during childbirth. SoMs are discussed in detail in Chapter 10.

Legal aspects of safeguarding

Primary legislation in the form of the Human Rights Act 1998 (HRA), Children Act 1989 and Children Act 2004 all impact upon safeguarding. While successive reports have reported failings in the system, the law has provided the legal framework for safeguarding. In addition, cases such as those of Victoria Climbié, Baby P and Daniel Pelka illustrate the nature and extent of harm that babies and children have been subjected to and the need for legislation to criminalise poor care. The legislation identifies the obligations that all health and social care workers have to identify and take action when they are concerned or consider children to be at risk.

Human Rights Act 1998

The Human Rights Act 1998 is based upon the European Convention on Human Rights. The HRA is primary legislation that has been enacted to ensure that the ethical aspects identified in the European convention are enforced. The key rights relevant here are:

- Article 2 The right to life;
- Article 3 Prohibition of torture;
- Article 8 The right to respect for private and family life;
- Article 9 Freedom of thought, conscience and religion;
- Article 14 Freedom from discrimination;
- Article 17 Prohibition of abuse of rights.

Children Act 1989

This was a significant piece of legislation (there are 108 sections) which overhauled approaches to children. Key significance of this Act is that rather than identifying the rights of parents regarding children, this Act reflected a new approach to the status of children. The Children Act 1989 introduced the notion of the role and responsibilities of parents (parental responsibility). A key principle of this Act is that in any orders, actions or provisions the child's welfare must be the first consideration. Section 1 identifies a welfare checklist to ensure that the child's welfare is the court's paramount consideration. In particular, it is necessary to identify each child's physical, emotional and educational needs. This is important, as children in the same family do not share the same needs. Note: linguistic background is specifically identified (along with religion, racial origin and culture) (Section 22 (5c)).

Part V Sections 43–52 concern the protection of children. 'Harm' is identified as ill treatment or impairment of health or development (Section 32 (9b)).

Specific new court orders are: Emergency Protection Order (EPO) Section 44, 45, 48; Parental Responsibility (PR) Section 2; Care Order (CO) Section 33; Child Assessment Order (CAO) Section 43.

The Children Act 1989 identify a statutory duty for a local authority to make such enquiries as they consider necessary to enable them to decide whether they should take action to safeguard or promote a child's welfare. This duty relies upon a local authority being informed (the child is in police protection or the subject of an emergency protection order) or having 'reasonable cause to suspect that a child who lives, or is found, in their area is suffering, or is likely to suffer, significant harm' (Children Act 1989, Section 47 (1)).

Children Act 2004

This required each local authority to establish a Local Safeguarding Children Board (LSCB) by 1 April 2006. The purpose of this is to coordinate the promotion of the welfare of children and safeguarding in every local area. The LSCB is a statutory board and agrees with relevant organisations how they will cooperate to safeguard and promote welfare in addition to ensuring the effectiveness of that process. Section 14 of the Children Act (2004) identifies the functions of the LSCB.

The Safeguarding Vulnerable Groups Act (2006)

This legislation does not provide a formal definition of 'vulnerability'. Pregnant women are usually considered to be vulnerable due to the healthcare needs associated with pregnancy. In addition, pregnant women are at increased risk of domestic violence (Bainbridge 2005: 717). Safeguarding vulnerable women and children is an important role of the midwife. Women have a lifetime risk of 1 in 4 of being a victim of domestic violence and pregnancy can trigger this (Barnett 2005: 702). Midwives undertake regular health assessments during pregnancy and childbirth and may be able to make a difference for vulnerable groups.

Statutory instruments

Nursing and Midwifery Order 2001 (SI 2002/253): this SI provides that a midwife can accompany the applicant in the risk assessment of a child. Working together and collaborating with other agencies enables midwives to uphold their responsibilities regarding safeguarding vulnerable babies and children.

Independent inquiries

There are numerous inquiries into safeguarding and many lessons to be learned. Two serious case reviews should be considered: Baby P and Daniel Pelka.

Baby P (Peter Connelly)

Peter Connelly died in London after suffering over 50 injuries over an eight-month period.

Baby P was born on 1 March 2006 and died 3 August 2007. Baby P's identity was revealed following a court anonymity order expiring on 10 August 2009. On 11 November 2008 two men were found guilty of the murder of Baby P. The mother had already admitted allowing or causing Baby P's death. There was insufficient evidence for a murder charge to hold. A summary of Peter's case can be found in the Appendices.

Baby P's case was widely reported for four reasons; first, the magnitude of Peter's injuries; second, criminal proceedings including a potential murder charge; third, because Peter lived in the London Borough of Haringey, the same authority that was involved in the case of Victoria Climbié. Victoria's death had led to a nationwide review of child protection services (Laming Report, 2000); fourth, there were a number of high-profile dismissals and resignations of staff. Senior government officials became involved and social media added to the publicity.

Laming published a progress report following the death of Baby P, which identifies that too many authorities had failed to adopt reforms identified in his previous review. This is significant as management of Child Services, in particular safeguarding procedures, continue to dominate professional concerns.

Daniel Pelka

Daniel Pelka was born on 15 July 2007 and died on 3 March 2012. The Serious Case Review (Coventry Safeguarding Children Board, 2013) identifies that the circumstances of Daniel's death suggested that he had been suffering abuse and neglect over a prolonged period of time. The review identifies the abusive experiences of Daniel and his siblings. The ethical issues for Daniel were around the sustained inhumanity and torture: his abuse was of all types. The legal issue was abuse and murder. However, it should also be remembered that also at issue were the abuse of his older sibling and the vulnerability of his younger sibling. Poor professional practice regarding communication, use of a sibling as an interpreter and reporter, as well as issues with record-keeping contribute to lessons that must be learned from Daniel's sad life. A summary of the case is provided in the Appendices. Daniel's mother and her partner were charged with Daniel's murder on 9 March 2012. They were convicted of his murder on 31 July 2013.

Daniel Pelka suffered and died as a result of a systematic failure of safeguarding strategy and the ability of his mother to hide his abuse, manufacture an illness (eating disorder) and isolate him from his family. This case is particularly worrying for midwives as Ms Luczak was able to present an image of being caring and concerned about her children while physically, psychologically and neglectfully abusing Daniel. Healthcare staff were involved in Daniel's health assessments but did not share concerns with others. Daniel's siblings were living in the same environment and it was not until the post mortem report revealed the extent of Daniel's neglect and injuries that the siblings were removed from the home and placed in foster care.

The serious case review identified 'confused and ineffective communication', 'inappropriate advice' and 'lack of referral', which prevented purposeful intervention which may have made a difference in assessing the family situation. The dilemma for midwives is that, having followed safeguarding procedures, can we trust our health and social care partners to take our concerns seriously? Compliance with safeguarding procedures is an important and essential role of the midwife. However, if the midwife does not feel comfortable with the inter-professional response, the midwife has a duty to escalate concerns and breach confidentiality if a child's welfare is at stake. The midwife has a duty of care 'if she is worried or concerned' to report and escalate those concerns.

Legal issues regarding safeguarding

Policy

The policy is working together, a shared responsibility, need for collaboration and an appreciation of the role and responsibility of partners.

The key legal issues are: safeguarding duties of health and social care professionals, best practice, professional practice and evidence.

Safeguarding duties

Working together to safeguard and promote the welfare of children and families is the current strategy (HM Government, 2010). Inter-agency working is intended to safeguard and promote the welfare of children. Everyone shares the responsibility for safeguarding (HM Government, 2010: 2.1). Many organisations work with children and while they share a commitment to safeguard, local authorities that are Children's Services authorities have specific duties. Specific roles and responsibilities are identified in Chapter 2. Fe, m/c – see Chapter 13.

Best practice

The integration of services is thought to enable health and social care workers to collaborate, communicate and, crucially, intervene when babies and children are at risk of harm.

While listening to children and young people is important, it is also vital that midwives listen to women. Recent evidence suggests that many women and young persons are reluctant to report abuse for fear that they will not believed. This is of particular concern as women who have been brave and shown courage in reporting abuse are further abused by healthcare professionals who are not alert and fail to make appropriate safeguarding referrals.

Midwives who have knowledge and information about the community in which women and families live are thought to help safeguard. There are strong links between domestic violence, substance misuse, alcohol consumption and child abuse. Midwives need to be able to recognise when a child is in need of help, services or at potential risk of suffering significant harm.

Midwives regularly undertake reflection to review and develop their practice. Considering data around birth and births attended can help midwives to maintain high standards of care.

Inter-professional working is key to safeguarding of babies, children and vulnerable women. Midwives need to have good communication skills to ensure that they are heard. Little is known about midwives' contributions to case reviews, but what is known is that for inter-professional working to be successful there needs to be good communication, collaboration and cooperation (Clarke, 1993).

Professional practice

Section 2.62 of HM Government's *Working Together to Safeguard Children* identifies that all health professionals working with children and young people should 'ensure that safeguarding and promoting their welfare forms an integral part of all elements of care they offer' (HM Government, 2010: 2.62). Midwives are required to provide a high standard of practice and care at all times (NMC, 2010a: 1), which includes keeping skills and knowledge up to date. Midwives have to be able to recognise the risks of abuse or neglect to an unborn child as well as existing children. In particular, midwives also need to be able to recognise the needs of parents who may need extra help in bringing up their children (HM Government, 2010: 2.63)

Evidence of abuse

Evidence of abuse is difficult to acquire as it relies upon health and social care sharing information, events, observations and contact. Professionals are reluctant to share information or notes resulting from patient encounters, often citing patient confidentiality as a reason to protect the client. Medical records, case notes and care provision are confidential, but if a child is at risk a healthcare professional must follow safeguarding procedures which include the core process identified in *What To Do if You Are Worried a Child is Being Abused* (Department of Health, 2010e). All professionals should be able to understand risk factors and recognise children in need of support or safeguarding. Working together identifies the general principles for all professionals and provider services. When it comes to evidence in safeguarding cases, the legal system uses 'experts'. Expert witnesses are used to demonstrate the nature, extent, value and accuracy of the evidence provided. It would seem reasonable and just to use medical experts to illuminate, clarify and validate information and materials to enable a correct and accurate conviction. The legal profession are trained to interrogate the accuracy of statements and the reliability of witness. However, the legal process is not foolproof; the Sally Clark case is an example of how evidence was used to secure a conviction, which was subsequently overturned.

Chapter summary

Best practice regarding safeguarding is thought to consist of inter-professional working, with professionals collaborating, communicating and always considering the baby/child as the focus of any safeguarding work. Safeguarding is not the main focus of any professional's work, but a fundamental part of it. All practitioners find safeguarding challenging and difficult. Repeated reports inform us about how we get safeguarding wrong, but there is little support for practitioners for inter-professional training, guidance or realistically time to undertake this work. There is a need for timely intervention to protect babies and children who are at risk of significant harm. Maternity services have an obligation under the Human Rights Act 1998 to identify and act when a baby is at risk of abuse. Midwives have a duty of care to protect or safeguard. There is a national shortage of midwives, high caseloading numbers and a priority for intrapartum care. Midwives who may be worried about a woman, baby or existing children need to be respected by and work with other agencies to safeguard them.

Case study: safeguarding

Samir has just given birth to a baby girl. Baby G has APGAR scores of 9 at one minute and 10 at five minutes. Baby G has been dried and has been skin-to-skin with her mum, Samir, for the last hour. Baby G has had an initial baby check by the midwife and is healthy and well. Samir has chosen to breast-feed Baby G. In Samir's notes there is a request that following delivery the social worker is informed of the birth and that Baby G will be placed on the safeguarding register.

Evaluation

The above case is an example of some of the complexities of working in a modern maternity service. There is a direct dilemma for the midwife. On the one hand, all is normal and healthy;

(continued)

on the other hand, there is fear and anxiety for the health and wellbeing of the baby. What could possibly be so serious that a social worker requires a midwife to disclose a birth and involve other government services that Samir may not want, wish or welcome? Should the midwife break the trust and partnership which she has established with Samir? Can the midwife ignore the request, maintain confidentiality and still uphold NMC guidelines? The dilemmas are numerous and the midwife may feel uncomfortable with reporting to social services so soon after the birth.

Analysis

From a professional perspective the midwife has a number of duties that she must fulfil. Providing care, notification of birth and supporting the new mother with her chosen method of feeding are priorities at this time. Midwives are autonomous practitioners and as such are accountable for actions taken as well as actions not taken. The midwife may not be aware of the specific circumstances that have led to concern regarding the safety and wellbeing of the baby. While the mother may not wish to discuss personal circumstances with the midwife it is hoped that during labour the midwife has been able to establish a relationship with the woman. Being 'with woman' and supporting her during labour should establish a trusting relationship – if the midwife then contacts social services it is likely that the woman will feel betrayed. Equally, if the midwife fails to inform social services that the birth has taken place the midwife will be failing in her duty to safeguard the baby.

What can be done?

While Samir is in hospital it could be considered that Samir and the baby are in a safe place. Hospital staff are able to keep a close watch on mother and baby and can supervise care if there is a risk of neglect. In addition, there is an opportunity for Samir to acquire and demonstrate parenting skills essential for baby health and wellbeing. Samir has chosen to breast-feed, which is considered best practice for a newborn baby.

Implications for practice

The midwife may break confidentiality and inform social services that Samir has given birth if there is cause for concern or worry about the baby's health and wellbeing. Theoretically, unless Samir threatens to or decides to leave hospital then both are safe and cared for. A midwife has a duty of care to both mother and baby.

The midwife also has a duty to do no harm to the patient (both mother and baby). It could be argued that separating a mother and baby is harmful to both. The midwife will be aware that successful breast-feeding relies upon physical and psychological mechanisms. It is likely that threatening contact with social services will increase anxiety and stress for all. Equally, social workers attending the labour ward is not appropriate either. However, a social worker visiting a postnatal ward is not confidential, sensitive or comfortable. The hospital may be a safe place for the baby while arrangements are made.

Conclusion

While safeguarding is not the primary role of the midwife, there is a duty to safeguard babies, children and vulnerable women. In order for midwives to uphold their clinical responsibilities and legal duty regarding birth notification, social services must work in partnership with maternity services.

Activity

1. What is the definition of parental responsibility? Do you know who has parental responsibility for a baby whose birth you have supported?
2. Parents with learning disabilities will need support to develop understanding, resources, skills and experiences to meet the needs of their children. Consider how the maternity services and midwife contribute to this support.

Practice check

1. Consider how you would feel if required to give evidence in court regarding safeguarding procedures and a baby which you have helped a woman birth.
2. What sort of things would make you worried about a baby? How would you manage and document this?
3. What is the procedure to follow if you are worried about the possibility of abuse for (a) a baby, (b) a young mother?

Useful websites

Department for Education and Skills: www.dfes.gov.uk
Children's Workforce Network: www.everychildmatters.gov.uk
Children First: www.childrenfirst.wales.gov.uk
Children in Northern Ireland: www.ci-ni.org
Children in Scotland: www.childreninscotland.org.uk
Four Nations Child Policy Network: www.childpolicy.org.uk
Legislation and Bills: www.legislation.gov.uk
National Service Framework for Children and Maternity Services:
www.dh.gov.uk/PolicyAndGuidance/HealthAndSocialCareTopics/ChildrenServices
Welsh Assembly Government – National Service Frameworks: www.wales.nhs.uk
Welsh Assembly Government – Children and Young People:
http://new.wales.gov.uk/topics/childrenyoungpeople
Office of the Children's Commissioner at www.childrenscommissioner.org

10 Supervision of midwives

Pre-requisites for this chapter

A good understanding of the role and responsibilities of the NMC as a regulatory body. It is anticipated that you will have access to the latest documents regarding supervision from the NMC. You should also be familiar with the role of the Midwifery Committee at the NMC.

Introduction

This chapter will focus on the supervision of midwives. Supervision is enshrined in statute and is a method of protecting the public from harmful practice as well as supporting midwives who are struggling to provide and maintain high standards of care. Supervisors of midwives (SoMs) have a statutory regulatory role, but they also have a supervisory role or governance of midwifery practice. SoMs support and guide midwives and provide help and advice for parents. Information for women regarding the role of SoMs and the support they provide (NMC, 2010f) is usually provided at the antenatal booking appointment. Supporting women with their birth choices and supporting midwives providing midwifery care is a balancing act for SoMs: 'Midwifery supervision is a statutory function, is highly valued by the midwifery profession and, indeed has been the envy of other professional groups' (Warwick, 2014c). While supervision of midwives may be envied, midwives' experiences of supervision and the process of supervision may be very different (McHugh *et al.*, 2013). Starting with the role and responsibilities of a supervisor, this chapter will consider the ethical basis for supervision, the legal aspects of supervision and the challenges that SoMs are currently facing in fulfilling their legislative function.

Supervision of midwives

Supervision of midwives can be traced back to the Midwives Act 1902. Statutory supervision of midwives enshrined in legislation is unique (Mannion, 2008). Midwifery supervision is highly valued by the midwifery profession (Stapleton *et al.*, 1998) and has been the envy of other professional groups (Warwick, 2014c). Statutory supervision of midwives is thought to have played an important role in driving up the quality of midwifery care (Department of Health, 2009). Supervision is considered to be an effective method for public protection as poor practice is identified and action taken with individuals and maternity services to support improvement. Mellor (2013) identified that at Furness General

Hospital the supervision of midwives system failed to identify poor midwifery practice in three separate cases where babies died.

What is the role of the supervisor of midwives?

The role of the SoM is to conduct a regular audit on midwives' note taking (Farrer, 1975). This outdated view of the role of the SoM is nonetheless an important aspect of clinical supervision. Following re-organisation of the NHS in 1972, the role of the non-medical SoM was confused (Farrer, 1975). There are a number of responsibilities in the role of supervisor. Namely, supervisory annual reviews, supervisory investigations and attendance at CNST incident reviews, submission of documents of supervisory investigations to the Local Supervising Authority (LSA), contact supervisor (rota) and the provision of professional advice and support. Given the number of responsibilities and the nature of those responsibilities (writing of reports, attendance at reviews, role model), it is safe to say that SoMs are busy. Midwifery supervision is thought to work by women and their families being protected from harm and midwives being supported in the delivery of the best possible care. The low numbers of midwives (proportionately) being referred to the NMC suggests that midwifery supervision is effective. In modern midwifery practice the role of the supervisor of midwives is to protect the public from harm. The supervisor protects from harm in the following ways (four pillars or four P's of supervision):

1. Promoting a safe standard of midwifery practice;
2. Providing support and guidance to every midwife;
3. Preventing poor practice;
4. Providing leadership.

How does supervision work?

The process of supervision is intended to ensure high-quality care is delivered and appropriate standards are met and that midwifery practice reflects the changing needs of women. The process of supervision is intended to not only identify poor midwifery practice but to support the development of good practice. In order to provide high-quality care the midwife provides evidence-based care. Midwifery practice is also influenced by policy, protocols, standards and guidelines developed by SoMs.

Originally, LSAs were responsible for enacting statutory supervision and reporting to the Central Midwives Board (CMB). Understandably, when control over midwives is exerted from another source (often perceived by midwives to be the medical profession) tensions exist. Supervision of midwives in the UK has had an interesting and chequered history. In 1981 the CMB reported that 85 midwives attended the four induction courses organised during the period under review (1980/1981). In 1995 the Association of Radical Midwives (ARM) identified specific recommendations for the future of midwifery supervision. The main recommendations of the ARM (1995) were around selection, preparation and education, communication, conflicting roles, clinical credibility and accountability of SoMs (ARM, 1995: 90–92). Since then, changes and improvements have been made to the process, procedures and the preparation for supervision of midwives.

Standards for supervised practice

Following an investigation or investigative report a midwife may be required to undertake a period of supervised practice. The NMC (2007c) identifies the standards for supervised practice. The supervised practice programme is an individualised plan based upon the issues identified in the investigative report. The alternative to supervised practice is a direct referral to the NMC regarding fitness to practise. There is limited understanding of the experiences of midwives who have undergone supervised practice. Anecdotal evidence suggests that the experiences for some is punitive (Flint, 1993), while others (Davidson and Raynor, 2012) suggest that midwifery supervision is 'gold standard'.

Midwifery supervision and finance

The maternity service is primarily intended to provide care and support for women during childbirth. Funding and time necessary for mandatory training, staff development or supervision activities will always compromise care. If these roles and responsibilities are built into the funding of midwifery care the real cost of midwifery provision might be calculated. In 2011, the Care Quality Commission (CQC) identified that many SoMs were overwhelmed with day-to-day difficulties, working in their own time to ensure that the statutory function of supervision was being provided to all midwives (CQC, 2011). Staffing levels in the NHS are an issue due to the national shortage of midwives. Staffing establishments need to take account of the broader educational activities associated with mandatory training, professional development, supervision of midwives and policy, guidelines and commissioning priorities. In 2010 the NMC raised concerns regarding the variations in the numbers of SoMs. A national survey of supervisors reveals that the structure, profile and remuneration of supervisors varies throughout the UK (Rogers and Yearley, 2013). While the survey focused upon recruitment and retention of supervisors, it was apparent that protected time (for supervisory duties), remuneration and on-call impacted upon the effectiveness of the role.

Is there any evidence that supervision works?

Supervision of midwives has changed, developed and evolved over the years. Skipworth (1996) reported on the development of local standards of supervision. In 1991, ten draft standards were circulated and audited as part of an amended quality cycle. The audit adopted a 'twinning arrangement' to enable supervisors from one district or trust to audit colleagues in their twin. The audit tool was used to identify whether the supervisors had the standards and were using them. A limitation of this study is that SoMs at this time were not all familiar with audit tools and some required additional support and training in their usage. There were also issues around the time taken to complete the audit and the change in the numbers of SoMs.

Duerden (1995) identifies that supervision of midwives has been 'operating in various fashions' for 93 years, and there has been scant research and very little recorded. She conducted an audit of the supervision of midwives in the North West Region, October 1994–October 1995.

Supervision to most people is linked with management (Barker, 2012) and something that the NMC seems to support, as SoMs are required to 'oversee the work of midwives' and meet with them regularly. Some SoMs (Barker, 2012) identify that they are trying to avoid the link and there has been an increase in the number of SoMs working in education. The term 'supervisor' usually means a person who is responsible for 'overseeing' the work of others. Barker (2012) suggests that midwifery supervisors are burdened with a title which does not depict the reality of a supervisor's work. Barker goes on to suggest that the NMC (2012d) reinforces the notion of overseeing the work of midwives to the general public in the document 'how they can help you'. The term supervisor is not considered to be a functional title (Barker, 2012)

In the previous chapter, supervision was identified as a legal requirement. Primary legislation in the form of the Midwives Act 1902 identified that midwives should be regulated under a system of supervision. This means that all registered midwives are allocated to an SoM who monitors their standard of care, ability to work and their professional development/education. It is thought that by supervising midwives in this way, members of the public are less likely to suffer harm from poor practice.

Ethical aspects

What are the dilemmas/issues for midwives regarding supervision?

There are a number of dilemmas surrounding supervision; namely, governance, finance, attitudes and effectiveness. The first dilemma regarding supervision is regarding governance, including the relationship between the supervisor and the midwife. The second dilemma is regarding financing of supervision and how the cost of supervising registered practitioners who are experiencing difficulties is funded. The third dilemma is the principle of fairness and equity. Finally, is supervision effective in protecting the public? Concerns regarding statutory supervision were highlighted in three incidents in the Ombudsman's report (PHSO, 2013).

Donnison's (1977) comparison with control of tradesmen was borne out in clinical settings when midwives became disillusioned with supervision. Claims that supervision was controlling and punitive stemmed from midwives' experiences of the process and procedure of supervision. A common complaint was that midwives did not know when supervisors were wearing which hat – was the midwife a manager or supervisor? Unfortunately, sometimes they were wearing both hats! Over the years terminology has changed; in 1937 the term 'inspector' was dropped in favour of 'supervisor'. In 1995, tensions regarding supervision of midwives, among midwives, were high. The ARM considered that there was an increase in the number of midwives being disciplined, either informally or formally. In 2012 the NMC and the CQC identified problems at Morecambe Bay around supervison of midwives and a number of maternal and neonatal deaths.

Midwifery supervision governance

In 1993 the ARM identified concerns regarding the quality of supervision. The ARM considered that the reasons for concern were around the dual role of supervisors (manager and supervisor), an apparent increase in the number of midwives being disciplined and the process of supervision (accusation, investigation, sanctions, discipline, no appeal and inability of the midwife to 'clear her name'). Downe (1994) was concerned that there was no mechanism for appealing against an accusation made by a supervisor, which does not subsequently get a hearing at a higher level. Flint (1993) went further and suggested that supervision of midwifery can be an oppressive tool based upon a nursing model of only having two ways of doing things – the right way and the wrong way.

Inequalities in the practice of midwifery supervision were identified by Stapleton *et al.* (1998). Standards of supervision were varied and experienced midwives were felt to be treated differently in different health authorities. In addition, personality had influenced outcomes and some supervisors were not supportive of midwives when clinical judgements had been made that they did not agree with. One concern was focused around the way in which SoMs were appointed. Some midwives felt that supervision was like an 'old boys network' or 'club' that some midwives belonged to and others were not invited to join. Concern was also expressed that some midwives were invited to become a supervisor and did not feel able to refuse.

Midwifery supervision finance

Walton (1995) considered that a particular problem of statutory midwifery supervision was that supervision was not timed, costed or funded properly. She also felt that audit of supervision and the 'monitoring of supervisory performance against national standards and criteria would reduce the feeling of powerlessness that many midwives feel about supervision' (Walton, 1995: 38). Financial inequalities are also a concern. Remuneration for supervision is not equitable and neither is the amount of time allocated for supervisory duties. According to Ashwin (2014), payments vary from trust to trust and the system of successful supervision relies upon the good will of SoMs.

Is midwifery supervision ethically based?

Ethical principles such as autonomy, reliability and equity may also be applied to supervision of midwives.

Autonomy

Do midwives have a right to choose their SoM? How far does the right to self-determination for midwives go?

When there is a difference of opinion regarding clinical care is the midwife able to act autonomously, or does the power exercised by the SoM reduce the agency of the midwife? The midwife may feel the duty to obey the SoM is greater than the duty of care to the woman when there are difficult choices to be made regarding choice and continuity.

SoMs may also feel that they are unable to act autonomously. Expectations upon their conduct, decision making and clinical skills are influenced by the responsibilities of being a supervisor.

Equity and fairness?

Is there any evidence that some midwives are treated differently by their SoM to others? Midwives who have been the subject of a supervisory investigation are informed of the outcome. The midwife may be required to undertake educational support or clinical supervision, or a combination of both. What may be unclear is if the midwife feels that the plan or outcome is fair, appropriate or excessive. In the application of ethical utilitarian theory it would seem justifiable if the outcome (improved patient care) or ends justified the means.

A further ethical dilemma regarding levels of support for midwives working as lecturers or researchers has been identified: the right of a midwife to fairness and equity – is the annual review with an SoM equitable? Most supervisors of midwives utilise a proforma for the annual review. Standards vary as to the structure of the proforma, but it is usual to find the following elements:

- discussion based around experiences, i.e. reflection of last year;
- audit of record-keeping;
- written reflections on practice – may also use some tools to achieve this;
- evidence of meeting PREP requirements;
- action plan or future plans.

Midwifery supervision: is it effective in protecting the public?

NMC records suggest that proportionally fewer midwives (than other registrants) find themselves the subject of an NMC hearing. An assumption could be that the mechanism of supervision means that midwives are clinically supervised and therefore less likely to make mistakes or fall short of the standards required of them. The NMC receives regular reports from each LSA regarding the activities and investigations being undertaken to protect the public. Certainly, in the fulfilment of the role of supervisor and the functioning of the LSA much work is undertaken. Evidence suggests that education, training, supervised practice, investigations and support for midwives is available at all times. The role of supervision in the identification of declining or poor standards has been questioned regarding events at Northwick Park, Morecambe Bay and Guernsey.

Legal aspects

Since the 1902 Midwives Act supervision has been part of midwifery practice. Subsequent legislation, development and implementation of national policies and guidance for supervisors, information technology and case rulings have developed and shaped supervision. Other legislation, such as the Health Act 1999 and the re-organisation of the NHS in 1974 have also impacted upon the organisation of midwifery supervision.

Supervision is governed by the NMC – the Midwives Rules identify the relationship and functions. The supervisory framework consists of national LSA and Local Supervising Authority Midwifery Officers (LSAMOs). Each SoM receives training and reports to an LSAMO.

SoMs are accountable to the LSA. All maternity services are subjected to an annual review by the LSA; the review consists of an audit of standards of supervision based upon the evidence submitted by each of the hospitals in the area. The LSA report informs the supervisory team of recommendations to drive up standards and enhance quality of the maternity services. The LSA report is shared with other regulators and interested parties such as the Royal College of Midwives.

An SoM (in keeping with the Midwives Rules), the same as other midwives, must always make women and their families the focus of their care. To this end supervisors are able to protect the public from a midwife whose fitness to practise has been questioned.

An SoM is available 24 hours per day to provide expert advice to midwives and as a point of contact for women and families with issues regarding midwifery practice. SoMs are considered to be independent advocates for women and their families. While the principles are ethical, the ability of an SoM to act as an independent advocate for a woman is questionable when the same midwife may also hold a managerial position in the service the woman is having issues with. Women who choose not to use the maternity services or undertake 'free birth' are acting autonomously but require the involvement of an SoM to provide independent, personalised and safe midwifery care.

Annual supervisory review

The annual meeting between a supervisor and midwife should not be confused with an annual performance review with a line manager. The annual meeting with a supervisor of midwives is a requirement which enables the LSA to monitor and provide evidence of midwifery practice annually. What is the benefit for the midwife? The meeting with a supervisor is an opportunity for a midwife to ensure that the professional portfolio, intention to practise and record-keeping are complete and to a professional standard. An SoM will use a proforma identified by the LSA, and the midwife brings to the meeting evidence which demonstrates professional practice (such as reflections, updates, training needs and concerns). SoMs utilise a number of strategies for exploration of the midwife's clinical experiences. For those midwives working in education, research, management or consultancy, different approaches may be necessary. An SoM needs to have an understanding of the different roles and responsibilities of supervisees to ensure that the annual review is meaningful and appropriate. A values-based approach can be used to focus the annual review. However, reliance on the six Cs alone is probably insufficient. Including continuity and complacency in the Cs ensures that the values that promote women's health during childbirth can be addressed. Barker (2013) identifies in her reflections on the annual review that it is an opportunity to support not only supervision and midwives, but additionally women and their families. To demonstrate how a supervisor of midwives may protect the public from potential harm is regarding the responsibility to ensure that the midwife is fulfilling duties of care such as safeguarding and referral when care is outside of a midwife's sphere of practice.

Statutory supervision

Statutory supervision of midwives was identified in the Midwives Act 1902. Subsequent legislation has not changed the concept of supervision but has enabled midwives to fulfil this role. The Nursing and Midwifery Order 2001 contains the powers for the NMC to set midwives rules which provide the existing rules regarding supervision, giving the status of statutory supervision. The NMC (2012a) Midwives Rules and Standards can be changed following consultation with the profession. The Nursing and Midwifery Order stipulates the establishment of a Local Supervising Authority (LSA).

Midwifery regulation

Following concerns regarding the effectiveness and the efficiency of the NMC as a regulatory body (Department of Health, 2012), a review of the regulatory body (CHRE, 2012) identified the need for changes. The Parliamentary Health Service Ombudsman report (PHSO, 2013) also identifies concerns regarding the NMC regulatory body regarding its abilities to regulate the nursing and midwifery professions. The PHSO recommended that midwifery supervision and regulation should be separate activities and that the NMC should be in direct control of the regulatory body. The Law Commission also published its review of regulation of health and social care professionals (2014). In 2014 the NMC responded to criticisms and identified a policy document of better legislation for better regulation. The process for legislative change is lengthy and the NMC asked Parliament to enable the legislative process to commence. The NMC also commissioned the Kings Fund to report on midwifery regulation in the UK. The recommendations of the Kings Fund were unsupportive of statutory midwifery supervision. No other healthcare professions shared this type of regulation and they found a lack of quantifiable evidence in the current system of supervision in protecting the public. In January 2015 (NMC/15/06) the NMC accepted the recommendations of the Kings Fund report and identified that they would be calling upon the government to provide an opportunity to amend the NMC's legislation. In addition, there was a decision to authorise the preparation of amendments to the standards component of the Midwives Rules and Standards. Consultation will now be required to initiate the changes to primary and secondary legislation.

Chapter summary

Midwifery supervision is enshrined in statute but not tablets of stone. The primary function of supervision is to fulfil the NMC's role in the protection of the public by actively promoting safe standards of midwifery care. NMC regulation of midwifery practice has recently been scrutinised and weaknesses have been found. Any changes made to the functions of supervision or the role of the SoM will require a change in the legislation. The supervisory system needs to be open and transparent so that all midwives understand the difference between regulation and governance. Supervision should not be punitive, but supportive, and there should be equity and fairness regarding those midwives under investigation for alleged misconduct. It is the author's opinion that clinical supervision could be supported through the Royal College of Midwives as and when the NMC are no longer responsible for statutory supervision. Professional bodies such as the RCM have clear understandings of the standards of clinical competence and care. Regulation and fitness to practise could be maintained by the regulatory body for midwives (whichever it might be).

Case study: Suzy's water birth

Suzy wants to use water for pain relief during labour and also give birth in it. At this time no water births have taken place in the maternity hospital. Suzy is happy to have the first birth in the pool in the maternity unit. If staff will not allow her to do this she would hire a pool and have the baby at home. The supervisor identifies that Suzy could use the pool at the hospital provided that a midwife who has undertaken a water birth before is available. If Suzy decides to have the baby at home and allow her partner at the birth and not a midwife, then she is 'breaking the law'. The supervisor offers a solution, have the baby at the maternity unit and she will undertake the delivery with a midwife who had studied water birth in attendance. If the supervisor was not available the option for a water birth would be withdrawn and Suzy must leave the pool! An agreement is drawn up and Suzy is asked to sign.

(continued)

Introduction

This case illustrates some common dilemmas faced by midwives around service provision, midwifery skills and maintaining professional development, defensive practice and an inability to provide choice. In addition it illustrates an incorrect belief that getting a client to sign a document constitutes consent. These key issues will be used to discuss the ethical and legal aspects of Suzy's case. Before addressing the issues around supervision in Suzy's case it is important to clarify the legal situation regarding midwives generally.

Evaluation

In considering the above case it should be remembered that many women are guinea pigs while accessing maternity services. The first ultrasound scan, the first electronic fetal monitoring and the first epidural will always raise issues regarding safety, risk assessment and what is best practice. Supervisors of midwives will be required to make preparations and training for midwives available to enable them to prepare as well as possible for providing proper care and attention. The midwife has a duty to learn as much as possible and act in a professional manner at all times.

The supervisor of midwives

Supervision of midwives is a statutory function that has evolved and developed over the years. The primary intention of supervision was to protect the public from 'the perceived dangers of the handywoman who attended women in labour at the beginning of the twentieth century' (Lewison, 1996). It is not possible to discuss SoMs in isolation as they are by definition also experienced midwives and often hold additional roles (such as team leader, manager or head of department/service). However, in 2011 the first full-time SoM was appointed in Barking, Havering and Redbridge University Hospitals NHS Trust (BHRUT).

Analysis

The aspects of supervision that are the most effective are likely to be those which demonstrate high standards of care and uphold the NMC (2010a) Code.

Annual audits of midwifery practice which include feedback from women can help to develop and enhance the maternity services. The requirement for Suzy to sign an agreement is unnecessary as it does not constitute a binding contract. In addition, a signature does not in itself constitute consent (see Chapter 6).

What can be done?

- Midwives need to be able to share good practice and learn from each other. Continuous professional development is not a luxury but a basic part of professional practice.

- Midwifery society, research lunches and midwifery newsletters can disseminate information, updates and trends in maternity care.
- Midwifery services should undertake an annual review of skills to enable the development of education and training needs.

Implications for practice

- Supervisors of midwives have a role to protect the public from harm. Any midwife providing care for the first time must be trained and supported regarding the skills required.
- Record-keeping is an important mechanism for identification of care provided and may subsequently be used as evidence in court.
- A signature on a form does not constitute consent.

Conclusion

Suzy's case was chosen to illustrate supervision in action. The case raised basic legal issues regarding the supervisor's belief that getting or coercing a patient to sign a document will prevent any chance of litigation. In addition, it demonstrates an unsavoury side of midwifery, namely that of control and lack of respect for the patient's wishes. Unethical midwifery practice may not be seen in that arguments presented may appear to be justified, reasonable or protecting one's registration. Midwives (and supervisors) whose behaviour and attitude do not respect the healthcare rights of women are controlling and limiting choices.

Additional case study

Stan is a newly qualified midwife and has accepted a job in a large maternity hospital. You have been asked to be Stan's supervisor of midwives. You have never worked with a male midwife before.

Use the framework (evaluation, analysis (ethical and legal issues), what can be done and implications for practice) to consider Stan's case.

Activity

The NMC is clear that supervision of midwives should contribute more to supporting women's healthcare. Publications (NMC, 2010f) are aimed at ensuring that members of the public recognise and use the role of supervisors.

Consider a recent episode of care you have provided and identify the following:

- Did the woman and/or her family know of or have heard of a supervisor of midwives?
- Have you seen a copy of the NMC patient information leaflet on supervisors?
- How can midwives use the process of supervision to better effect?
- When do midwives complete their annual intention to practise?

Practice check

- When did you last meet with your supervisor of midwives? What was the purpose of the meeting (e.g. annual review, identification of development needs, discussion, clinical audit, support)?
- What sort of evidence do you use to 'inform' your meeting with a supervisor?
- How helpful is your supervisor in identifying your learning and development needs?
- What is the difference between supervised practice and a student being supervised in practice?
- Consider the possibility that the NMC 'audited' your professional portfolio. Does it contain evidence of supervision and professional development?

Practice check (supervisors of midwives)

- Practice standard: what should your professional midwifery portfolio demonstrate?
- As a supervisor of midwives what do you understand by the NMC's statement that you should oversee the work of midwives and meet with them regularly? What ethical dilemmas does this requirement present?
- In your professional portfolio is there any evidence that service users have contributed to your development?

Activities

- Access the NMC website (www.nmc.org.uk) and consider how midwives could use the mechanism of supervision to better effect.
- Registered midwives should seek/use opportunities to demonstrate annual notification of intention to practise to students and service users.

Useful websites

Association of Radical Midwives (ARM): www.midwifery.org.uk
Local Supervising Authority (LSA): www.nmc-uk.org/Nurses-and-midwives/Midwifery-New/
Contact-a-LSAMO1/Local-Supervising-Authority-Midwifery-Officer-contacts-England
Nursing and midwifery council (NMC): www.nmc-uk.org
Supervisory Guidance and Investigation: www.lsa.westmidlands.nhs.uk

11 Birth environment

Pre-requisites for this chapter

Take time to identify the home birth rate and Caesarean section rate in the NHS trust near to you. You should have a good understanding of the ways in which fear, anxiety and stress impact upon labour. Childbirth may also act as a trigger for painful memories associated with abuse, female genital mutilation or other abusive experiences.

Introduction

For centuries women have given birth at home, but in the UK numbers of home births have declined. Successive government reports have supported the principle of home birth but have also recommended hospital birth as being safer. The dilemma for the mother and the midwife is: how can home birth be safe if the majority of births are taking place in hospital?

This chapter considers birth environment from an ethical and legal perspective. This chapter is concerned with the rights of women to a birth environment which is safe, appropriate and acceptable to them. The legal right to a home birth is considered and the effect of the law regarding midwifery practice is addressed. What rights do women have around home birth? Do midwives control the birth environment? What choices are there for home birth? Is home birth a realistic option in a cash-strapped NHS?

Loss of home birth skills

Historically the number of home births have declined. This decline has been attributed to the power and control exerted over the maternity services by the medical profession. It could be argued that since the medical profession relinquished their control over the regulation and control of midwives that their energies have focused upon controlling childbirth through the hospitalisation of childbearing women:

> obstetricians would clearly like a legal embargo on any alternative to hospital intra-natal care if this were politically and practically feasible. In Britain, the Royal College of Obstetricians and Gynaecologists has suggested to successive Government Committees reviewing the maternity service that recommendations in this direction would be welcome.
>
> (Tew, 1990: 25)

Tew goes on to suggest that despite a monopoly on childbirth care, obstetricians the world over would prevent the slightest competition 'however offensive' to human rights. In addition, successive government reports and mortality statistics are thought to have been influential in increasing hospitalisation. If ever there was an argument for midwives to become political-minded or politically active, then choice of place of birth is one to lobby for. Resource management also impacts upon the choice of birth environment for women. In 2012, new legislation identified a new process for commissioning of healthcare services (Health Service Act, 2012, part 1, numbers 25–28). Closer examination of the maternity services reveals that there is great variation between the numbers of consultant obstetric units and midwifery-led units and birth centres in England (Beake and Bick, 2007). It would seem that women have accepted that hospitalisation of birth is normal (Edwards, 2008). Women's acceptance and midwives' lack of ability to provide and support choice (Hollins Martin, 2007) would suggest that home birth, midwife-led care and birth centres are not likely realistic choices. Even if there is choice and equity of choice, the amount of choice is not fairly distributed or available. These childbirth injustices further demonstrate that ethical-based maternity care remains an aspiration. *Maternity Matters* (Department of Health, 2007a) suggested that women would have increased access to services and continuity of care by 2009.

Ethical issues

The dilemma for the midwife is how to maintain high levels of clinical skills for all birth environments. Regularly working in a particular area ensures that skills are up to date and confidence is high. A midwife who works in the community is comfortable with flexibility and maintains good relationships with acute and emergency services. A midwife who works in a hospital environment is comfortable with routine policies, maintains inter-professional working relationships and hierarchical control. The two midwifery environments are not mutually exclusive but do require refreshers and reminders about the differences. If the maternity services are organised such that midwives rotate too frequently or infrequently, there is a risk that the culture does not support safe care. Midwives are required to maintain high standards of care in all environments and at all times. Providing care for women in labour is a challenge as childbirth outcomes are measured and women's experiences are felt for a lifetime. For example, a woman may be able to cope with a change to her birth plan, an emergency delivery or a stillbirth if she has experienced compassionate care, dignity and respect. Equally, a woman who has experienced roughness, feels uncomfortable, rushed, threatened or assaulted may not be able to cope even though she achieved her plan to birth a baby at home. Birth environment is so much more than venue, geography and ambience. It is about the culture within the environment. Compliance with outdated or routine procedures and complacency regarding poor standards are just as unethical as lack of confidentiality. Whatever the birth environment, women need to be included in the decision-making process.

Women's childbirth rights

The section focus upon the specific rights associated with childbirth. The healthcare rights of women are generally a neglected area (WHO, 2002). The rights of women during childbirth are no exception in England. Despite the rise in the number of births in the last decade, an increase in the proportion of complex births and a shortage of midwives, the rights of women during childbirth are being generally ignored. Repeated reports have identified that maternity services in England are at breaking point (logistically, financially and staffing). Despite the stress and difficulties, midwives have tried to develop innovative and supportive services for women. Women's memories of their experiences during childbirth are thought to last a lifetime (White Ribbon Alliance, 2014). Significantly for some women, the experience is so traumatic that they do not go on to have any further children. Fear of birth, post-traumatic stress and maternal suicide are examples of how childbirth experiences affect women.

A charter of seven fundamental rights for childbearing women has been identified (White Ribbon Alliance, 2014). These childbirth rights are:

1. freedom from harm and ill treatment;
2. information, informed consent;
3. privacy and confidentiality;
4. dignity and respect;
5. equality and freedom;
6. right to healthcare;
7. liberty and autonomy.

Women have the right to choose where and how to birth their babies. Choices in childbirth range from variety of environments to position, tranquil to clinical, as well as different types of care.

Women who choose to exercise their right to choice during childbirth may cause a dilemma for the midwife as the risks associated with the choice may be perceived to be untenable. In spite of information, advice and explanations, women sometimes make choices that seem risky or unsafe. Providing capacity is not an issue, the midwife is required to support that choice and continue to provide the best possible care.

Rights of the fetus and baby

Fetal rights are only able to be considered after upholding of maternal rights. For example, a fetus cannot have an absolute right to a healthy gestation as it is not possible for women to control the uterine environment.

While theoretically babies have the right to be born in a safe environment, the location of the birth (home or hospital) cannot be forced upon the woman. The potential is that if a woman does not accept or choose the birth environment, she may decide to free birth (Edwards and Kirkham, 2012). Free birth is the term given whereby the woman plans to deliver her baby away from hospital, without medical care and without the care and support of a midwife. The removal of any professional support during childbirth is associated with poor fetal and maternal outcomes.

Right to choice

When utilising a business model for the maternity services (and who would not, given the cash-strapped NHS, spiralling costs and increased workloads?) it would seem logical to consider the views of Henry Ford, who said that you could have 'any color of car as long as it was black'. By limiting the choice for his customers he was able to keep up the supply. By offering specific packages of healthcare the private sector has managed to turn healthcare into a profit-making business. Reduction of choice is the way forward for ensuring cost efficiencies and effectiveness. Encouraging all women to birth their babies in hospital should enable a safe, effective and efficient solution to having a baby. This argument does not hold on two accounts. First, hospital delivery is financially expensive; second, repeated reports (Department of Health, Expert Maternity Group, 1993; Department of Health, 2007, 2010c; RCOG, 2008) identify that women want choice, continuity and culturally sensitive midwifery care.

The right to choose where to birth your baby is flawed, as for many years women have been led to believe that hospital births are safer and that having a home birth is at best risky and at worst dangerous. Opportunities for discussing birth environment are limited to short antenatal appointments. Maternity services are commissioned by local commissioning groups (H&SC Act 2012) and may not include choices or different birth environments. The NHS is structured and focuses upon hospital birth. Current austerity measures mean that for some women lengthy travelling to city units is necessary. While 80 per cent of women in a 2005 poll identified that they were happy with midwifery care, they also identified that they wanted more choice. The dilemma for midwives is how to support choices made by women while there is a midwifery staffing shortage.

Right to safe care

In 1970 the Peel Report identified that provision should be made to enable 100 per cent hospital confinement. The rationale was that hospital births would reduce maternal mortality. Medical staff suggested that hospital birth was safer and persuaded the government that hospital births would improve maternity care. Unfortunately, at that time the report was interpreted to mean that 100 per cent of women should give birth in hospital. Between 1970 and 1990 the percentage of women giving birth increased and the number of obstetric units and maternity hospitals increased to cope with the number of women 'choosing' to deliver their babies in hospital. The effect of the hospitalisation of women in childbirth has been an erosion of midwifery skills regarding home birth. Floyd (1993) found that midwives had little experience of home birth and lacked confidence and skills. Midwives working in community settings were encouraged to rotate to labour wards in hospitals to increase confidence in providing care during labour.

Since the 1990s government policy for the maternity services has been around offering childbearing women choice. *Changing Childbirth* (Department of Health, Expert Maternity Group, 1993) clearly identified that women should have choice, continuity and control over childbirth. Edwards (2008) questions whether subsequent policy (NSF and *Maternity Matters*) is any different and whether it is likely to be successful when other policy has failed to ensure that childbearing women get choice, especially with regard to place of delivery. The Health and Social Care Bill (2011) sets out the new process for commissioning healthcare. Will commissioning consortia enable women to have more choice for the place of delivery?

Duty of care

The professional standards for care during labour apply regardless of the environment. That said, there is a clear and fundamental difference in that in the home environment there is a desire to keep labour normal, reduce interference and empower women to birth their babies how they wish. The midwife is a professional visitor to the home and maintains professional boundaries and upholds NMC guidelines. In a hospital environment there is anticipation of abnormality, expectation of risks and the woman and her partner may feel part of a 'work load'. NHS hospitals talk about delivery rates, bed occupancy and time constraints.

Legal aspects regarding birth environments

The laws relating to the environment of birth in the UK are varied. There is no one statute that covers the legality of birth and there is no statute that identifies a woman's right to a home birth or alternatively preventing a home birth. Equally, there is no legislation which forces women to go into hospital to birth their baby. There is legislation which protects the role and responsibilities of a midwife regardless of the location of birth. The place of birth is thought to be a cultural issue and in the UK the main culture is for childbirth to take place in hospital. Following identification of relevant statute, this section will consider relevant case law. The main issues regarding birth environment stem from the concept of safety.

National Health Service Act 1977

NHS Act 1977 Section 3 (1d) identifies that facilities for maternity services are to be determined by the Secretary of State.

Human Rights Act 1998

The Human Rights Act 1998 (HRA) is primary legislation, which has been enacted to ensure that the ethical aspects identified in the European convention are enforced. The key rights relevant to midwifery here are the following.

Article 2 The right to life

This refers to the right of all individuals to live their lives as they see fit. It gives responsibility for others to make sure that they do not shorten or prevent that life.

Article 3 Prohibition of torture

Obstetric torture and inhuman treatment during childbirth are grave concerns. Expecting women to birth babies while restrained or subjected to painful experiences is not associated with good care. The rights of childbearing women have been clearly identified by the White Ribbon Alliance.

Article 8 The right to respect for private and family life

Article 8 of the European Convention on Human Rights concerns the right to private and family life. If this article is applied to childbirth it concerns or protects the woman's right to choose where to give birth. The dilemma in England is that while the woman may choose where to birth her baby, having a baby in any environment does not guarantee safety of mother and baby. In other words, there are risks associated with childbirth that medical practitioners wish to control. The defensive position based upon an old report (Peel Report) is that it is safer to give birth in hospital, whereby medical practitioners would be able to deliver to the latest medical standards. The question for women in 2014 is: why would you want to birth your baby in hospital when your risk of intervention and specifically Caesarean section can be as high as 28 per cent?

Article 9 Freedom of thought, conscience and religion

Childbearing women are entitled to their views, opinions and religion. A midwife needs to be able to support women with their choices and preferences.

Article 14 Freedom from discrimination

Supervisors of midwives (SoMs) provide support for women in making choices around childbirth. Women are given information at booking regarding the role of the SoM (NMC, 2010f). SoMs are in a key position to ensure that the basic human rights detailed above are fulfilled for all birth environments. During the antenatal booking appointment the woman should be given information regarding choices for place of birth of her baby. It could be argued that not offering a choice of place of birth is discriminatory. The level of choice available to women in practice is restricted when maternity units have to be closed for short periods to safeguard the quality and safety of care when demand might outstrip capacity. Over one-quarter of maternity units had to close to admissions for half a day or more between April and September 2012. The main reported reason for these closures was a lack of either physical capacity or midwives.

Article 17 Prohibition of abuse and rights

Childbearing women have a right to safe and compassionate care. Pregnancy is not a time for restricting existing rights or an opportunity to degrade or humiliate.

All of the above articles have been incorporated into the Code so that midwives are reminded of the standards and the requirements of ethical-based midwifery care.

National Health Service & Community Care Act 1990

The National Health Service & Community Care Act 1990 stemmed from the government's white paper (Department of Health, 1989). In the white paper minimal reference is made to the maternity services – they are not included in the list of core services. Midwifery is mentioned once as an example of cost-effective resource management.

This Act introduced:

- Self-governing hospitals (NHS trusts) which enable the management team to determine what and how many services they will offer. The effect of the legislation is to further restrict choice with regard to birth environments.

- The GP contract, which identifies the services which a GP will provide. As GPs no longer are required to attend home births this part of the legislation does not impact upon the birth environment.

Health and Social Care Act 2012

This Act comprises seven chapters and 457 pages, including schedules! It established the National Health Service Commissioning Board or Health and Wellbeing Board (NHS HWB). This Board is important, as the Secretary of State no longer has a duty to promote a comprehensive health service. The HWB and the commissioning boards now have the legal duty to improve the quality of services, reduce inequalities, promote autonomy, research, education and training, reporting and the reviewing of treatment providers. Midwives and midwifery are not mentioned specifically in the Act. The purpose of the Act was to strengthen public health services.

Standards/safety

Historically, the number of home births has declined. The reasons for the decline in home births is multifactorial (government agenda, numbers of multiple births, complex pregnancies, women with pre-existing medical conditions, lack of service provision).

A frequently used argument to support hospital birth is that statistics prove that hospital birth is safer as maternal mortality and morbidity has decreased following hospitalisation. Other arguments are that home birth is less safe because there is insufficient time to get expert medical intervention (emergency LSCS, management of haemorrhage and resuscitation of the asphyxiated baby).

The birthplace study (BECG, 2011) identifies that the risks for home birth are low. However, the number of women choosing a home birth is approximately 3 per cent of the total births. Making home births safe for midwives is an important aspect of the role of the SoM. It is important that lone working policies are developed to ensure that a midwife's personal safety is upheld.

Is there a legal right to home birth?

The legal situation would seem to be clear. The NHS is required to provide maternity services and all areas provide a home birth service. However, the nature and extent of the service is not prescribed and each NHS trust may vary the provision of a home birth service. For example, some NHS trusts have birth centres or midwifery-led units for those women whose pregnancies are low risk. While these facilities are not strictly a home, they are presented (decorated and equipped) in a home-like way. The benefit of midwifery-led units and birth centres are that women have close proximity to a hospital labour ward if an emergency should occur.

Can home birth be illegal?

Birthing a baby at home is not illegal in England. However, if a woman chooses to birth her baby at home and uses her partner, husband, relative or doula to provide midwifery care, monitor progress of labour or condition of the baby (midwifery services) this is illegal as it breaches section 44 of the SI 2002/253 (Nursing and Midwifery Order 2001).

Unassisted birth: the legal position

If a woman chooses to birth her baby without the assistance of a midwife or medical practitioner, is this illegal? Free birth (Edwards and Kirkham, 2012) is not illegal in itself, but midwives should do all that they can to ensure that a woman has professional support during childbirth. It is thought that supervision provides a safety net for these women. If the woman chooses to arrange for an inappropriate person to 'stand in' for the midwife to give her the birth experience she wants, then the woman is acting illegally (Nursing and Midwifery Order 2001 SI 2002 235 Part IX Section 5, Article 45).

What is the legal status of a birth plan?

The birth plan identifies a woman's preferences for birth. Women who wish to identify in advance of labour what they wish to happen or choices to be made usually write birth plans. As the plan is written by one person it cannot be a contract as the care provider has not signed the agreement, and even if there was a midwife's signature (witness to the birth plan) it does not constitute consent or agreement. Equally, the opposite is true: if a woman signs a birth plan which indicates that she does not want a particular intervention it does not mean that the intervention may not be offered. Consent or refusal has to be obtained at the time and is part of a process (Chapter 6).

Chapter summary

Constant changes in society, childbearing practices and increased numbers of women with complex healthcare needs creates a demand for maternity services and high-quality midwifery care. In the UK there are low rates of maternal mortality but increasingly high rates of dissatisfaction with maternity services. Removing choice and continuity of midwifery care leaves women upset and deeply disappointed with their childbirth experience. Mothers, babies and families have a fundamental human right to quality maternity care to enable them to have a healthy start to family life. While there is no legal right to a home birth, there is a legal obligation to provide emergency care. A midwife has a duty of care to attend a labouring women wherever she may be.

Case study: Scott

Scott is a male midwife and is employed to work in the community by an NHS trust. Home deliveries account for approximately 3 per cent of the trust's annual deliveries. Due to a shortage of staff the NHS trust has suspended the home birth service. Scott has a home birth booked (Sherie) as part of his caseload. Sherie informs Scott that she has gone into labour. Scott decides to attend the home birth.

Evaluation

Discussions about home birth often focus on safety and emotional wellbeing. Inch (1982) suggests that safety and emotional wellbeing are not mutually exclusive. For some women it will feel safer to go into hospital to deliver their baby, especially if they have complex medical needs. For other women birthing their baby at home feels safer as they can control the environment and receive one-to-one midwifery care. Sherie has booked for a home birth and has received continuity of care from Scott. The head of midwifery and the supervisor of midwives are aware of the home birth caseload and have agreed that Sherie can plan for a home birth. Measurements of safety usually focus upon detection of emergencies and the time it takes to gain expert or emergency care. It is not the purpose of this case study to argue the advantages or disadvantages of home and hospital births. The premise is that women have the right to choose, but in making that choice they are informed so that their safety and emotional wellbeing are paramount. The expectation is that the standard of care, safety and professional services of a midwife are upheld in all childbirth environments.

Analysis

The Midwives Act 1936 (consolidated in the 1951 Act) made it compulsory for local authorities to provide sufficient midwives to attend women confined at home in their area. While the Act has not been repealed, local authorities have been replaced by Area Health Authorities. The NHS and Community Care Act 1990 made provision for local NHS trusts to provide healthcare services.

Childbirth rights are based upon attitudes and behaviours such as respect, dignity, honesty and autonomy. Childbirth rights regarding location, environment or specific pain relief are not guaranteed.

Providing continuity of care, planned care and meeting Sherie's expectations regarding childbirth are important. Scott has a moral and legal duty to provide care during labour. The dilemma is that he has to ask Sherie to attend the hospital, which was not her wish, plan or intention. Is this right to home birth absolute?

In attending a home birth when the service is suspended, the midwife is in breach of contract with the employer (NHS trust). Scott may feel strongly that the NHS trust is failing to provide a home birth choice as they have suspended the service. Scott may also be aware that NHS trust hospital services are struggling to cope with labour ward workloads. He may also feel that morally it is not right to withdraw the possibility of a home birth at the last minute. Midwives who face dilemmas should discuss the issue with a supervisor of midwives, who provides support and

(continued)

information at this time. The role of the supervisor is primarily to protect the public, so Scott may feel that the supervisor would automatically advise him to ask Sherie to come into hospital.

What can be done?

Scott has to attend the home birth. He must ensure that he delivers high-quality care and follows home birth procedures and protocol. As he is in breach of his contract with the NHS trust, it is likely that following the delivery there will be an NHS trust management investigation and a decision made regarding his employment.

Implications for practice

- accountability
- supervision
- investigation
- professional misconduct.

Conclusion

Scott conducted a home birth during an NHS trust suspended home birth service and without informing the supervisor of midwives. Scott acted illegally in that he deliberately failed to follow his employer's guidelines and procedures; he was in breach of contract. Scott's ethical stance (upholding a right to home birth) was in conflict with ethical principles regarding beneficence and non-maleficence and effectively put a patient's choice above a patient's safety. Midwives, due to the nature and extent of their work, often face dilemmas in clinical practice. A breach of contract puts Scott and his patient at risk as he is no longer insured.

Practice check

1. How do you keep up to date/informed regarding your employer's policies, procedures and protocols?
2. Do you have indemnity insurance? If you are employed in the NHS you will have indemnity insurance, but if you choose to work outside the NHS you are required under European and UK law to arrange for indemnity insurance.

Activity

1. How does the NHS keep patients informed regarding accessing and receiving healthcare services?
2. The NMC is routinely informed of any illegal activities of midwives. There is no right of confidentiality. In light of Scott's breach of contract, what do you think might happen?
3. Determine your plan of action should you be faced with a woman who declines midwifery care.

Useful websites

Birthrights (UK): www.birthrights.org.uk/library/factsheets/Unassisted-Birth.pdf
Home birth information: www.nct.org.uk/birth/faqs-home-birth
Indemnity insurance: www.nmc-uk.org/registration/professional-indemnity-insurance
Midwives Rules and Standards: www.nmc-uk.org/Publications/Standards/The-code/Introduction
Nursing and Midwifery Standards and Fitness to Practise: www.nmc-uk.org/Hearings/Information-for-those-whose-conduct-is-under-investigation
Respectful maternity care: http://whiteribbonalliance.org

12 Abortion

Pre-requisites of this chapter

It is assumed that your knowledge and understanding of abortion is around techniques and interventions to terminate a pregnancy. You should be familiar with the latest professional regulatory standards (NMC, 2010a) *The Code: Standards of Conduct, Performance and Ethics for Nurses and Midwives*. The terms abortion and termination of pregnancy are both used and explained in this chapter.

Introduction

This chapter considers the ethical and legal issues surrounding abortion. While abortion is illegal in England, the practice is permitted and tolerated if certain criteria are proven (grounds) and two doctors sign to that effect. Assuming that the legality or grounds for abortion are present, the contentious issue regarding the abortion limit is a dilemma for healthcare. Advances in technology and the ability of some babies to survive birth under 24 weeks' gestation provides a moral dilemma. Are abortions being undertaken on healthy fetuses which could survive? Bainbridge (2008) considers that the argument between abortion limits and the viability of very premature births should not be mixed up. The costs of caring for a very premature birth are emotional, physical and financial. The cost to the NHS of doing everything for a much-wanted healthy baby is ethically different from not terminating pregnancies on the basis of gestation. The 20-week scan may be the first indication of severe abnormality and thereby a small window to make care plans exists. This leaves very little time to identify and talk through concerns and consult with relevant healthcare professionals. Consideration will be given to the notion that abortion is available 'on demand' in England and Wales. Ethical issues around sanctity of life, personhood and human rights are paramount throughout the chapter. Conflict between the rights of the woman, partner or father and the potential rights of the baby are addressed. It is assumed that the reader has a good understanding of the methods for procuring an abortion and the impact of those techniques on professional practice. Readers will be aware that personal values and beliefs will influence attitudes to abortion and that also includes the author. Abortion may be justified (or not) by individuals on religious grounds, validity and health reasons. Newspaper articles frequently use headlines that are emotionally charged to activate responses of anger or support for abortion services. Strong use of language such as 'murder', 'violence' and 'perfect', and emotional language such as 'beautiful', 'anger' and 'frustration' impact upon an individual's perception of abortion. Other factors influencing abortion include age, status of a relationship and financial health. Abortion is a sensitive topic and everybody has opinions regarding the practice. It is also acknowledged that some opinions remain fixed throughout a lifetime and that for others opinions may be challenged, modified or altered.

Ethically, individuals may object to abortion and some conscientiously object to abortion. The legal situation is focused upon primary legislation, namely the Abortion Act 1967. However, it is also necessary to make reference to other legislation, for example the Human Fertilisation and Embryology Act (HFEA) 1990 (which has the effect of amending the Abortion Act 1967). In 2008 the proposal to reduce the time to 22 weeks was rejected during the passing of the HFEA 2008.

Whatever our personal views are, modern healthcare services provide and undertake abortions, and healthcare practitioners are required to provide sensitive and appropriate care for those women who require this service.

The main legal issues are around the number of abortions, control and regulation of the process of abortion and upholding of standards of professional conduct.

Defining and quantifying abortion

Abortion may be defined as unlawfully procuring a miscarriage. Therefore, performing an abortion when the terms and conditions of the Abortion Act 1967 are fulfilled effectively means the legal termination of a pregnancy. Abortion refers to the illegal termination of a pregnancy. Miscarriage refers to the spontaneous loss of pregnancy. To terminate a pregnancy is then a criminal act unless performed within the constraints of the Abortion Act 1967 (as amended by the HFA Act).

How many abortions take place?

Abortion rates are a cause for concern. Evidence suggests that the number of abortions carried out for women resident in England and Wales in 2011 was 189,931, which is an increase of 0.2 per cent on 2010 and 7.7 per cent on 2001 (Department of Health, 2012d).

This year-on-year increase in the number of abortions has led to the perception that abortion is available 'on demand' and that women are using abortion rather than contraception. In 2011, 96 per cent of abortions were funded by the NHS. Of this, over half (61 per cent) took place in the independent sector under NHS contract, up from 59 per cent in 2010 and 2 per cent in 1981. Ninety-one per cent of abortions were carried out at under 13 weeks' gestation. The under-16 abortion rate was 3.4 per 1,000 women and the under-18 rate was 15.0 per 1,000 women, both lower than in 2010 (3.9 and 16.5 per 1,000 women, respectively) and 2001 (3.7 and 18.0 per 1,000 women, respectively). Medical abortions accounted for 47 per cent of the total, up from 43 per cent in 2010 and 13 per cent in 2001. There were 2,307 abortions (1 per cent) carried out under ground E (risk that the child would be born handicapped). Given the increasing number of abortions in the UK it could be argued that the law pertaining to abortion is abused. It has been argued (Worth, 2006) that the intention of the Abortion Act was to reduce illegal abortions and strictly control the numbers of abortions undertaken. Worth (2006: 338) identifies how doctors and midwives have (in the past) been required to 'clear up the mess after a bungled abortion'.

Table 12.1 Illustration of abortion rates for women resident in England and Wales

	2001	2002	2010	2011	2012
Overall abortion rate for women aged 20	33 per 1.000 (20 years)	30.7 per 1.000 (18–19 years)	33 per 1.000 (20 years)	33 per 1.000 (20 years)	31 per 1.000 (21 years)
Total number of abortions	176,364	175,900	189,574	189,931	185,122
Age-standardised abortion rate	17.1 per 1,000 resident women (15–44 years)	18.6 per 1,000 resident women (15–44 years)	17.5 per 1,000 resident women (15–44 years)	17.5 per 1,000 resident women (15–44 years)	16.5 per 1,000 resident women (15–44 years)
Number of weeks	78 per cent under 10 weeks	57 per cent under 10 weeks 87 per cent under 13 weeks	77 per cent under 10 weeks 91 per cent under 13 weeks	78 per cent under 10 weeks 91 per cent under 13 weeks	77 per cent under 10 weeks 91 per cent under 13 weeks
Under 16 years	3.7 per 1,000 women	3.7 per 1,000 women	3.4 per 1,000 women	3.4 per 1,000 women	3.0 per 1,000 women
Ground E (child would be handicapped)	N/K	1,900 (1 per cent)	2,290 (1 per cent)	2,307 (1 per cent)	2,692 (1 per cent)

What are the risks of abortion?

Legal abortions are generally considered to be safe, but the risk of complications are increased with increasing lengths of gestation. Abortions have been associated with haemorrhage, shock, infection and depression. Conversely, women who have been unable to procure an abortion have attempted suicide to avoid the shame of an unwanted pregnancy (Worth, 2006). Mental health following an abortion has also been a concern, with some women experiencing extreme guilt and regret regarding their decision to terminate a pregnancy.

Ethical abortion issues

The ethical issues around abortion are complex. There are no right or wrong answers as everybody has their own opinions and beliefs regarding when life begins. In addition, beliefs often change over time and depending upon circumstances. In Chapter 2, ethics were suggested to be beliefs and values owned by society or a section of society, whereas morals are considered to be owned by an individual. A dilemma is a situation where 'one is faced with two alternative choices, neither of which seems a satisfactory solution to the problem' (Campbell, 1984: 2). For some women their moral standing is revisited when they become pregnant and question their ability and desire to parent. When financial status, relationship status and circumstances of conception are added to the situation, it is easy to understand the dilemmas facing women.

The main ethical issues are around the sanctity of life, a woman's autonomy, rights and beliefs around whether or not the fetus is a human being or a number of cells with the potential to develop into a human being. Knowledge about fetal development, perception of fetal movements and ultrasound pictures have all contributed to the perception of a baby and in many cases of specific gender (a son or daughter). Reinforcing the notion of a baby (as opposed to a fetus) increases the potential for bonding and relationship building early in a pregnancy.

Objections to abortion may be religious, humanitarian or moral. Supporters of abortion promote the autonomy of the woman, misery of unwanted babies and unnecessary suffering. Objections to abortion are mainly around the belief that all life is precious and that the fetus has a right to life. This brings forth the question of when life begins.

When does human life begin?

Does human life begin at conception? When all major organs are formed? When the fetus can survive? The moment of birth? Human anatomy and physiology teaches us that there are specific stages of embryonic development to which we can ascribe significance. These are:

- fertilisation
- implantation
- fully formed but immature fetus
- viability
- birth/delivery.

Each of the above stages may have psychological, legal and/or social significance, and as such impact upon the way in which a woman approaches abortion. An example of this is that for some women it is not abortion to prevent the fertilised ovum from embedding in the lining of the uterus, whereas other women find the use of an intrauterine device an abortifacient as there is a belief that from the moment of fertilisation human life has begun. For some individuals human life begins when the fertilised ovum embeds in the lining of the uterus and the cells differentiate into what is visualised as a fetus and placenta.

Abortion: the dilemma for midwives and midwifery

Abortion is a dilemma for midwives, midwifery and the maternity services. Ethical issues (autonomy, rights, beliefs) and attitudes (morals) are relevant to individuals and may or may not be shared by your profession or employer. For example, a midwife may personally be against abortions but while working as a midwife recognises that women accessing healthcare may choose to terminate the pregnancy. The local health trust may identify or determine that at certain times (gestations) a termination of pregnancy or abortion (under the Abortion Act 1967) should take place in the maternity unit (delivery suite).

This policy may result in women terminating pregnancies being cared for in the same environment as those women labouring with live births. Midwives working in maternity services may believe that they will be caring for women during childbirth and not participating in terminations of pregnancy for abnormality. The counter argument is that in the interests of safety the care is best provided in an environment and location where safety and high-quality (one-to-one) care is available.

Terminology and interpretation regarding abortion are also a dilemma for midwives as often termination, abortion and sometimes miscarriage are used interchangeably or meaning is different depending upon the environment (public or health service).

Abortion is also discriminatory. Abortion on the grounds of physical or mental abnormalities (to be born with a serious handicap) limits the number of persons in communities with disability. It is suggested that abortion due to fetal abnormality is discriminating and further increases the lack of tolerance of difference in the UK.

Ethical theories applied to abortion

A utilitarian approach to abortion surrounds the desire to create the greatest benefit for the majority of people. A utilitarian approach would uphold the principle of utility. Utilitarian theory supports actions which create the greatest good and diminish harm. Therefore, utilitarianism would tolerate abortion for fetal abnormality on the grounds that, while harm is incurred, in the long term pain and suffering of a baby with abnormalities are diminished. However, the assumption here is that all babies born with abnormalities will incur pain and suffering.

A deontological approach to abortion would focus upon the woman's choice and her autonomy. With consideration of the woman's autonomy there is conflict with the ethical principle of the sanctity of life. The sanctity of life relates to the fetus and the inherent need to preserve and protect fetal wellbeing.

Abortion is wrong in certain circumstances as a means to an end. For example, an abortion for fetal abnormality: consider that it would be an immoral act to destroy all fetuses with abnormalities.

When considering the ethical principle of respect for autonomy (Beauchamp and Childress 2013) then midwives have the right to conscientious objection. In the case of Doogan and Wood (2012) the court ruled against the midwives as it was deemed that working on a hospital labour ward in a supervisory capacity did not constitute 'participation' in abortions. It would seem that the right to conscientious objection to abortion only extends to the actual medical practitioner medically or surgically causing the abortion. Midwives' autonomy has been lost to the environment in which the practitioner works.

Ethical principles applied to abortion

Rights to abortion

A woman's right to determine what happens to her body is based upon autonomy. The right to self-determination for childbearing women is in direct opposition to the father of the baby. If the woman's right is upheld then the rights of the father to become a dad are diminished. If a potential father was afforded rights regarding supporting or refusing abortion of the woman it would mean that her right to determine what happened to her body would be removed.

What about the right of the fetus?

While the fetus has no legal rights in utero, if a fetus shows signs of life (live birth) following abortion the fetus is afforded basic human rights. The charity organisation LIFE identifies that all fetuses should have a right to life. In support of this principle it provides care and support for women who actively choose not to terminate the pregnancy and ensure that following the birth the mother can make choices regarding the baby's future welfare.

Principle of the sanctity of life

Sanctity of life is the principle that suggests that all life is sacred and precious. The fetal right to life is supported by this principle. Sanctity of life is to value life regardless of the quality (suffering, disadvantage, discrimination). The principle of sanctity of life does not discriminate regarding gender (boys being worth more than girls).

Right to terminate for abnormality

The woman's right to choose overrides those of her partners. This ethical principle has been clarified by case law. A woman does have the right to terminate a pregnancy even if the father of the baby wishes for the pregnancy to continue. An individual cannot remove the woman's autonomy to terminate a pregnancy on the grounds of severe abnormality. Although the interpretation of severe is varied. See the case of *Jepson* v *The Chief Constable of West Mercia Police Constabulary 2003*.

Right to conscientious objection

Health and social care staff have the right to conscientious objection to abortion. The Abortion Act Section 4 stipulates that staff cannot be made to participate in a practice to which they morally object. While some may argue that the choice to participate or not should depend upon the circumstances (for example, was the pregnancy as a result of rape, failed contraception or lack of contraceptive use?), this flexibility cannot be managed in a healthcare setting. Employers need to know how many of their staff conscientiously object in order to provide a healthcare service. If staff were to pick and choose which care they wished to participate in based upon their perception of the rationale for abortion it would not be possible to provide a service. Many midwives feel that their role with pregnancy and childbirth is focused upon promoting health, saving lives and sharing the joy of childbirth, and that abortion does not sit comfortably with this philosophy. Some midwives also hold religious beliefs that impact upon their personal and professional lives. In line with most adults, it is not uncommon for midwives to uphold religious celebrations, attend prayers or participate in fasting. Midwives have moral obligations to women they provide care for. Management have the right to expect staff to fulfil their professional roles and responsibilities. Conscientious objection is when an individual identifies that they object to an action or event on the basis of their moral beliefs or on religious grounds. Under the Abortion Act 1967 midwives are able to conscientiously object to abortions. However this objection is limited, as in an emergency the right is lost and the duty of the midwife is to provide care in these circumstances.

Midwives who wish to pursue conscientious objection need to know how to object in order to maintain their rights. The case of a medical secretary (*Janaway* v *Salford AHA*) gives a good example of how a healthcare worker with clear objections to abortion could not exercise her right to object. The RCM position paper No. 17 identifies conscientious objection and how this works. Further information is also available from the NMC (2012e).

A dilemma for midwives can occur in clinical practice when a patient requires an abortion on medical grounds. The abortion may take place in an NHS hospital, possibly as an urgent or emergency case and staff may not wish to participate in the abortion

While midwives have the right to conscientiously object to abortion, their role as a healthcare provider may require them to be involved with legal terminations of pregnancies. As an employee they are responsible for identifying their objections (and they may be required to provide evidence of them). Conscientious objections should be provided at the earliest opportunity, as early identification enables managers to allocate staff and manage healthcare provision effectively.

Right to respect of family life, the right to a family

Sometimes having a right restricts or removes another person's right. While both men and women have a right to respect of family life, a man cannot enforce his right to a family when that right is limited by the consent or willingness of a woman to engage in childbirth.

Maternal vs fetal rights are usually considered to be a lost cause as a individual (fetus or unborn baby) cannot make legal demands upon another person. The mother's right to autonomy is paramount.

Legal aspects of abortion

Abortion in England is a criminal offence. Two Acts of Parliament make abortion a crime. The statutes are the Offences Against the Person Act 1861 and the Infant Life Preservation Act 1929. However, times change and attitudes and lifestyles also change. There are now two Acts of Parliament which permit abortion in certain circumstances. These statutes are the Abortion Act 1967 and the Human Fertilisation and Embryology Act 1990. Consideration will now be given to the legislation in the order of enactment.

The Offences Against the Person Act 1861

This Act identifies in Section 58 that 'Anyone who does something to themselves to procure an abortion can be prosecuted'. A third party who does something to another to procure an abortion can be prosecuted under Section 59. However, Section 59 was challenged in the courts in 1939 in the case of *R* v *Bourne* (1939). Dr Bourne was charged with procuring an abortion (Section 59 Offences Against the Person Act 1861). The judge advised the jury that abortion was lawful when done for therapeutic reasons (the patient was a 14-year-old rape victim). Consequently, precedent was set that suggests that an abortion is not a criminal offence if undertaken for 'therapeutic reasons'. This common law case is said to have paved the way for the Abortion Act 1967.

The Infant Life Preservation Act 1929

This Act identifies that anyone who does anything to a child in the womb which is capable of being born alive, causing it to die before it has an independent existence of his mother, will be guilty of child destruction (Section 1).

- Capable of being born alive means viable.
- The Act was brought about to fill a gap in the law, e.g. if a head of the baby is born and it is killed, is it child destruction? (No – is it viable?). Is it murder? (No – it is not capable of a separate existence.)

The Abortion Act 1967

This is the key and primary legislation regulating and controlling the circumstances which allow abortion in England. The Abortion Act 1967 is technically the defence to the criminal act of abortion, that is to say it decriminalises abortion in England and Wales. The Abortion Act 1967 is particularly interesting as it started its journey as a Private Members Bill. The passage of a Private Members Bill is always going to be challenging as it does not have the support or weight of the government, and Members of Parliament may choose how they vote and which aspects to support. The legislation that a government can pass is also affected by the amount of parliamentary time, the number of amendments and the amount of support. Private Members Bills that do not have the support of the government will also be less likely to succeed. Some issues such as abortion are so important and have ethical implications that political parties may not provide support. The Private Members Bill is described as 'a lottery' (Jones and Jenkins, 2004: 7).

The progress of the Abortion Act 1967 through Parliament has been well documented (Jones, 2000a: 112; Pattinson, 2006; Mason and Laurie, 2006). Understandably, many people had differing views and many objections were raised. Activists such as the anti-abortion group LIFE actively opposed the Bill, whereas human rights supporters supported it. Following is a summary of the key elements of the Abortion Act 1967.

Section 1(i)

> a person shall not be guilty of an offence under the law relating to abortion when the pregnancy is terminated by two Registered Medical Practitioners (RMP) if two RMPs are of the opinion, formed in good faith...

Two registered medical practitioners (RMPs) are used as a double check, though one doctor is sufficient in an emergency. The Royal College of Nursing (RCN) has challenged the notion of participation in an abortion. The case of *RCN* v *DHSS* (1981) clarified what was meant by 'participation'. This case was significant as nurses are not trained to undertake abortions and are not able to prescribe drugs to induce an abortion. The House of Lords ruled that providing *the doctor remains in charge* of the treatment, it is acceptable for properly trained nurses acting *under the doctor's guidance* to carry out procedures. Care is necessary to ensure the correct level of clinical supervision.

Section 1 (1a)

> The continuance of the pregnancy would involve risk, greater than if the pregnancy were terminated, of injury to the physical or mental health of the pregnant woman or any existing children of her family, then the pregnancy may be terminated at any time before the end of the 24th week of the pregnancy.

Section 1 (1a) uses distinct wording: 'The continuance of the pregnancy would involve risk, greater than if the pregnancy were terminated' and 'injury to the physical and mental health of the pregnant woman' and 'existing children of the family'. This distinct wording may initially appear clear. However, the practitioner may be concerned that there is room for interpretation and subjective views. Concerns are that risk, injury and existing children could be widely interpreted. This has led to the perception that Section 1 (1a) of the Abortion Act is justifying minor therapeutic or social reasons for abortion. While theoretically there is no social ground for termination of pregnancy the interpretation of Section 1 (1a) is that this ground, unlike other grounds, is widely interpreted and accounts for the vast majority of legal terminations.

Section 1 (1b)

> The termination of the pregnancy is necessary to prevent grave permanent injury to the physical or mental health of the pregnant woman.

One would expect a narrow interpretation regarding grave permanent injury. However, in 2003 our understanding of 'grave permanent injury' was challenged. In *Jepson* v *The Chief Constable of West Mercia Police Constabulary* [2003] EWHC 3318 a trainee vicar reviewed medical records and established that an abortion had been carried out as the fetus had a cleft palate.

Section 1 (1c)

> The continuance of the pregnancy would involve risk to the life of the pregnant woman greater than if the pregnancy were terminated.

This section of the Abortion Act is narrowly interpreted. However, when raised blood pressure in pregnancies threatens maternal wellbeing this ground may be used. Midwives should consider:

- How would you interpret 'the risk to life' of the pregnant woman?
- What is the difference between this section and the previous section?

Section 1 (1d)

> There is substantial risk that if the child were born it would suffer from such physical or mental abnormalities as to be seriously handicapped.

This section of the act clearly identifies birth physical and mental abnormalities. However, the broad interpretation of serious handicap has caused concern. What does serious handicap mean? Is it possible to measure the potential of pain and suffering prior to birth? Does this include cleft palate?

Serious handicap can be narrowly (major heart defects) or broadly (cleft palate) interpreted. A scientific definition would not relate to perceived minor definitions. A medical or sociological definition could include minor abnormalities but with life consequences. Midwives may find themselves providing care for women whose pregnancy is terminated for serious handicap which they perceive to be significant but not serious or life threatening. In *Jepson* v *The Chief Constable of West Mercia Police Constabulary* the courts were asked to clarify if a cleft palate was eligible under Section 1 (1d) of the Act. From an ethical perspective one would need to consider if the cleft lip causes suffering (significant harm) or impairment (disability).

Section 4

This concerns conscientious objection to abortion. As identified earlier, the ability for healthcare professionals to object to abortion is an important right. However, the right could be considered to be narrowly interpreted as in an emergency the healthcare professional must provide care and attend to the woman's needs. If someone believes that abortion is morally and ethically wrong then they should not be forced to participate in the abortion. This right to conscientiously object comes with the responsibility of the practitioner to declare the objection and to demonstrate in their lifestyle and conduct that the objection is genuine. The reason for this is to ensure that the right is solid and does not vary or change to suit the practitioner. For example, the midwife cannot decide that on one day she or he objects to abortion but on another that objection is removed because she or he believes that abortion is justified when rape has produced the pregnancy. Providing abortion services is a controversial aspect of healthcare. Sometimes it is not obvious or clear that a maternity service is engaged in this activity. Student midwives are not usually exposed to caring for women undergoing a termination of pregnancy and may not be comfortable, following registration, participating in this care. Labour ward managers need to have the skills to ensure that staff do not avoid or make judgements which can compromise high-quality care for all patients. For many midwives, choosing to work in a maternity hospital means that they are unlikely to be required to participate in an abortion. However, maternity hospitals or departments are licensed to undertake abortions and from time to time women do require a termination of pregnancy, which necessitates care.

Participation in termination of pregnancy has been challenged in the courts. What does participation mean? Over the years practitioners have debated the nature and extent of participation. In 1989 a medical secretary refused to participate in the typing of medical records/letters for a lady who required an abortion (*Janaway* v *Salford Health Authority* [1989]). More recently two midwives in Scotland refused to participate in abortion on a labour ward.

In summary, the right to conscientious objection is an important right of healthcare professionals, including midwives. However, this right is narrowly interpreted and does not apply in emergency situations. All midwives must continue to fulfil their role and responsibilities to women undergoing a termination of pregnancy in an emergency.

The Human Fertilisation and Embryology Act 1990

The Human Fertilisation and Embryology Act 1990 amends the Abortion Act as follows. The age of viability was reduced from 28 weeks' gestation to 24 weeks' gestation. This is important as babies' survival rates at 24 weeks have vastly improved due to advances in and quality of neonatal care. The arguments to reduce the age of viability to 22 weeks are strong as there are a number of babies born at this gestation who have survived. The difficulty is that proportionally more babies born at 22 weeks' gestation die, fail to develop normally and require long-term medical care.

As identified, there are two Acts of Parliament – the Abortion Act 1967 and the Human Fertilisation and Embryology Act 1990 – which regulate the provision of abortion in *England, Wales and Scotland*. The legislation does not extend to Northern Ireland. It is useful here to consider the effect of the legislation. The first effect is a social effect in that women can travel to another country to gain access to health services. Healthcare tourism is not confined to abortion, but other patient choices as well, such as assisted suicide. Frequently when citing legislation, writers will refer to The Abortion Act 1967 (as amended) meaning as amended by the Human Fertilisation and Embryology Act 1990.

The Abortion Act 1967 (as amended by HFEA 1990)

The HFEA 1990 provides four legal grounds which are defences for the criminal act of abortion. These four grounds effectively legalise abortion in England when they are present. The HFEA 1990 provides detail regarding the four grounds.

The first ground is often referred to as the 'social' ground (continuation of the pregnancy would involve risk, greater than the risk if the pregnancy was terminated or injury to the woman's mental health or that of any child in her family). The HFEA 1990 identifies that an abortion is allowed if the pregnancy is under 24 weeks. Most abortions are authorised under this category. There is concern that while the Act stipulates 24 weeks it does not identify if the 24 weeks is calculated from the first day of the woman's last period, date of implantation or date of fertilisation (McHale and Tindle, 2007).

The remaining grounds (Section 1 (1b and 1c) are not subject to a time limit. Basically the Act makes provision for the pregnancy to be terminated at any time if it is (a) necessary to prevent grave and permanent injury to the physical or mental health of the pregnant woman (maternal ground); (b) if continuing with the pregnancy involves a risk to the life of the pregnant woman greater than if the pregnancy were terminated (maternal ground).

The final ground which legalises abortion in England is a fetal ground and there is no time limit here. This ground makes it possible to terminate a pregnancy on the ground of serious handicap. Unfortunately the legislation does not quantify serious handicap. This ground has been tested in the courts (*Jepson* v *Chief Constable of West Mercia* [2003]).

Case law

The following cases provide insight and legal clarification regarding abortion.

Jepson v Chief Constable of West Mercia (2003)

West Mercia police decided not to investigate an allegation that a fetus had been aborted because otherwise it would have been born with a cleft palate. The decision was based upon the fact that two medical practitioners had provided evidence that they had acted in 'good faith'. Jepson challenged that a cleft palate constituted 'serious handicap'.

Paton v Trustees of BPAS (1978)

With regard to women's rights, case law has established that the biological father of the fetus has no right to prevent his partner from terminating the pregnancy. In the summing up, Justice Baker identified that 'Not only a bold, brave judge … but a foolish one who would advise otherwise'. Paton appealed to the European Court of Human Rights.

Paton v UK (1980) (ECHR 408)

In this case Paton cited Article 8 of the ECHR (the right to respect for family life). The ECHR ruled that the right to respect for family life was not breached. In a similar case, C v S (1987) the ruling in *Paton* v *UK* was followed.

Re B. (The Independent 22 May 1991) (Family Division)

This example of case law is with regard to children (minors). It appears that parents cannot prevent abortions if the minor has the support of their doctor. Having said the abortion cannot be prevented, the child must be held to be Gillick competent for an abortion to be allowed. The Gillick case is discussed in detail elsewhere (Chapter 6, concerning consent). Gillick competency requires consideration regarding abortion as a young person's understanding and beliefs regarding abortion may be immature or lacking detail. Fraser guidelines (after Lord Fraser) are applicable to minors requesting family planning, and are also applied to requests for termination of pregnancy. This would seem to be a good application of case law as it supports ethical principles of autonomy and justice.

The following two cases are used to illustrate the difference between homicide and murder.

R v Anderson (1975)

Anderson shot his pregnant girlfriend. The child was injured in the womb as a result of the shooting. It was born alive by Caesarean section and died. Anderson was found guilty of murder (the child was born alive) and is serving life imprisonment.

Keeler v Superior Court of Amador County (1970)

In comparison, the case of *Keeler* v *Superior Court of Amador County* (1970) is focused on Keeler's behaviour, but with a different result. Keeler kneed his pregnant girlfriend in the abdomen, intending to kill the child. The child was injured, died in the womb and was delivered by Caesarean section. The mother was well. The court ruled that as the baby was stillborn, Keeler was not guilty of murder as the baby was not capable of being born alive. The Infant Life Preservation Act is only relevant if a child is capable of being born alive. On reflection, the judgements do not appear to be fair. It could be argued that the law protects those who cause an intrauterine death but criminalises those who cause a delivery which results in a live birth. To secure a conviction in the Keeler case it would have been necessary to deliver a live baby at Caesarean section.

Janaway v Salford Health Authority (1989)

In 1989 a medical secretary refused to participate in the typing of medical records/letters for a lady who required an abortion, citing conscientious objection. Her case failed as Janaway tried to object on the grounds that the doctor whose letters she was typing was undertaking abortions. If a healthcare worker wishes to exercise his or her objection to abortion then it must be undertaken in a specific way (Ferguson, 1987).

Doogan and Wood v Greater Glasgow & Clyde NHS (2012)

In 2012 two Roman Catholic midwives objected on religious grounds to participating in abortions. The case is unusual as the midwives were employed as labour ward coordinators in a Scottish hospital. The two midwives had exercised their right to object and refused to be involved in terminations. In 2007 the hospital decided to move all medical terminations of pregnancy to the labour ward (it is not uncommon for women to require midwifery skills and care as well as obstetric support in such circumstances) (BBC News, 29 February 2012).

Chapter summary

This chapter has considered the ethical and legal issues around abortion. Abortion is a controversial issue and has ethical and legal implications for all healthcare practitioners. Midwives are in a difficult position as there may be conflict with personal beliefs about abortion and the decisions made by women to request an abortion. Midwife means being 'with woman' and in doing so the midwife may find providing healthcare during a termination of pregnancy a challenge when it conflicts with personal beliefs. Midwives need to be able to make the woman (patient) her first consideration and recognise that personal beliefs and attitudes will impact upon care given. It has been argued that personal opinions may make it difficult for a midwife to provide effective care. It is significant that midwives are not autonomous practitioners in the therapeutic use of abortion as it is outside their sphere of practice.

The legal situation identifies when an abortion may be carried out legally in England and Wales. The case study demonstrates application of ethical and legal aspects to that of Sara, who has requested an abortion.

Case study: Sara

Sara presented at an antenatal clinic, pregnant at 22 weeks' gestation with her fifth baby. Two days earlier, during a scan performed to investigate irregular menstruation, Sara had been informed that she was pregnant. The ultrasound scan suggested a 21+ weeks singleton with no abnormalities detected. The midwife working in the community had provided maternity care throughout Sara's four previous pregnancies, all of which had been straightforward births resulting in four healthy children. Sara has identified to the midwife that this pregnancy is unplanned and unwanted by both her and her husband. She feels that it would put a strain on her and her family, physically, emotionally and financially. Sara discloses that she is going to terminate this pregnancy.

Evaluation

Sara has been cared for in all of her previous pregnancies by the same midwife. Continuity of care and continuity of carer are important cornerstones of midwifery practice. It is likely that Sara and the midwife have a good relationship and that Sara trusts the midwife well enough to disclose the decision to have an abortion. The rapport between Sara and the midwife should be established and based upon sharing of information, trust and confidence. Sara felt comfortable in sharing her intention to terminate this pregnancy. It is not known what the personal beliefs and attitude of the midwife are, but regardless of these feelings the midwife is required to provide safe and evidence-based care. The midwife must be careful not to let her feelings and views influence and affect Sara's care. The midwife must also not be tempted to try to influence or inflict personal views upon Sara. The midwife's loyalty is to Sara, even though the midwife may feel or believe that the fetus should have the right to life.

Sara's case is not uncommon. Many women find it necessary to make difficult choices during pregnancy, but the decision to terminate a pregnancy is very emotional and also impacts upon other family members. Abortion and termination of pregnancy have always been controversial, but the complexity of abortion has also increased over the years. As human rights have expanded, the rights of partners and family members mean that what was once a personal decision to terminate a pregnancy is challenged and becomes the subject of discussion and debate, guilt and erosion of the woman's individual rights. It is difficult to resolve different opinions about terminating a pregnancy, especially when others may feel that it is their potential son, daughter, grandchild or sibling.

Analysis

The respect for a woman's autonomy is a key principle regarding abortion. There have always been women who want or need an abortion (Worth, 2006). The decision to have an abortion is not usually taken lightly. In the past, women have been driven to extreme lengths to procure an abortion – for example, travelling abroad, self-harm to induce an abortion and using illegal and unregistered services. Prior to the 1902 Midwives Act it was also thought that some midwives or 'handy women' were able to procure abortions (Worth, 2006). Sara's decision to have an abortion also impacts upon midwives, who need to ensure that they 'enable women to make decisions about her care based on her individual needs, by discussing matters fully with her' (NMC Rules and Standards, standard 4). The feelings of the midwife in the above case may also be forgotten. It is often assumed that the midwife is not affected by choices that clients make and that personal feelings do not need to be addressed. Psychological support for midwives is necessary to ensure that they can continue to provide care even when the decisions made by clients are not always agreed with.

(continued)

An argument to undertake abortions is around the principle of beneficence. This can be argued from a service provision (late terminations) or resources (intensive care and long-term health needs of babies with abnormalities) aspect.

What is the difference between termination of pregnancy and abortion?

Abortion is often used by the public to identify the termination of an unwanted pregnancy. Termination of pregnancy as used by the medical profession relates to all pregnancies when they are ended and the intention is to ensure that the fetus is not alive. Abortion has been defined as the intentional termination of pregnancy with the resultant death of the embryo or fetus (Hope *et al.*, 2008).

Does Sara have the right to terminate this pregnancy?

Sara's case is interesting as there are a number of ethical aspects around confidentiality, consent, advocacy and ensuring Sara's autonomy. The main ethical issues in the above case are around rights, namely the rights of Sara and the rights of the fetus. While it might be perceived that terminating a healthy pregnancy with a normal fetus when the fetus might survive should not be allowed, morally a woman is not under an obligation to carry a pregnancy to full term.

Is Sara's abortion a crime?

If Sara decided to go to any means to terminate the pregnancy, or in other words procure an abortion, then she could be committing a crime. The whole point of the Abortion Act 1967 was to reduce the numbers of illegal abortions. The 1967 Act enables pregnancies to be legally terminated in specific healthcare environments by registered practitioners whose practice standards and safety measures are monitored. Sara can be confident in her healthcare providers and does not need to risk seeking a termination illegally. Abortions in England are criminal if not conducted by licensed practitioners who are registered and working in an approved environment.

Is Sara's abortion legal?

Sara's pregnancy is 22 weeks' gestation; therefore in theory she meets the criteria for abortion under Section 1 of Abortion Act 1967 as amended by the Human Fertilisation and Embryology Act 1990. Sara has also stated that if the pregnancy continued it would 'put a strain on her and her family, physically, emotionally and financially'. This would seem to meet the criteria of Section 1 (1a) of the 1967 Act.

Should Sara's abortion take place?

The fetus has no legal right and although it has the ability to become a human being it is not considered viable at this gestational age. It does not acquire 'personhood' until it is separated from its mother and therefore does not have the same legal rights as a human being. Sara's rights are paramount and the abortion statute and legislation allows Sara to do what she believes is right for her and her family at this time and in these circumstances.

An important concept in midwifery is autonomy. Midwives are said to be autonomous practitioners, which means that they are 'personally accountable for their own actions (and inactions) and are legally permitted to oversee the total care of women with normal pregnancies and labours' (Tiran, 1997: 19). As an autonomous practitioner, the midwife needs to ensure that Sara has choice, continuity and control during her pregnancy (Department of Health, Expert Maternity Group, 1993). The dilemma is that the midwife could compromise Sara's autonomy if an approach is adopted whereby the midwife does not act quickly in referral to an abortion service, or makes an inappropriate referral (to an obstetrician who opposes abortion).

Clarke (2004) identifies that being an autonomous practitioner is deep in the psyche of midwifery. Clarke suggests that autonomy and independent practice is a perception that midwives hold and that it is not borne out in reality. How can a midwife be an autonomous, independent practitioner when working in maternity services is as confined as the women they attend? Midwives are controlled and dominated by policies, protocols and contractual obligations. Clarke (2004) identifies four areas (clinical practice, clinical learning environment, ownership of patient and clinical judgement) which may compromise autonomous midwifery practice.

What can be done?

Sara's request to terminate this pregnancy can be an expression of her right to make decisions about her healthcare. The World Health Organization (WHO) identifies that for some groups (including women) rights to healthcare are not equal. While the above case does not identify Sara's age it would seem reasonable to assume that Sara is an adult. Adults make choices that other adults may not agree with. The midwife may feel that having looked after Sara previously and having got to know her and her husband that Sara should have this baby. After all, previous pregnancies have gone well and Sara's other four children are all healthy. Looking after one more baby when you already have four should be easy? However, the application of personal views and attitudes does not help the situation.

Implications for practice

The midwife cannot use his or her feelings to influence the discussion. Sara's autonomy is important; her right to determine what happens to her body and confidentiality surrounding her healthcare must be respected. Midwife means 'with woman' and Sara's midwife needs to be with her emotionally and support her decision making.

(continued)

The dilemma for Sara is that parents are expected to take responsibility for their children. Mothers, in particular, are expected and required to provide for their children. In our society maximising potential, promoting health and wellbeing of our children is considered to be good. Having more children than you can look after, care for or feed is associated with poor mental health and wellbeing. Sara is wishing to avoid the negative effects of another child upon her family.

Practice check

1. What is the legal status when an aborted fetus is found to be breathing?
2. What responsibilities does a midwife have in these circumstances?
3. What should be done to prevent this?
4. What other statute specifically allows conscientious objection?
5. Which clause of the NMC Code of Conduct pertains to conscientious objection?

Reflection

The following clinical cases are intended to enable the reader to use ethical pathways to consider if abortion is ever justified.

- Case study 1. An unmarried mother (32 years) with two children seeks an abortion on the grounds that she was raped. Discuss the legal position and identify any ethical issues you may have.
- Case study 2. Following an amniocentesis, a pregnant woman is informed that the fetus has Down's syndrome. Identify the ethical issues and critically analyse the implications.

This clinical case is intended to enable the reader to consider the legal situation:

- Case study 3. A woman requires assisted fertility and following a healthy pregnancy delivers a normal healthy baby weighing 3.43 kg. While checking the placenta the midwife identifies an abnormality and the labour ward coordinator identifies a papyraceous fetus.

How would you define grave permanent injury to the physical or mental health of the pregnant woman?

Reader activity

Give examples of how each of the following phrases could be interpreted:

- serious
- risk to life
- doctor's guidance.

Ask to see the documentation which has to be completed when an abortion is requested. Consider whether it is clear what criteria are being used.

Reflection

What effect does the judgment in *RCN* v *DHSS* (1981) have on midwifery practice?

Useful websites

British pregnancy advisory service: www.bpas.org/bpaswoman
Human Fertilisation and Embryology Authority: www.hfea.gov.uk
Women's rights: http://rightsofwomen.org.uk

13 Female circumcision, cutting and genital mutilation (FGM)

Pre-requisites of this chapter

It is assumed that you have a good anatomical knowledge of normal female genitalia and perineum as well as the physiology of menstruation, micturition and the female sexual response. You should also be utilising the latest professional regulatory standards. You may wish to access some background reading regarding cultural childbirth issues. The terms FGM and female circumcision are both used and explained in this chapter.

Introduction

Before considering ethical and legal aspects of female cutting or circumcision, I wish at the outset to identify a personal belief that FGM/circumcision is an infringement of human rights, children's rights and the right to health, and therefore consider that FGM should be abandoned and eradicated. FGM/C is physical abuse and as such I am concerned regarding the psychological aspects of this practice. As a member of the FGM National Clinical Group (www.fgmnationalgroup.org) I actively seek to improve the lives of women and their daughters at risk of FGM. I recognise that, as a white, married, employed mother in a European country, it could be argued that my interest in FGM is prejudiced. I am familiar with this criticism and understand its origin. As a midwife who has seen and witnessed the adverse health consequences of FGM during childbirth, my interest and attitude is based upon the need to provide a high standard of care to all women during childbirth and to ensure that women, babies and children are not subjected to physical abuse. My compassion is with babies, girls and women who are unable to choose not to be subjected to FGM. My attitude is that babies and girls have the right to genital autonomy and it is the role of the midwife to provide sensitive and compassionate care to all women during childbirth. Women and girls who have experienced FGM are victims of physical abuse, and should not be subjected to any further types of abuse. British midwives who are challenged about intolerance of FGM while living and working in a country that tolerates genital surgery, piercing and others forms of alteration to the female appearance have a dilemma. Should the midwife tolerate FGM on the basis that he/she lives and works in a country that tolerates other forms of genital alteration? Or should the midwife work with communities to inform and educate regarding the severe and specific adverse health outcomes of FGM? The author's concern regarding FGM is on the basis of the physical, psychological and health detriments caused by FGM and the disrespect to women and a desire to control sexuality of girls.

Women who choose to undergo surgery, piercing and other forms of alteration to the appearance of their genitalia do so with consent, explanation and knowledge. Information is available to them to make an informed choice and anyone who forces or makes a woman undergo genital surgery against her wishes risks a criminal allegation of FGM. Women who have experienced female cutting or circumcision also deserve explanation, knowledge and consent to intervention (deinfibulation) to ensure future care is appropriate and does not result in further abuse. This chapter should be read on the understanding that I have declared an interest and my views regarding FGM. My bias and stance obviously influence the writing of *Law and Ethics for Midwifery*!

This chapter starts by defining FGM; consideration will be given to the types of FGM and the context of FGM in the UK. Following definition and clarification regarding the traditional practice of cutting, the focus will be around the ethical issues of rights, moral judgements, autonomy and physical abuse. The legal aspects of FGM include primary legislation and lack of successful prosecutions under the legislation. Relevant guidelines and the use of safeguarding will be identified and explained. The illegality of FGM in the UK is considered and discussed within the context of modern healthcare. It is not possible here to address the global legal aspects, so this chapter is written from a UK perspective, where the pressure to secure a prosecution is seen as paramount.

What is female genital mutilation?

A simple definition of FGM is the cutting of the female genitalia and the subsequent stitching up of the raw edges. Various commentators (Shandall, 1967; Verzin, 1975; Mahran, 1981; El Dareer, 1983; Cutner, 1985; Shaw, 1985) have defined and described FGM. The justification of FGM varies, as does the amount of tissue excised and method used during the procedure. FGM comprises all procedures that involve partial or total removal of female genitalia and/or injury to the female genital organs for cultural or any other non-therapeutic reason (WHO, 1996).

FGM is a collective term for 'a range of procedures which involve partial or total removal of the female genitalia for non-medical reasons' (Crown Prosecution Service, 2012). FGM is defined as 'all procedures involving partial or total removal of the external female genitalia or other injury to the female genital organs, whether for cultural or other non-therapeutic reasons' (RCOG, 2009a).

Terminology can be misleading; interchanging words such as Sunna, Islamic circumcision and infibulation can confuse and create emotional barriers to meaningful discussion. Communities who undertake female cutting or circumcision do not like, understand or consider the term female genital mutilation. Yet activists such as Dorkenoo (1994) prefer to use the term FGM as it conveys the severity of the practice. The term female circumcision itself is misleading; it implies that female cutting is similar to that of male circumcision, which it is not (see Table 13.1). Male circumcision is a religious ceremony and practice which involves the removal of skin from the end of the penis. Female circumcision/ FGM is not a religious requirement and may involve skin, tissues, nerves, glands and organs (clitoris). Supporters of male circumcision suggest that anecdotally male circumcision improves male sex lives; the

Table 13.1 Contrasting circumcision

Female genital mutilation	Male circumcision
No religious requirement	Religious
May include removal of organ, skin, nerves, ducts and glands	Removal of skin only, to expose the glans penis
No health benefits	Health benefits (reduction in penile cancers)
No medical indications	Medical reasons
Unhygienic (infections are common)	Hygiene
No pain relief offered	Topical analgesia safe and effective (if used)
Girls to adulthood (usually pre-pubescent)	Newborn male babies
Illegal in the UK	Not Illegal in the UK
Risk of criminal prosecution and fines	Not regulated in the UK
Professional misconduct	Not restricted to professional practice

same cannot be said of female cutting, which can be (depending upon the type of FGM) psychosexually, emotionally and physically harmful.

FGM/C (see WHO classification) is not a religious requirement, does not share any similarity with male circumcision and involves the removal and damage to highly sensitive organs, occlusion of the urinary meatus and vagina and a predisposition to infection, pain and suffering for the rest of her life. Dorkenoo (1997) refers to FGM as 'the wound that never heals' and goes on to suggest that the only cure is prevention.

The WHO (1997) classifies FGM into types:

- Type 1 – excision of the prepuce with or without excision of part or all of the clitoris (clitoridectomy);
- Type 2 – excision of the clitoris together with partial or total excision of the labia minora;
- Type 3 – excision of part or all of the external genitalia and stitching/narrowing of the vaginal opening (infibulation);
- Type 4 – unclassified – pricking, piercing or incision of the clitoris and/or labia;
  - stretching of the clitoris and or labia
  - cauterisation – burning of the clitoris and surrounding tissue
  - interocision
  - scraping (angurya cuts) or cutting (gishri cuts) of the vagina or surrounding tissue.

The WHO classification has been updated (2008) and also includes the introduction of corrosive substances or herbs into the vagina, in addition to any other procedures that fall under the definition of FGM given. The above definition may be helpful from a theoretical perspective in drawing attention to the changes to female anatomy. The classification of FGM using a grading system, whereby the most altered anatomical appearance is Type 4, may be confusing. In reality Type 1, which involves clitoridectomy, has severe life-long consequences around mental health and wellbeing (this is a neglected area of NHS healthcare). Regardless of the type of FGM, the young person may experience the above without any pain relief (WHO, 2008) as part of a ceremony into womanhood (Momoh, 2005) or for social reasons (RCN, 1994). The circumcision or cutting is often undertaken by a female relative or family friend. All practitioners who are required to document and collate data and analyse research regarding types of FGM should be mindful that accuracy may be difficult. In reality, for the midwife providing care the classification or type of FGM may be difficult to assign; the woman may not know what type has been performed; she may have been subjected to repeated cutting; physical appearance may not be a good indicator of the nature or extent of the infibulation.

The WHO classify FGM as a traditional practice that should be eradicated (WHO, 2008). Communities that perform FGM do not usually consider FGM to be physical abuse and do not normally use or refer to the term genital mutilation. Communities who believe in female circumcision or cutting believe it to be a traditional practice associated with their culture. Any attempts to stop communities undertaking FGM are branded culturally intolerant. In order to justify the traditional practice it is considered appropriate to use the term circumcision, which is widely associated with culture and justified on that basis. This confusion of terms (female circumcision) with male circumcision is not justified from a physical, religious or health paradigm as they are not similar in any way.

What is deinfibulation?

Deinfibulation is the term given to the procedure to 'reopen' a vaginal opening. In the UK, deinfibulation often takes place during the antenatal period. Information regarding deinfibulation is available from the FGM National Clinical Group, British Medical Association and Royal College of Obstetricians.

What is reinfibulation?

Reinfibulation is the term given to the practice of re-stitching, re-sewing or re-closure of the labia or tightening up of the vaginal orifice (following childbirth). For some women reinfibulation is undertaken after every childbirth. There is debate as to whether reinfibulation is covered in the British legislation. Guidance to healthcare professionals (RCOG, RCM, RCN) is unclear.

What is the difference between male and female circumcision?

The term circumcision may be applied to both males and females. Using circumcision to describe the cultural practice of cutting the female genitalia, closing the labia or removal of the clitoris is incorrect and inappropriate. There is no similarity in the circumcision of males and females. Farooqui (1997) suggests that female circumcision equates more with penile amputation as the clitoris constitutes a primary ergogenic zone and FGM involves removal of sexual organs, damage and scar tissue. Therefore the female sexual response is affected by the amount of tissue removed or damaged, the sensitivity of the scar tissue as well as the pain and degree of healing that has taken place. Circumcision in the male is clearly defined and limited to skin at the end of the penis. There are thought to be health benefits of male circumcision and some religions advocate its use. Female circumcision consists of a number of types and involves additional structures such as nerves, organs and glands. There are no known health benefits – on the contrary there are clear health risks. In addition, there is no religious requirement for female circumcision.

Male circumcision is the removal of skin from the penis. The so-called foreskin is removed exposing the glans penis. Male circumcision is thought to be beneficial to health as infections may be reduced.

Male circumcision does not damage or remove any structures or nerves. Male circumcision is not thought to interfere with the male sexual response other than on a temporary basis around the time of the procedure. Male circumcision is advocated and promoted by some religions.

Female circumcision is also performed in different circumstances, dependent upon the traditions of the community. Communities who advocate female circumcision do not usually provide analgesia, sterility of equipment or have access to emergency healthcare. The procedure is often undertaken on many girls in succession and associated with celebration (singing and music). The memories of the circumcision stay with them for life.

Female circumcision is the removal of skin, soft tissues, nerves and genital organs. The aim is to close the urethra and vagina so that they cannot be seen, giving a smooth, flat surface to the genital area. Female circumcision is not advocated by any religion. Female circumcision has specific and life-threatening health implications. Mortality and morbidity are associated with FGM/C. A comprehensive account of the rationale for FGM/C is provided by Momoh (2005).

What is the difference between FGM and other surgical procedures such as vagino-plasty and designer vaginas?

FGM and cosmetic genital surgery have similar origins in that they are concerned with control of a woman's genital appearance and sexuality. The main differences can be summarised as ethical, environmental, educational and financial. FGM/C and designer vagina/laser vagino-plasty will be contrasted as they illustrate ethical and legal issues around consent and ethical issues regarding the evidence base used to justify the health purposes.

Ethical issues and FGM

The main ethical issues are around autonomy, rights, control of women, women's experiences, intolerance of all forms of FGM and provision of services which are sensitive to the needs of FGM victims.

Autonomy

In recent history campaigners have identified a right to genital autonomy. The right to genital autonomy is for all persons not subjected to any form of genital alteration. Specifically, the right of all baby boys and girls not to be circumcised. Genital autonomy would also be relevant regarding gender reassignment, cosmetic surgery and operations to remove malignant tumours. With regard to the WHO classification of FGM/C, all types of FGM/C breach the rights of females to genital autonomy.

Cultural rights

Communities have practised female circumcision for hundreds of years. For centuries tradition, ritual and culture have attempted to control the sexuality and status of women. FGM is usually practised in countries where there are inadequate healthcare facilities, illiteracy, poverty and inequalities. Any attempts to change a pattern or way of life are threatening to those communities. Female circumcision provides a divide between those who feel that female circumcision is a cultural and traditional practice, which defines and is the right of a community to practise, and those who feel that an individual's autonomy should be respected and upheld. There are strong arguments that a society which tolerates physical violence towards specific members is uncivilised and abusive. Here is the difficulty; communities which practise FGM do not consider it to be abusive. On the contrary, it is viewed as a positive prevention of teenage pregnancy, reduces promiscuity and is a traditional practice which has been followed for hundreds of years. Disturbingly, women may be recircumcised following each birth of a child, following the death of a husband or following a divorce. Women who allow, encourage or enable their daughters to be circumcised do so in the belief that circumcision is a benefit for their daughter. There is an argument that to circumcise a daughter is an act of love and not an act of cruelty (Whyte, 1989). In some areas not having a daughter circumcised brings shame on her family, limits her ability to find employment, reduces the likelihood of a husband and increases the community's perception of the woman's purity. A concern is that when women move to another country they continue to uphold cultural practices (preservation of identity) which are not the norm in the host country. Respecting cultural traditions and practices is not acceptable if they are illegal or abusive.

Children's rights

The Convention on the Rights of the Child (1989) identifies in Article 19 that all children should be protected from 'all forms of physical or mental violence, injury or abuse, neglect or negligent treatment'. While most people understand that FGM is physical violence, others recognise that the mental ill health (depression, anxiety, fear, post-traumatic stress) is seldom addressed. The psychosexual issues around feelings, responses and sexual arousal are seldom discussed due to fear and embarrassment.

The Convention on the Rights of the Child goes further; in Article 24 it identifies that effective and appropriate measures should be taken to abolish traditional practices prejudicial to the health of children.

A more contentious issue is the families that argue that rather than being neglectful 'FGM is "an act of love" not cruelty' (Whyte, 1989). The premise here is that by circumcising a daughter she is more likely to get married, the family reputation is honoured and she is more likely to be clean and get a job.

Health rights

FGM is thought to breach basic human rights regarding sexuality, health and reproductive rights for women and children. Phrases like 'live and let live', professionals not engaging in the strategy to eradicate FGM and ignoring the health consequences of FGM for fear of being seen as racist or judgemental are unethical. Ethical behaviour demonstrates care and compassion for others and failing to engage in the discussions on the grounds of not offending someone is not a valid argument. It is possible to discuss FGM respectfully and compassionately. However, I acknowledge that routinely informing postnatal women who have a daughter that FGM is illegal is a challenge to midwifery communication skills. Specific training and excellent communication skills will be required to enable healthcare workers to provide this information. Morally the issue is around the right to cultural self-determination and the right to a culture and tradition, which here causes harm to women and children.

Research regarding FGM also needs to be treated with care. Any research that concerns sensitive issues, such as different values, beliefs and attitudes to that of the researcher, requires caution. The basic human right to genital autonomy is not a universally shared right. When 'research' is undertaken regarding a controversial practice by those who do not share the same view, care should be taken to ensure that offence or anxiety is not created. In addition there is evidence that undertaking research which requires self-reporting, potential embarrassment or anxiety must be ethically approved and steps taken to protect the participants from further harm.

Victims of FGM also have a right to confidentiality and support. Healthcare must ensure that both physical and mental health issues for FGM are addressed.

The author recognises that the term FGM may be perceived as offensive to some individuals, but the term is widely used in the context of British culture whereby physical violence and abuse of women is not acceptable. Justification for use of the term is that in the UK context FGM is the accepted legal term. In this country FGM has been criminalised and many people (FORWARD, REPLACE, RCM, FGM NCG, L.B.M. Women's project) are all working hard to eliminate this traditional practice. The British government have also recognised the need to engage in the elimination of FGM.

Discrimination against women

The United Nations Convention on the Elimination of All Forms of Discrimination Against Women (UNEDW), in Article 5 (a), calls for all parties to 'modify the social and cultural patterns of conduct of men and women, with a view to achieving the elimination of prejudices and customary and all other practices which are based on the idea of the inferiority or the superiority of either of the sexes or on stereotyped roles for men and women'. While 'social and cultural patterns of conduct' is not defined in the convention, female cutting is undertaken with a desire to control sexuality and sexual behaviours.

Childbirth rights

Childbirth or reproductive rights are promoted as part of the Convention on the Elimination of All Forms of Discrimination Against Women (1981). The convention considers that the role of women in procreation should not be a basis for discrimination. The treaty affirms women's rights to reproductive choice and considers rights regarding family planning, maternity as a social function and shared responsibility for child rearing. From an ethical point of view if 'fully shared responsibility for child rearing' (UNEDW, 1981) is taken seriously this means that fathers who allow their daughters to be genitally cut are just as responsible and accountable as the mother.

As midwives, it is important to provide a high standard of care to all women during childbirth. It is vital that midwives are not only able to meet the needs of circumcised women but to be able to understand the impact that FGM has on the woman's reproductive experiences. A variety of psychological and psychosexual problems associated with FGM have been reported and may impact upon the birth experience. Failure to understand the emotional and social aspects of circumcision means that compassionate, empathetic and respectful care cannot be achieved. All women have the right to birth their baby in a way that is acceptable to them (White Ribbon Alliance, 2014). Obstetricians who advocate elective Caesarean sections for FGM women as a safe option are failing to take account of the long-term effects upon mother and baby.

FGM has major health implications and obstetric consequences (Berg and Underland, 2013); it is important that the NHS provides information and care for all women. Improving the health and wellbeing of women and girls who have been subjected to FGM is a priority at this time. Maternity services need to be informed and provide appropriate clinical care for these women. Clinical standards for FGM services are available (see the useful websites list at the end of this chapter). Additionally, it is paramount that health and social care professionals work inter-professionally to provide a safeguarding service which meets high standards of care for these vulnerable women, girls and female babies. Readers who wish to know more about the eradication of FGM in communities should familiarise themselves with the intercollegiate recommendations (RCM *et al.*, 2013) and resources such as toolkits for working with communities (REPLACE, 2012).

Human rights

Basic human rights are fundamental to all aspects of health and social care. Since the Human Rights Act, government departments, agencies and hospitals are required to comply and support human rights as identified in the European Convention on Human Rights. FGM has been the subject of political interest. Globally the WHO and UNICEF have campaigned for the eradication of FGM.

Nationally there have been professional guidelines regarding the management of FGM (RCN, 2015; RCOG, 2009a; BMA, 2011). There are currently no guidelines regarding general education or education and training for the medical profession, midwives or allied healthcare professionals in the UK.

Adults' versus children's rights

The UK is signed up to the Convention on the Rights of the Child and as such needs to honour its commitments to children's rights. The Convention on the Rights of the Child identifies that the child has a right to enjoy the 'highest attainable standard of health' (Article 24 (1)). In addition, 'parties shall take all effective and appropriate measures with a view to abolishing traditional practices prejudicial to the health of children' (Article 24 (3)). Articles 2, 12, 14 and 19 of the Convention are also particularly relevant.

In addition to the Convention on the Rights of the Child, the 2012 Helsinki Declaration identified the right to genital autonomy. The Helsinki Declaration declares that it is 'the fundamental right of each human being a Right of Genital Autonomy, that is the right to: Personal control of their own genital and reproductive organs; and protection from medically unnecessary genital modification and other irreversible reproductive interventions'.

While adults/parents may wish to uphold their rights (such as cultural identity, right to family life, etc.), when these conflict with the rights of a child there is a dilemma. In England the right to family life which includes FGM conflicts with the law. Those families who choose to continue to undertake FGM are acting illegally. Criminalisation of FGM prioritises children's right to health and genital autonomy. FGM is considered physical abuse of girls and women and as such is subject to safeguarding procedures in the UK. For many communities, keeping cultural traditions alive is essential to their sense of identity and wellbeing. In modern Britain the tradition of FGM conflicts with the right of a child to be safe and not subjected to abuse. FGM is illegal in the UK and subjected to criminal investigation. This results in the dilemma for all agencies, professions and individuals around safeguarding.

Women's experiences of FGM

Much of the research conducted regarding FGM suggests that women are suffering and are in pain as a result of the circumcision, cutting and trauma (Rushwan, 1980; WHO, 2008). The literature refers to immediate, short-, medium- and long-term effects of the practice, all of which can be from physical, psychological and social aspects. It is often difficult to talk to women about this traditional practice as some people find it hard to understand why FGM should ever happen. Unhelpful attitudes towards cultures which support FGM/C – such as having a moral high ground, feeling superior or intelligent – are insensitive and can cause hostility and resentment. It is unlikely that communities will abandon the practice of FGM if researchers or health workers lack understanding.

Female circumcision, like male circumcision, is associated with tradition and is argued to be culturally required. Circumcision is associated with a purification rite.

Healthcare professionals and FGM

Healthcare professionals in the UK would not contemplate undertaking FGM as it goes against medical codes of conduct, violates healthcare rights and fundamentally violates the ethical principle of 'do no harm'. On any ethical level FGM is not considered acceptable. The WHO (2008) banned and is intolerant of all forms of FGM. In addition, there is pressure to eradicate all forms of cultural childbirth practices which are associated with harm.

Intolerance and eradication of FGM in the UK

Internationally, 6 February is designated International Day of Zero Tolerance for Female Genital Mutilation. The UK strategy for eradication of FGM is based upon education, safeguarding and working with communities to provide information and appropriate culturally sensitive healthcare. The government strategy (HM Government, 2014) identifies the case for a national action plan and confirms that the government is unequivocal that, in the UK, FGM is a criminal offence and that they are committed to eradicating it.

There is no merit in debating whether FGM should be criminalised or not. FGM in the UK has been criminalised. The effect of criminalisation of FGM/C in the UK has effectively ensured that FGM/C has gone underground. FGM/C is a misunderstood practice which the media have reported, and created fear and anxiety for individuals, communities and professions. Communities are silent and reluctant to engage with healthcare professionals for fear of accusations of abuse, fear of criminal proceedings and discrimination. The lack of understanding, denial and embarrassment associated with FGM/C further isolates and compounds the suffering of FGM/C women. Language barriers do not help and the use of the term FGM is offensive to some communities. *Tackling FGM in the UK* (RCM *et al.*, 2013) are intercollegiate recommendations for identifying, recording and reporting of FGM. This strategy is intended to bring about changes in the UK to help eradicate FGM. The Home Affairs Select Committee (July 2014) identifies that tackling FGM requires a comprehensive approach, including prevention, punishment, enforcement, support and protection measures. At the Girl Summit (22 July 2014) a global movement to end FGM identified pledges from around the world committing to the elimination of FGM. The UK government announced a package of domestic measures to tackle FGM in the UK and highlighted that everyone has a responsibility to end FGM. The Home Office workstreams include mandatory data collection, reporting of FGM, safeguarding and education. The FGM Prevalence Data Set is a monthly return of data from acute hospital providers in England (HSCIC, 2014a). It is an aggregated return of the incidence of FGM (includes women previously identified and currently being treated for FGM- or non-FGM-related conditions) and newly identified women within the reporting period. This data set has been a mandated collection since 1 September 2014 (HSCIC, 2014b).

Legal aspects of FGM

As a registered midwife my duty is to provide appropriate and compassionate care (physical, psychological and emotional) to all women during childbirth. This responsibility of appropriate care means that cultural aspects and sensitive care is paramount for all, including the specific care of FGM women during labour. In the UK two pieces of legislation address the issues around FGM. In 1985 the Prohibition of Female Circumcision Act made FGM an offence. This legislation was considered unsuccessful as it failed to prevent circumcision and also permitted FGM on specific physical and mental health grounds. Following immense pressure the government passed the Female Genital Mutilation Act 2003.

The Prohibition of Female Circumcision Act 1985

This makes FGM an offence, except on specific physical and mental health grounds.

Female Genital Mutilation Act 2003

This strengthens and amends the 1985 legislation. It makes it an offence for the first time for UK nationals or permanent UK residents to carry out FGM abroad, or to aid, abet, counsel or procure the carrying out of FGM abroad, even in countries where the practice is legal. The 2003 Act also increases the maximum penalty for committing or aiding the offence from five years' to fourteen years' imprisonment.

Section 5 identifies that it is an offence for any person to:

Excise, infibulate or otherwise mutilate the whole or any part of a girl's labia majora, labia minora or clitoris

Aid, abet, counsel or procure the performance by another person of any of those acts on that other person's body

Aid, abet, counsel or procure a person to excise, infibulate or otherwise mutilate the whole or any part of her own labia majora, labia minora or clitoris.

FGM Act [2003] introduced the concept of extraterritoriality making it an offence to take any girl who is a UK national or UK permanent resident to any other country for purpose of FGM

Penalty for carrying out FGM or arranging to carry out is 14 years imprisonment or a fine or both.

Female Genital Mutilation Act 2003

CHAPTER 31

CONTENTS

Figure 13.1 The Female Genital Mutilation Act (2003)

Practical distinctions

FGM Act [2003] Section 1 (2), surgery necessary for physical or mental health. Mental health assessment – no account can be taken of any belief that the operation is necessary for her physical or mental health. FGM cannot legally occur on the grounds that a girl's mental health would suffer if she did not conform to the custom of her community.

FGM Act [2003] Section 2(b)

This allows a surgical operation in any stage of labour for the purposes of labour (deinfibulation) that must be carried out by an approved person (doctor, registered midwife or student midwife) *but* reinfibulation is unlawful. It is likely that reinfibulation, repair and control of bleeding will remain controversial, especially when experts, clinical judgements and anatomical abnormality are questioned.

RCOG and RCM interpret this to include the re-stitching of a previously infibulated woman following vaginal delivery. This means that a perineum, which has been torn or been cut to facilitate delivery, may be repaired, but not to the extent that intercourse will be difficult or impossible.

Midwives should be mindful that other terminology such as that used in cosmetic or plastic surgery (designer laser vaginoplasty, G-spot augmentation) could be considered to be female genital mutilation. One difference is that cosmetic and plastic surgery is undertaken with consent. FGM as defined by the WHO (with or without consent) is a criminal offence.

Serious Crime Act 2015

Received Royal Assent 3rd March 2015. See sections 70–75.

Prosecution

There have been no prosecutions under the FGM Act 2003 to date (time of going to press), but the CPS has scheduled a case of a London-based doctor and a woman's husband to court in January 2015. There is an argument that as there are no prosecutions then the 2003 Act is an ineffectual law. The CPS identifies that there has been a lack of referrals of FGM to them. The CPS suggests that there is a lack of referrals due to a reluctance to refer to them by healthcare professionals for fear of being considered

Table 13.2 Difficulties in securing a prosecution

	Political	Educational	Social
Identification	Lack of funding for women's health	Healthcare practitioners unfamiliar with types of FGM	Disclosure of FGM
	No specific 'codes' for NHS	Healthcare practitioners not aware of FGM	
Referral	Fear of being labelled racist	Confidentiality	Fear of being labelled racist
	Who to refer to (direct referrals to the police from healthcare practitioners are not common)	Reluctant to invoke safeguarding procedures Do not wish to jeopardise relationship	Difficulties of inter-agency working
	Lack of cases recorded Lack of cases known by CPS	Police difficulties regarding investigating	
Process	Pressure on CPS to secure a prosecution	Professional malpractice Safeguarding procedures	High profile of FGM cases
	Large caseloads of social workers Publicity	Data collection (referral of all girls born to FGM women)	Media attention Investigative journalism
Outcome	No prosecution = ineffective law	No prosecution = FGM legislation not taken seriously	Communities willing to continue with FGM

racist. The CPS also identifies that there are no statutory guidelines on FGM to aid practitioners regarding reporting of FGM. Mandatory reporting of FGM is currently under consultation and results will be known in spring 2015.

The CPS monitored and evaluated cases from September 2011 to September 2012 (Strategy & Policy Directorate). The standard of evidence and the nature of evidence make it difficult to secure a prosecution. There are a number of difficulties associated with securing a prosecution under the legislation (Table 13.2).

The CPS acknowledges that there are major difficulties with all aspects of the prosecution process regarding FGM.

Box 13.1 The CPS process

Complaint
Provision of evidence
Cooperation of victim
Nature and extent of victim support

Complaint

According to the CPS prior to 2010 there were no referrals regarding FGM. Since 2010 the CPS has been asked to demonstrate follow-up regarding all reported incidents of suspected FGM. Many victims of abuse do not report the abuse for fear of (a) not being believed; (b) shame; (c) not knowing how to or who to disclose the abuse to. It is hoped that the NSPCC help line (telephone: 0800 028 3550) will enable victims to seek support and disclose their worries regarding FGM. The victim of FGM is unlikely to disclose the abuse as she is usually living with her family, who arranged and paid for the FGM. Reporting your parents to a statutory agency (police, health or education) does not facilitate good relations.

Evidence

Evidence required – international evidence, experts, local authority and victim evidence. A major problem is securing the evidence regarding where, when and who undertakes FGM. Identification of the type of FGM may be difficult to obtain. No one would wish to subject an individual to further abuse in order to obtain evidence. Consent for intimate examination, especially for young girls, is complex and risks further trauma.

Continued cooperation

Given the length of time it may take to investigate, assemble evidence and present at court, there is adequate opportunity for the victim to change her mind, be reluctant to continue or be afraid of breach of confidentiality.

Victim support

Standards – Victim's Code and Prosecutors' Pledge. In 2013 the CPS published standards regarding the treatment of victims and the aspects of the service to be improved.

Professional misconduct

While there have been no successful criminal prosecutions (at the time of going to press) under FGM legislation, there have been investigations into suspected circumcisions in the UK and some success regarding removal of practitioners from registers.

In 1993 the GMC struck off a Harley Street Doctor Farooque Hayder Siddique for agreeing to carry out a female circumcision (*Sunday Times*, 7 November). The CPS had not pressed criminal charges as there was 'insufficient evidence to proceed' (Dyer, 1993) The CPS is not able to proceed with criminal prosecutions where there is difficulty with the acquisition, process, standard or type of evidence. Registered practitioners are more likely to be referred to their regulatory body where their fitness to practise will be called into question.

The Foundation for Women's Health Research and Development (FORWARD, 2004) identified the case of a doctor in the North East London Strategic Health Authority who was struck off the GMC register for serious professional misconduct for offering to carry out FGM for £50 per time. In April 2012 there were arrests in Birmingham of two men (one a dentist and the other a doctor) thought to be offering to circumcise girls. The difficulty with the case revolved around the way in which the information was obtained. An undercover journalist was referred by a GP to a dentist. The dentist was filmed allegedly offering to circumcise her 'nieces'. The case was referred to the CPS but did not progress to court. The CPS will only progress cases where it is in the public interest and if there is the required standard of evidence. Coverage of the allegations were published in the press and the dentist was struck off the General Dental Council Register for undertaking a medical examination (not a dental examination) and the medical practitioner was referred to the GMC.

In 2014 medical practitioners united in support of Dr Dharmasena from the London Whittington Hopsital who had been accused of performing FGM on a young mother who delivered in November 2012.

Contrasting FGM and female genital surgery (FGS) or cosmetic gynaecological treatment

Cosmetic gynaecological treatments are similar to FGM from an anatomical perspective, in that the genital structures may be surgically changed. Similarities with FGM are that payment is private, details of techniques or procedures are scant and women do not usually discuss the experience. FGS does not share the same illegality as FGM. FGS is usually undertaken on those over 18 years (but increasingly less so) and is associated with enhancing self-esteem and confidence. Terminology is not similar to FGM in that classification is not based on types and the surgery is not limited to removal and may involve augmentation and allegedly rejuvenation. There is no regulation regarding cosmetic genital surgery. Culturally, FGS is considered acceptable in the UK, whereas FGM has been criminalised. British women are felt to have double standards when criticising women for tolerating FGM while allowing FGS to go unchallenged, unregulated and involving vulnerable women. Is it ethical to allow one form of genital surgery and not the other?

Contrasting episiotomy and FGM

While theoretically episiotomy and FGM are very different, the concern is that for the woman's health the physiological aspects are similar (pain, bleeding, difficult healing process, risk of infection and uncomfortable sexual intercourse). The legal situation is also very different. FGM is illegal in the UK while it is legal for a midwife to perform an episiotomy.

It can be argued that episiotomy is a cultural childbirth practice in the UK. FGM has been justified through culture and tradition (WHO, 2008). Interestingly, midwives have also justified episiotomy in cultural terms, as well as protecting a child's right to a safe delivery.

FGM is not usually performed during childbirth; on the contrary, it is used as a way of controlling sexual activity and preventing pregnancy. Other arguments are that episiotomy is a surgical procedure and therefore is undertaken by a skilled and registered practitioner: episiotomy does not involve other organs (clitoris); episiotomy is conducted under hygienic conditions and consent is gained. The main argument that episiotomy is not mutilation rests on the assumption that the episiotomy is doing good in the prevention of more extensive trauma and the perception that a surgical cut heals better than a tear.

The use of episiotomy is regulated and controlled through secondary legislation and the NMC (2004, 2008d). The European Directives (EMD 80/155/EEC) provide that student midwives must gain clinical experience of episiotomy and suturing.

Deinfibulation, repair and tightening operations

Midwives in the UK provide midwifery care and support to women from a multicultural perspective. Increasingly, birth partners are present at delivery and sometimes fulfil the role of advocate for the woman. Supporting women's choices is a fundamental role of the midwife. Sometimes requests may be problematic as they may put the midwife in a difficult position. For example, the tradition of tightening operations of the vulva after delivery, when the woman wishes to be stitched up.

The tradition of tightening operations of the vulva after delivery has been described by Berggren *et al.* (2006: 407). A concern is that some women who had not previously experienced FGM and some who had undergone an LSCS were subjected to vaginal tightening operations (reinfibulation) and surgery which could be considered as female genital mutilation. The research was carried out in Sudan, where reinfibulation is illegal. Berggren *et al.* (2006) found a prevalence of 61 per cent of postpartum tightening operations in Sudan.

In 2014 the CPS alleged that a London doctor (Dr Dhanuson Dharmasena) had conducted a reinfibulation of a young woman (referred to as AB) in November 2012. The announcement by the Director of Public Prosecutions (Alison Saunders) made headlines news as 'The first female genital mutilation prosecutions announced' (BBC, 21 March). At Southwark Crown Court in February 2015 Dr Dharmasena was cleared of the allegations.

Safeguarding against FGM

Following extensive media coverage regarding FGM, the Department of Health (2012c) circulated a letter in May 2012 asking all health professionals to 'familiarize themselves with the actions they need to take where they have reason to believe that a girl has undergone, or is at risk of, Female Genital Mutilation (FGM)'. Multi-agency guidelines were issued in 2011.

Midwives are usually the first health professional to be informed or identify that a woman has undergone FGM. Midwives are therefore key to ensuring that women who have experienced FGM are provided with appropriate care and that their right to health is promoted at every opportunity. The midwife is also best placed to initiate safeguarding (Gardner, 2012b). When a woman who has undergone FGM gives birth to a daughter, she should be provided with clear information that FGM is illegal in the UK and should not be performed on her daughter. This should be done in a sensitive way and recorded. The baby notes should be clearly marked with the fact that the genitals have no abnormality detected (NAD).

Chapter summary

This chapter considered the ethical and legal issues surrounding FGM, often known as cutting, piercing or female circumcision. This chapter has defined FGM, considered the reasons for FGM, compared and contrasted FGM and other traditions and surgical procedures, identified the difficulties with consent and demonstrated that in providing ethically based care midwives should ensure that an appropriate clinical care pathway is in place, alongside culturally sensitive patient care. Male and female circumcision have no health or religious similarities and should not be compared. Deinfibulation requires informed consent, confidentiality and psychological preparation and support both before and following the procedure. The legal aspects of FGM were identified and explained. The illegality of FGM in the UK was considered and discussed within the context of modern healthcare. The case study (Sylvie) is used to consider ethical and legal aspects of FGM illustrating the vulnerability of women during childbirth.

* FGM is a criminal offence in the UK (and other countries).
* Safeguarding is a professional requirement.
* Criminal prosecutions in the UK are difficult to achieve, as family members are unlikely to testify against each other.
* Elimination of FGM requires a multidisciplinary approach.
* There is a lack of knowledge of FGM (public and all professionals).
* Midwives have an important role to play not just in the care and management but also the education and support of communities.
* Criminalisation of FGM means that lack of trust and fear makes communities protective and reluctant to accept 'interference' with health issues.
* Evidence of FGM is often unobtainable.
* Midwives must provide physical, psychological and emotional support for FGM women, as well as fulfilling health promotion and educational roles.

Key learning

* Attention should focus on the difficulties associated with effecting a prosecution.
* Midwives need to be mindful of the imminent changes to reporting, recording and legalities around FGM.

Case study: Sylvie

Following an antenatal deinfibulation, Sylvie has given birth to a healthy baby girl. The midwife present at the birth congratulates Sylvie on her beautiful daughter. Sylvie intends to leave hospital as soon as possible to return home. The midwife is concerned as she has heard about FGM and is worried that Sylvie may want her baby to be 'circumcised' as well.

This case illustrates the dilemmas experienced by many midwives when providing care to women during childbirth. Dilemmas are around: health assessments, legal aspects associated with birth, procedures and length of hospital stay. On the one hand, there is an understanding that childbearing women wish to be home with their families as soon as possible; on the other hand, there are health assessments and certain legal requirements which take time to complete before they leave the hospital. The duty of care is complex: the midwife ensures records are made and maintained, birth to be notified and policy and procedures to be undertaken, while also providing help and support, care and risk assessments and ensuring that the health and wellbeing of mother and baby are maintained.

Evaluation

There are guidelines regarding safeguarding which the midwife should follow. There is no evidence that because a woman has been circumcised that she will automatically want the same for her daughters. Risk assessment is important as the midwife needs to understand the risk (likelihood) of Sylvie wishing to mutilate her daughter. Sylvie must be provided with information regarding the illegality of FGM in the UK and its legal effect upon British citizens. The midwife owes a duty of care towards the baby girl and must ensure that the birth records identify normal genitalia at birth.

Analysis

Midwives are the most senior person present at the majority of births in the UK. They have a moral obligation to provide sensitive and compassionate midwifery care. Midwives need to be able to balance the responsibilities of duty, confidentiality and safeguarding with the provision of a sensitive and appropriate service for FGM women. Women affected by FGM need to be cared for by health professionals who are able to meet healthcare needs as well as providing psychological support. Women need to be informed that midwives have a role in safeguarding and as such will initiate referrals that seek to protect girls and women from FGM.

Safeguarding is an important role of the midwife and all midwives are required to undertake mandatory training on an annual basis. As Sylvie has given birth to a girl she should be provided with information about FGM. The opportunity to discuss FGM with Sylvie may be initiated on the basis of the deinfibulation that Sylvie experienced antenatally.

Some cultural childbirth practices (episiotomy) are legal and some (FGM and tightening operations) are illegal in the UK.

What can be done

Current approaches to eradicating FGM are empowering women to challenge the practice through education of specific communities where FGM is practised.

Implications for practice

- provision of information to Sylvie;
- records to identify that genitalia were normal at birth;
- safeguarding procedures.

If Sylvie is a UK citizen and was subjected to FGM after 2003 a criminal act has occurred. Technically the midwife is required to refer this to the police. Safeguarding adults is an important role of the midwife. The midwife should discuss and document her concerns with a supervisor of midwives.

Practice check

1. Do you enquire about FGM? If so, do you communicate with women in a sensitive and culturally appropriate way?
2. Do you record 'normal genitalia' on birth records, discharge notes and the 'red book'?
3. Are you familiar with the latest safeguarding guidelines?

Activity

1. Having read this chapter, take the opportunity to discuss your views regarding cosmetic surgery with a colleague.
2. Consider what information should be provided to communities regarding FGM.

Guidelines and policy

British Medical Association (2011) *Female Genital Mutilation: Caring for Patients and Safeguarding Children*. BMA, London.

European Institute for Gender Equality (2013) *Female Genital Mutilation in the European Union and Croatia Report*. EIGE, Belgium. Available at: http://eige.europa.eu/content/female-genital-mutilation

HM Government (2011) *Multi-agency Practice Guidelines: FGM*. Department of Health, London.

HM Government (2014) *Female Genital Mutilation: The Case for a National Action Plan*. December, Secretary of State, London.

Royal College Obstetricians and Gynaecologists (2009) *Green Top Guideline No 53 FGM and its Management*. RCOG, London.

Royal College of Midwives (1998) *Position Paper No 21: Female Genital Mutilation*. RCM Welsh Board, Cardiff.

Royal College of Midwives, Royal College of Nursing, Royal College of Obstetricians and Gynaecologists, Equality

Now and UNITE (2013) *Tackling FGM in the UK: Intercollegiate Recommendations for Identifying, Recording and Reporting*. RCM, London. Available at: www.rcm.org.uk

Royal College of Nursing (1994) *Female Genital Mutilation*. RCN, London (at the time of writing this is being reviewed).

International Centre for Reproductive Health (IRCH) (2009) *Responding to FGM in Europe: Striking the Right Balance Between Prosecution and Prevention*. IRCH, Ghent University, Belgium.

REPLACE (2012) *FGM Toolkit for Working with Communities: Researching Female Genital Mutilation (FGM) Intervention Programmes Linked to African Communities in the EU*. Available from: www.replacefgm.eu/toolkit

World Health Organization (2008) *Eliminating Female Genital Mutilation: An Interagency Statement*. WHO, Switzerland. Available from: www.who.int/reproductivehealth

Useful websites

FGM resources: http://www.fgmnationalgroup.org
FORWARD (information regarding FGM): http://www.forwarduk.org
NHS Choices and FGM at: http://www.nhs.uk

14 Episiotomy

Pre-requisites for this chapter

It is assumed that the reader has a good understanding of the anatomical structures of the female genitalia and perineum and the physiology of labour.

Introduction

In a previous chapter the concept of consent and refusal of treatment was considered. This chapter identifies a specific midwifery intervention and considers the ethical and legal issues surrounding episiotomy. While most episiotomies are performed urgently in the second stage of labour, women frequently identify in their birth plans that they do not wish to have an episiotomy. If an episiotomy is performed by the midwife, should written consent be gained to 'override' the refusal identified in the birth plan? The use of episiotomy during childbirth is controversial. According to Sleep (1983: 81) the term 'episiotomy was coined in 1957 by Braun, who condemned it as unadvisable and unnecessary (Nugent, 1935 in Sleep, 1983: 81). Since 1983 midwives have been permitted to perform episiotomies and it is thought that undertaking an episiotomy is a 'respectable way of avoiding a tear' (Enkin *et al.*, 1989). Normal childbirth in the UK has been characterised by a number of midwifery practices and obstetric interventions which have been challenged. Cameron and Rawlings-Anderson (2001) suggest that healthcare beliefs and practices without adequate explanation or consent can cause distress and suffering.

Consideration will be given to contrasting the ethical issues around episiotomy and those of female genital mutilation/circumcision (FGM/C) and laser vaginoplasty as they illustrate ethical and legal issues around consent. The author will also suggest that episiotomy is a form of FGM that is accepted as legal in the UK. Ethical issues around the gaining of consent and the dilemma or conflict between the rights of the woman and the potential rights of the baby are addressed. Repair of episiotomy is also considered as suturing is usually undertaken by the practitioner performing the episiotomy.

A midwife undertaking episiotomy repair is required to have received training and demonstrated clinical skills. Readers will be aware that much has been written and research undertaken around the practice of episiotomy; it is against this backdrop of changing midwifery practice that this chapter is written. Is episiotomy justified? That is a current dilemma facing midwives (see Chapter 10). Midwives undertaking perineal repair also need to consider the possibility of an accusation of FGM if they do not demonstrate the standard of perineal repair that is required by a registered practitioner. Reinfibulation is 'the tightening and mimicking the narrow interoitous of a virgin' (El Dareer, 1982; Ahmed Mageed, 2000a,b; Almroth-Berggren, 2001, all cited in Berggren *et al.*, 2006).

What is an episiotomy?

Episiotomy has been defined as 'a surgical incision of the perineum which is carried out prior to the delivery of the infant' (Verrals, 1980). The reality for the woman is that there is cutting of the skin, muscles and vagina to enlarge the birth canal. Prior to 1967 episiotomy was regulated and mainly undertaken by obstetricians, after which the Central Midwives Board (CMB) permitted midwives to undertake an episiotomy in an emergency. By 1983 the CMB allowed midwives to repair the incision. Types of episiotomy are medio-lateral, midline and anterior. Serious complications with midline episiotomies have been reported in America. In the UK a medio-lateral episiotomy is the preferred method. An anterior episiotomy is an American term for an operation used to separate perineal tissue following FGM/C. Anterior episiotomy is not a term used in the UK. The separation of perineal tissue in a woman who has experienced FGM is called deinfibulation. Episiotomy is the most common cause of perineal damage and is associated with pain, discomfort and scar tissue.

Student midwives are currently required to observe episiotomy and receive instructions on perineal repair. The current midwifery professional body, the NMC (2009b), identify that if students are unable to witness episiotomy they should receive clinical simulation in the procedure.

Normality of episiotomy

The high incidence of episiotomies performed during the 1970s and 1980s suggest that episiotomy was the norm for primigravida. Sleep *et al.* (1984) report an episiotomy rate of 61 per cent and 52 per cent during spontaneous deliveries in their hospitals prior to undertaking a randomised trial. By 1987 the rate of episiotomy was 20 per cent. Current rates of episiotomy are around 8.2 per cent (HSCIC, 2011). Women's experiences of episiotomy are well documented (Kitzinger and Walters, 1981). In the hand-held pregnancy notes (Perinatal Institute, 2012) records are made regarding integrity of the perineum in previous pregnancies.

Garcia *et al.* (1985) report that the majority of maternity units in their study did not have a policy on episiotomy, and that those that did 'could allow a wide interpretation'. When it came to suturing the perineum, Garcia *et al.* (1985) also found that by 1984, 55 per cent of midwives were suturing and a further 7 per cent of units' midwives were suturing but with restrictions such as first degree tears only.

The decision to perform an episiotomy is a professional clinical judgement and will vary according to evidence and experience. Midwifery textbooks (*Myles*, *Mayes*) identify a number of risk factors for perineal trauma ranging from tissue type to size of the baby. The indications for an episiotomy are not absolute and clinical discretion must be used. Rigid perineum, fetal compromise and prevention of severe perineal trauma are all mentioned. The dilemma for midwives is clear: should I perform an episiotomy to expedite delivery of a distressed/compromised baby and in doing so perform surgery associated with risk of infection and pain, or should I restrict the use of episiotomy and risk a perineal tear and a baby born with low APGAR scores?

How is consent gained for episiotomy?

Pregnancy and childbirth in the UK are characterised by antenatal preparation. Healthcare professionals such as midwives and doctors provide information and explanations around childbirth practices.

Episiotomy is usually discussed in birth preparation classes and women are informed that in an emergency an episiotomy may be undertaken. During labour the midwife will have ascertained the woman's wishes and choices. Labour ward policies and guidelines identify that the midwife will discuss the possibility of episiotomy with women. By the second stage of labour the midwife will have verbal agreement from the woman that if it becomes necessary an episiotomy will be undertaken. The consent is usually verbal and rarely in writing.

What happens if the woman chooses not to have an episiotomy? The legal situation is clear, if an adult can make a decision to accept treatment, the same adult can also decline treatment. The standards for acceptance are the same as for declining. So if a woman chooses not to agree to an episiotomy then the midwife may not perform one. This is a fundamental human right to self-determine what happens to our bodies, assuming that capacity is not an issue – capacity cannot be questioned just because the midwife does not like the woman's answer.

What do women feel about episiotomies?

The *British Way of Birth* (1982) was a BBC survey of 6,000 mothers. The strongest comments from mothers about episiotomy were around the time women had to wait for a doctor to come along and put the stitches in; the insertion of the stitches was painful; gratitude to midwives who allowed slow and gentle stretching and avoided the need for an episiotomy; women who wished they had been cut rather than acquire a perineal tear. Women's experiences of episiotomy are important; if we know what their concerns are, midwives can act as advocates for the women. Understanding the woman's views also enables midwives to question policy and procedures which do not meet women's needs or expectations. Childbirth is a challenging time without having to wait for hours to have an episiotomy repaired. Fortunately, midwives are trained to repair perineal trauma and women should not have to wait for a repair to be undertaken. However, this provides another dilemma for the midwife in terms of prioritising care. Does perineal repair take precedent over skin-to-skin contact, newborn checks and birth records?

Childbirth rights

During childbirth the rights of the woman may be considered to clash with the rights of the baby. Morally, some people believe that a baby is a person from the moment of conception, implantation and throughout pregnancy. Psychologists suggest that the bonding process starts early in pregnancy. Culturally, Western antenatal care reinforces the notion with pictures and images of the baby in utero. Knowledge around the sex of the baby enables women to plan and focus their attention on gender issues. Families anticipate the arrival of baby girl or boy and often have named the baby prior to delivery. In other words, the fetus has acquired personhood and identity in the eyes of the woman and her family. In legal terms it is only when the baby is born that it acquires the status of a baby with its specific identity and needs. The moment of birth is when the baby also acquires rights associated with the moral obligation to meet those rights.

Dilemmas occur when the rights of the woman (mother) are potentially compromised by another (fetus/baby). For example, should a woman be required to have an episiotomy to expedite the delivery of a baby who has fetal distress? An episiotomy to protect the delivery of a pre-term baby? An episiotomy to speed up the delivery of the baby? An episiotomy to enable the birth attendant to perform manoeuvres? An episiotomy to enable an birth attendant to undertake an assisted (forceps, ventouse) delivery?

Could episiotomy be a form of genital mutilation?

On first consideration episiotomy cannot possibly be FGM and there are midwives who may believe that to consider the two practices together is inappropriate. While theoretically episiotomy and FGM are very different, the concern is that for the woman's health the physiological aspects are similar (pain, bleeding, difficult healing process, risk of infection and uncomfortable sexual intercourse). Culturally, midwives are able to justify episiotomy as a childbirth intervention in the UK. FGM has also been justified as culture and tradition (WHO, 2006). Interestingly, midwives have also justified episiotomy in cultural terms.

On second consideration, episiotomy may be considered to be genital mutilation if consent is not sought, valid or reliable; if an episiotomy is not performed correctly; or cutting involves the labia as well as perineum. FGM is a collective term for a range of procedures which involve partial or total removal of the female genitalia for non-medical reasons (Crown Prosecution Service, 2012). It is defined as 'all procedures involving partial or total removal of the external female genitalia or other injury to the female genital organs, whether for cultural or other non-therapeutic reasons' (RCOG, 2009a). FGM is not usually performed during childbirth; on the contrary, it is used as a way of controlling sexual activity. Other arguments are that episiotomy is a surgical procedure and therefore is undertaken by a skilled and registered practitioner: episiotomy does not involve other organs (clitoris); episiotomy is conducted under hygienic conditions; and consent is gained. The main argument that episiotomy is not mutilation rests on the assumption that the episiotomy is doing good in the prevention of more extensive trauma and damage, whereas FGM does not do any good, is traumatic and has not been shown to have any health benefits – on the contrary, it has been associated with ill health (infertility, infections, haemorrhage and shock).

Episiotomy, then, is supported as it is thought to prevent complications and reduce the risk of unnecessary trauma to the baby's head and prevent a third or fourth degree tear. Episiotomy is thought to be mutilation 'if used without good cause' (Verrals, 1980: 38).

Episiotomy may be considered to be genital mutilation if consent is not sought. When a patient does not consent to an intervention or treatment, midwives are risking an allegation of assault. If a midwife attempts to perform an episiotomy and does it poorly, or does not follow the correct procedure and the woman sustains injury/damage/trauma, this could also be considered to be genital mutilation.

Episiotomy repair and tightening operations

Reinfibulation is defined as the re-stitching of scar tissue after delivery, resulting from infibulation (Verzin, 1975). Midwives in the UK provide midwifery care and support to women from a multicultural perspective. Increasingly, birth partners are present at delivery and sometimes fulfil the role of advocate for the woman. Supporting women's choices is a fundamental role of the midwife. Sometimes requests may be difficult as they may put the midwife in a difficult position. For example, the tradition of tightening operations of the vulva (vaginoplasty) after delivery if the woman wishes to be stitched up tighter. The tradition of tightening operations of the vulva after delivery to mimic the narrow or small interoitus of a virgin has been described by El Dareer (1982). A concern here is that some women who had not previously experienced FGM and some who had undergone an LSCS were subjected to a tightening operation which equates to FGM. In more recent research carried out in Sudan, where reinfibulation is illegal, Berggren et al. (2006) found a prevalence of 61 per cent of postpartum tightening operations. In the UK reinfibulation or any tightening or stitching up of the vulva is considered FGM. Episiotomy repair has to be undertaken carefully and documented clearly to reduce risk of accusation of FGM.

Chapter summary

Some childbirth practices (episiotomy) are legal in the UK and some (FGM/C and tightening operations) are illegal. Midwives are the most senior person present at the majority of births in the UK. They have a moral obligation to provide sensitive midwifery care. Cameron and Rawlings-Anderson (2001) suggest that midwives should use the same methods for eradicating episiotomy as for FGM. Current approaches to eradicating FGM are empowering women to challenge the practice through education of specific communities where FGM is practised. Using this approach with antenatal women and providing them with episiotomy rates for trusts, birth centres and birth units would enable them to make an informed choice regarding place of delivery. It has been argued that antenatal preparation classes should include this information.

This chapter has defined episiotomy, considered the rationale for episiotomy, compared and contrasted episiotomy with female genital mutilation, considered the difficulties with consent and demonstrated that in providing ethically based care midwives should ensure that, prior to undertaking an episiotomy, informed consent is obtained and adequate explanations have been provided. The case study (Sophie) will be used to consider ethical and legal aspects of episiotomy illustrating the vulnerability of women during childbirth.

Case study: Sophie

Sophie is a primigravida in established labour. She has chosen to deliver her baby at home. Sophie was unable to obtain a home birth service from her local NHS trust and has employed the services of an independent midwife. Spontaneous labour progresses well until the second stage of labour. Following spontaneous delivery of the baby's head, normal restitution is not observed, the baby's face is congested and the midwife recognises the emergency situation of shoulder dystocia. The midwife recognises that the fetus is distressed and desperately tries to perform an episiotomy to facilitate delivery of the shoulders.

Evaluation

There has been a steady decline in the number of home births. The Department of Health suggests that 1–2 per cent of all births are at home. There are professional arguments to be had around lack of choice, lack of service provision and in some countries the criminalisation of home birth. The focus of Sophie's case is the professional care and accountability of the midwife. In an emergency situation the midwife is required to undertake all necessary measures while awaiting

(continued)

medical support, and the expectation is that medical help is readily available. With a home birth not only is the midwife the professional attendant, but medical help is likely to be some time away and/or transport to access help is some time away.

Analysis

Sophie has been unable to secure the midwifery services from the local NHS provider (NHS Foundation Trust) and has employed an independent midwife. This is not an uncommon situation for home births. Not all NHS midwives are experienced with home births or are comfortable working away from labour wards where most of their labour management has been experienced. An independent midwife who regularly attends home births maintains clinical skills and expertise.

In deciding to undertake an episiotomy the midwife must gain consent prior to the procedure. Consent is necessary if the midwife wishes to avoid a possible negligence claim. In addition, consent is necessary to secure the cooperation of Sophie.

What can be done?

- The midwife must summon medical aid; this is an emergency situation which requires the help and support of other healthcare practitioners.
- The midwife can undertake the manoeuvres associated with the emergency management of shoulder dystocia.
- Any decisions made with regard to episiotomy must be taken on the basis of previous experiences, skills possessed and the consent of the woman. The midwife must not panic and undertake random cutting as the standard performed will be scrutinised. There is a danger that the fetal head may become damaged if there is substandard care when undertaking an episiotomy.

Implications for practice

- Emergency situations require clear communication with other healthcare professionals.
- Skills drills are an important method of maintaining fitness to practise.
- Midwives should not harm their patients; if you are not trained and skilled to do something then it is outside your role and responsibility.
- FGM carries a custodial sentence.

Conclusion

While it is not possible to predict the risk of shoulder dystocia, the midwife must be competent in recognising shoulder dystocia and undertake emergency measures. In emergency situations the midwife fulfils a professional duty of care. The midwife must maintain good communications and take 'reasonable' actions associated with professional practice.

Practice check

Undertake a self-audit to identify your episiotomy rate.

Activity

1. Reflect upon the last vaginal birth at which you were present and identify aspects of communication which impacted upon the woman's decision making.
2. Record-keeping: what standards are demonstrated in regard to perineum?

Useful websites

Explanations for women about episiotomy:
www.nhs.uk/Conditions/pregnancy-and-baby/Pages/episiotomy.aspx
NICE guidelines regarding episiotomy:
http://publications.nice.org.uk/intrapartum-care-cg55/guidance#normal-labour-second-stage
Womankind: www.womankind.org.uk

15 Caesarean section

Pre-requisites of this chapter

It is assumed that you have a good anatomical knowledge of the normal female reproductive system as well as the physiology of labour, micturition and the digestive system. You should also be utilising the latest professional regulatory standards (NMC, 2015) (consultation regarding a new edition is in progress). You should be familiar with the CNST standards regarding 'decision-to-cut times'.

Introduction

This chapter reaffirms the right of all women to accept or reject treatments and interventions. The ethical principle of autonomy is fundamental and the legal status of birth plans will be considered. Caesarean sections are a major surgical procedure for delivery of a baby via the abdomen, usually undertaken by a doctor in a hospital environment. It is generally accepted that there are two types of Caesarean section:

1. emergency (see CNST classifications);
2. elective Caesarean section (patient choice or care pathway).

It is outside the scope of this chapter to consider the clinical procedures and practice of Caesarean section; for this refer to traditional midwifery textbooks such as *Mayes' Midwifery* or *Myles Midwifery*. The reader should consider the CNST criteria regarding the type of Caesarean (time from decision to undertake LSCS to surgical incision and time of birth) before considering the ethical and legal issues of the case studies. There are a variety of reasons and clinical indications for undertaking a Caesarean section. In all cases written consent is required for this surgical method of assisting the delivery of a baby.

A common reason for advocating a Caesarean section is that it is in the 'best interest' of mother or baby. Care needs to be taken with the use of the phrase 'best interest' as medical, legal and social meaning of 'best interest' varies. Childbearing women also have specific understanding of their own 'best interest'. Equally, there may be occasions when the best interest of the mother and the best interest of the baby are not the same.

Research (Churchill and Benbow, 2000) suggests that type of delivery and an active role in decision making are important factors with regard to maternal satisfaction with care. It is likely that the decision to undertake a Caesarean section has far-reaching implications and unintended outcomes in the future. The key issues around lower segment Caesarean section (LSCS) are around court-ordered LSCS, 'on demand' LSCS, emergency LSCS for fetal distress and the potential for sterilisation during Caesarean section.

Caesarean section: ethical dilemmas

Typical ethical dilemmas regarding Caesarean section are:

- the woman does not want to have an operative delivery of her baby;
- medical advice is that a Caesarean section is strongly recommended thereby potentially removing the right of autonomy;
- there is undue pressure or coercion applied to secure agreement for Caesarean section;
- maternal condition is such that a Caesarean section is necessary to save the life of (a) mother, (b) baby or (c) both;
- mental ill health, lack of capacity, loss of capacity;
- court-ordered LSCS.

The ethical issues around Caesarean section are usually about patient rights, autonomous decision making, advocacy and the potential for paternalism. Caesarean section is an intervention and is a solution to a number of obstetric problems. While surgery is a radical procedure for enabling the delivery of a baby there are risks for both mother and baby. There is a danger in assuming that all women would be prepared to undergo a Caesarean section regardless of the indication for the surgery. For some women having a surgical delivery of the baby brings a feeling of disappointment and fear, in addition to anxiety, which can extend into the rest of their lives. Women may also feel that it is confirmation of their inadequacy and increase their sense of loss and low self-esteem.

Autonomy is an ethical principle that it is the right of a patient to make decisions about their treatment free from any pressure, influence or control from others. The right of autonomy is not absolute in healthcare as it conflicts with equity and fairness when considered from a service provision point of view. With absolute autonomy it would mean that others might be denied healthcare in order to prioritise existing patients or resources. Making decisions and choices often impact upon others in ways that are not apparent. An example of this is that if significant numbers of women choose to have elective Caesarean sections then there may be a delay in providing theatre space for an emergency Caesarean section.

Paternalism is the opposite of autonomy, in that paternalism is when a doctor decides what is best and carries out a Caesarean section with minimal consent or agreement. Paternalism is no longer the basis for patient–healthcare provider relationships. Modern NHS healthcare is based upon key NHS values (Department of Health, 2013: 5). The NHS values provide a common ground for cooperation with patients, staff and organisations. Expectations are such that childbearing women have the right to be involved in, contribute to and make choices regarding their treatments and interventions. Healthcare practitioners are required to work together for patients, value every patient by respecting their aspirations, choices and commitments, demonstrate compassion in giving comfort and time for patients and improving their health and wellbeing by the type of care provided. In the past women may have accepted paternalistic approaches to childbirth, but this is no longer the case according to the report *Changing Childbirth* (Department of Health, Expert Maternity Group, 1993). In many ways paternalism has been replaced by the term 'partnership', whereby women are actively encouraged to discuss care options and share in the decision to undergo Caesarean section.

Caesarean section: legal issues and principles

The main legal issues are around gaining consent to surgery, court orders and potential for trespass. There is a risk of an allegation of negligence if the surgery is not conducted to a good standard or there is a clinical error. Negligence and malpractice are discussed in Chapter 18. Trespass is considered in detail in Chapters 6 and 18. In Chapter 6 the author identified that there is no law of consent in so much that no single statute covers consent. Consent guidelines (Department of Health, 2003c; RCOG, 1997, 2009b, 2015; NMC, 2008d) identify the ways in which consent should be obtained.

Consent to Caesarean section usually takes place as an emergency during labour. Two clear dilemmas are evident. The first dilemma is whether consent obtained in an emergency can be valid. The second is whether consent that has been obtained during labour (when a patient is in pain, may have been receiving medication or is stressed and anxious) is reliable. Midwives regularly working on delivery suites and labour wards will be familiar with the speed and urgency necessary when a Caesarean section is required. Opportunities to provide detailed explanations and discussions are not available. The midwife will be reliant upon trust, inter-professional team working and demonstrating good communication skills to enable safe surgery to take place.

In an emergency it could be argued that there is insufficient time to provide informed consent and that an agreement to surgery is made based upon the 'best interest' principle. The midwife should ensure that the woman understands the reasons for surgery and where possible written consent is obtained. The surgeon would be undertaking the surgery in the interests of saving life (usually the baby's, but maybe both mother and baby). However, the woman cannot be forced to have a Caesarean section against her will and if she does not wish to have surgery (even if it seems unreasonable) her wishes must be upheld. However, if capacity is lost or compromised (patient is not conscious) the surgeon is undertaking the surgery in the best interest of the woman (there is a greater risk of her dying than the risk of a Caesarean) then the ethical basis for surgery is sound.

If a woman will not consent to a Caesarean section can the surgery take place on the basis that her partner consents to the surgery? No.

Would it be possible to declare that the woman lacks capacity and that in her best interests the Caesarean section is necessary? The Mental Health Act 1983 cannot be used when the woman does not like/does not wish the treatment offered. Only in an emergency can 'best interest' be used

Mental Health Act 1983

In the past the Mental Health Act 1983 has been used to secure or compel a woman to undergo a Caesarean section. If the ability of the woman to make a decision is compromised (fatigue, pain or contraction) or attention is lost (contraction, breathing techniques) the midwife will need to wait until the woman is able to listen and consider the options available to make a decision. The midwife cannot use temporary loss of capacity to claim/force/coerce a decision to be made.

Mental Capacity Act 2005

The Court of Protection may be used to determine mental capacity and also whether Caesarean section is in the woman's best interests. It is not for the midwife to make that decision.

Chapter summary

Ethical midwifery care demonstrates respect for childbearing women by enabling them to question options available to them, consider the recommendations made and make informed choices based upon good communication. Midwives play an instrumental role in the type of delivery experienced and need to ensure that women are well informed, choices are identified and the best interest is from the woman's perspective and not the best interest of the service or the midwife.

Case study: Sienna

Sienna is married to a professional cricketer. She is pregnant with their first baby and has undergone routine antenatal screening. Sienna's baby is a boy and she is looking forward to resuming her career (she is 'the face' of a well-known cosmetic company) after the baby's birth. Sienna has already agreed a contract with a national magazine to allow pictures of their new family in their home following the birth. Sienna attends an antenatal appointment and identifies that she is a frightened of labour and would like an elective Caesarean section.

Evaluation (ethical principles)

Tokophobia or fear of birth is not uncommon and is thought to affect one in six women. Sienna would appear to be making informed choices regarding her pregnancy. The dilemma for the midwife surrounds Sienna's choice of elective Caesarean section. The following questions identify the ethical dilemmas in Sienna's case. Is this Sienna's choice or has she been coerced into the decision? Is it Sienna's right to have an elective LSCS? Is elective LSCS available to NHS patients? What are the role and responsibilities of the midwife for the LSCS care pathway? Can the midwife provide sufficient support to Sienna to enable her to overcome her anxiety, reduce her fear and gain confidence in her ability to birth her baby boy?

Analysis (application of ethical theory)

Throughout all care episodes, the midwife will require excellent communication skills to enable the woman and her partner to be comfortable and confident regarding midwifery care. Midwives are able to provide a variety of information to women making choices regarding their care. What happens when a woman makes a choice that seems to be unreasonable or different from the majority? If a woman makes a choice that is less common, such as elective LSCS, should the midwife address this? When and how should the midwife discuss the issue of elective Caesarean section?

What can be done?

There are a number of dilemmas here for the midwife. When is the best time to discuss the issue

(continued)

of elective Caesarean section? Is a Caesarean section an option for Sienna? When should and to whom should the midwife refer the Sienna?

Implications for practice

It is likely that midwives will not always be aware of or informed of women's motivation and beliefs regarding childbirth choices. Partnership working requires excellent communication skills and a respect for others whose opinion is different from our own. It is likely that expectations of childbearing women may be unrealistic given the lack of funding for the maternity services. Interventions such as Caesarean section usually have a short-term solution but may provide long-term healthcare needs. The WHO (1995) recommends a 10–15 per cent LSCS rate.

Conclusion

Women have to make numerous choices regarding pregnancy and childbirth. Sometimes the rationale or decision-making process is difficult to understand. Sienna has made a decision based upon what she feels is best for her. The role of the midwife is to ensure that Sienna receives sufficient information to be able to weigh up the pros and cons for herself and make a decision. The midwife will need to ensure that facts are reported accurately and any personal bias is parked away from the discussion.

Case study: Sally

Sally is a young mum with learning difficulties. She has a daughter, called Susie (18 months old) and is currently expecting her second baby. Sally's mother (Mrs S) has parental responsibility for Susie and is concerned that she will struggle to look after this new baby. Mrs S has requested that when Sally undergoes an elective LSCS the doctor sterilises Sally at the same time. Mrs S could not possibly cope with looking after Sally as well as potentially three children.

Evaluation

It is outside the scope of this case study to consider the clinical indications and decision to undertake an elective Caesarean section. The focus here is regarding sterilisation of a person with learning difficulties. It is stated that Sally has learning difficulties, which suggests that Sally may not have capacity to consent. Mrs S, who has parental responsibility for Sally, agrees to the elective Caesarean section. It is unclear if Sally understands that in addition to the Caesarean section sterilisation is also planned. Patients with learning difficulties are at greater risk while accessing healthcare (Flemming, 2013). Government policy with regard to those who have learning difficulties is also clear in that there should be no decision about them without involvement regarding decisions on care (Department of Health, 2000). The dilemma is regarding the nature and extent of understanding that Sally has, her reproductive rights and her right to safe and effective healthcare. There can be no consideration regarding the potential or otherwise to be a good parent or judgement made regarding the skills or otherwise required for parenting.

Analysis

Unless there is a court order, the doctor may not sterilise Sally. The midwife has a role and responsibility to ensure that sterilisation does not occur during the Caesarean section. Sally lacks decision-making ability and therefore any healthcare decisions must be made under the auspices of the Mental Capacity Act 2005. Best interests should be determined using the checklist of factors identified in the Mental Capacity Act 2005. Any treatments for Sally can only proceed if it is in her best interest.

What can be done?

The midwife has a duty to improve the health and lives of those with learning disabilities. In fulfilment of this duty the midwife can be alert regarding situations when rights, interests and the safety of Sally are at risk.

Implications for practice

- Midwives are advocates for women.
- Midwives are in a position to safeguard vulnerable women.
- Inter-professional working is essential to ensure that the rights of vulnerable women are not compromised.

Conclusion

The right to self-determination for Sally means that she has the right to determine what is done or undertaken to her body. Individual autonomy is a basic principle upon which healthcare is based. Sally lacks the ability to make decisions and the Mental Capacity Act 2005 identifies principles to be upheld to ensure that Sally's rights and interests are upheld. As Sally's lack of capacity is permanent there is need to identify lasting power of attorney or court of protection deputy (public guardian).

Additional case study: Shona

Shona is a 37-year-old lawyer. She is in established labour with her first baby. The midwife caring for Shona is compliant with Shona's birth plan. While undertaking routine assessment of labour the midwife detects a variation in the fetal heart rate. The midwife gains consent from Shona to commence electronic fetal heart rate monitoring. The electronic monitoring reveals that the fetal heart rate is abnormal. In line with hospital guidelines a doctor is summoned and identifies that an emergency Caesarean section is required as the baby is very distressed.

Please use the framework below to complete this case study:

- Evaluation
- Analysis
- What can be done?
- Implications for practice
- Conclusion

Practice check

1. What is the current LSCS rate in your NHS trust?
2. When 'booking' place of birth are women informed of the LSCS rate?
3. When capacity is a concern, what guidelines are available to help you promote a woman's autonomy?

Useful websites

Confidential Inquiry into Premature Deaths of People with Learning Disability (CIPOLD):
www.bris.ac.uk/cipold
Improving Health and Lives Learning Disabilities Observatory (IHL):
www.improvinghealthandlives.org.uk/
Information about consent: www.dh.gov.uk
Information for people with learning disabilities: www.mencap.org.uk
Improving Public Health: www.gov.uk/government/organisations/public-health-england
Legal guidance on the Mental Capacity Act 2005: www.justice.gov.uk

16 Surrogacy

Pre-requisites for this chapter

Identify your own attitude to surrogacy and consider how it might influence your care.

Introduction

Surrogacy may be defined as 'the practice whereby one woman (the surrogate) becomes pregnant with the intention that the baby should be handed over to the commissioning couple (or individual) after the birth' (Jackson, 2006: 872). Dimond (2006a: 549) simplifies this to the use of another person for the production of a child. Partial surrogacy uses the surrogate's own eggs and the commissioning couple's sperm (or donated), whereas full surrogacy utilises assisted reproductive technologies (ARTs) in the form of embryo donation. The focus of this chapter is not physiology, clinical care or midwifery services, but the ethical and legal dimensions of surrogacy.

Surrogacy is a controversial subject with many opponents as well as supporters who believe that this may be the only way in which they can have a family. Ethical issues focus on attitudes and beliefs around motivation for becoming a surrogate, psychological aspects of caring for and then 'giving' away a baby, emotional attachments; legal issues are centred around commercialisation, contracts and status of the participants (birth mother, biological mother and parental responsibility).

Midwives have found themselves caught up in the emotional aspects of surrogacy as well as having concerns regarding possible conflict and care needs of the commissioning couple. The Royal College of Midwives (RCM) produced a position paper in 1997, *Surrogacy: Defining Motherhood*, in an attempt to address the concerns of its members. Some midwives may feel that surrogacy, like abortion, should be considered as grounds for conscientious objection.

Surrogacy first came to public attention in the 1980s after Kim Cotton became the UK's first surrogate mother. As a result of this there was adverse publicity, with the *Sun* newspaper calling it 'rent a womb'. Public attention was focused around the apparent lack of control over the process and the possible commercialisation and exploitation of infertile couples. As a result the Warnock Commission was set up which gave rise to the Human Fertilisation and Embryology Act 1990.

Ethical aspects of surrogacy

Having a baby may be viewed as a fundamental human right and that for those couples who are unable to conceive that right has been denied. There are many reasons for couples not being able to conceive naturally, and surrogacy has been considered one solution to being childless. Surrogacy relies on a third party and the first objection to surrogacy is based on the premise that the motivation of the third party may not be honest, permanent and without financial benefits. The second objection to surrogacy is that of risk – obstetric and medical risks to the surrogate and the baby. Another risk is that of psychological concerns around emotional stress, anxiety and possibly depression. Opponents feel that the risks of the birth mother declining to hand over the baby are great. The argument is: how can you possibly carry a baby for nine months or the duration of the pregnancy and then hand the baby over to the commissioning couple? If the surrogate has a partner he may not agree to the arrangement. For everybody, the anticipation of a baby may be an anxious and exciting time. Surrogacy has been made possible because of the skills and techniques used in assisted conception, embryo research and artificial insemination. It does not necessarily follow that because something is possible that it is morally right to do so. On the one hand, being able to fulfil the right to a family has to be considered against the inequality that some women cannot afford to pay for the services of a surrogate. Surrogacy raises a number of ethical-based questions such as:

- Should women be able to buy babies?
- Should a woman 'rent her womb'?
- What should the birth certificate say?
- Depriving children of the right to obtain knowledge of their personal identity is a violation of the European Convention on Human Rights (Article 8).
- What happens if the baby is abnormal?
- What if the baby is compromised during labour and an emergency LSCS is advised?
- How do other siblings feel?
- How does surrogacy 'fit' within the wider debate about adoption services and reform?
- Exploitation.
- Infertile couples, poor families.
- Baby selling schemes.
- Transatlantic infant adoption schemes or reproductive tourism is also a concern.
- The Hungarian geneticist Dr Endre Czeizel found guilty in Budapest of violating Hungary's Family Act in 2002.

Surrogate

Another ethical concern is around consent and surrogacy. Questions may arise about whether or not a woman is coerced or has been subjected to unreasonable pressure to carry a child. Sometime the pressures could be from a sister or other family member and the potential surrogate may feel obliged to offer her womb, go through pregnancy and childbirth to fulfill a relative's dream.

Consent is required by both the mother and father of the reproductive products.

There have been several high-profile cases of people who have donated reproductive products and their relationship has since come to an end (see the Natalie Evans case in the appendices). The Court of Appeal (2005) has upheld the 'father's right' to have such products destroyed (see Natalie Evans case).

Children's rights with regard to knowing one's origins have significance and importance to their psychological and emotional wellbeing. Sperm donor anonymity has been removed and the UN Convention on the Rights of the Child (1989) is clear that under Article 7 the child has a right to know its parents.

Artificial insemination by donor is not covered by the Human Fertilisation and Embryology Act

1990 and there has been concern that sperm can be purchased over the internet. In addition, there has been uncertainty of the father's situation (donor anonymity). The charity Childlessness Overcome Through Surrogacy (COTS) is not regulated and original concern regarding its activities and funding led to the need for legal provision to ensure that surrogates were not paid (so-called womb rental) so that COTS was a not-for-profit organisation.

The cost of surrogacy is also an ethical dilemma. At present there is a cost involved in IVF treatment and couples who bypass IVF treatment and go it alone using surrogacy may find the costs involved are very different. Is this justice? There is an argument that science should be used to enhance fertility and not to 'rent' a womb! If so, should all have equal access rather than just those who can afford to pay?

Assuming that surrogacy is a solution to the problem of childlessness and that it is ethically acceptable, are there any other concerns? The answer is yes. What happens when the child is born to a surrogate mother and has an abnormality or is less than perfect?

Issues have been raised regarding commissioning parents wanting a 'perfect child'. It could happen and has in America, whereby neither surrogate mother or commissioning mother wanted the baby – it then becomes a burden on the state!

Legal aspects of surrogacy

Primary legislation in the form of the 1985 Surrogacy Arrangements Act is the key statute. This was an emergency legislative framework to address the main concerns of the Kim Cotton surrogacy case. Subsequent legislation has sought to control and regulate the process of surrogacy. The Kim Cotton case first alerted the government to the need to regulate and control surrogacy arrangements. Surrogacy cases continue to make headlines and in June 2014 Louise Pollard from Plymouth was jailed for fraud when she posed as a surrogate mother and took money from two couples and subsequently claimed to have miscarried (BBC, 2014)

The Surrogacy Arrangements Act 1985

The Surrogacy Arrangements Act makes it a criminal offence to make commercial arrangements for surrogacy. Surrogate mothers are allowed to claim 'expenses' that are incurred via being a surrogate, but these expenses have to be reasonable. In some cases these are found to be excessive and unlawful. Other legislation which impacts upon surrogacy is as follows.

Human Relations Act 1998

This Act has previously been identified as containing basic human rights that everybody should be entitled to.

Adoption Act 1976

This Act makes provision for the legal adoption of babies and children. It identifies the specific requirements for the adoption.

The Adoption and Children Act 2002

This Act ensures that adopted children are able to know their origins.

Children Act 1989

Key aspects are around parental responsibilities. The birth mother automatically has parental responsibility. It can be shared and can be 'ordered' by the courts.

Children Act 2005

This Act focuses on safeguarding.

The Human Fertilisation and Embryology Act 1990

The HF&E Act 1990 established the Human Fertilisation and Embryology Authority (HFEA), which keeps under review and regulates the care of embryos. This Act is significant in that it ensures that gametes and embryos are stored and used appropriately. Consent is important regarding use and the HFEA are required to regularly review their procedures.

Section 27(1) Definition of mother

> The woman who is carrying or has carried the child as a result of the placing in her an embryo, sperm and eggs, and no other woman is to be treated as the mother of the child.

This also states who the father is:

> S.28(1) where a child is being or has been carried by a woman as the result of the placing in her of an embryo or of sperm and eggs or her artificial insemination if...
> a) At the time of the placing in her of the products as listed above the woman was party to a marriage and
> b) The creation of an embryo carried by her was not brought about with the sperm of the other party in the marriage.

Section 38

This section makes the provision that people are allowed to make conscientious objection (as with the Abortion Act). Both of the sections were influenced by the Roman Catholic Church.

The Human Fertilisation and Embryology Act (2008) (HF&E Act)

The HF&E Act 2008 has further changed the legal situation. The 2008 Act makes provision for the surrogate to have the legal right to change her mind and keep the baby, even if the baby is not 'biologically' hers (genetically related or implanted embryo). Section 54 of the HF&E Act 2008 provides the detail regarding parental orders. The HF&E Act 2008 also clarifies that the HFE Authority does not regulate or license surrogacy arrangements as such.

Chapter summary

Surrogacy is a controversial topic and midwives will have personal views regarding surrogacy. Ethically, surrogacy provides a solution to the human right to have a family. The dignity of a child and the confidentiality of the arrangements may be a challenge. The right to know one's biological origins is upheld provided that the surrogacy arrangement is legal. Legally it complicates the registration of births and the status of children. Surrogacy has attracted specific legislation to ensure non-commercialisation of the process. A midwife needs to be clear regarding focus of care, status of the biological mother and possible safeguarding issues.

Case study: Siân

Siân is a 32-year-old multiparous lady with three children (ages 5, 7 and 11). All three previous pregnancies were normal and the children are healthy. Siân and her husband (Ray) have made a joint decision for Siân to become a surrogate for her sister and her husband. Mr and Mrs H have undergone two unsuccessful courses of IVF treatment and feel that surrogacy is the only option for them now. Siân is now pregnant with a baby which resulted from assisted insemination (utilising Mr H's sperm)

Evaluation

Siân's situation may be regarded by some as brave as she is willing to put her own health at risk for her sister and her partner to have a baby. The motivation may be sympathy or compassion; either way the surrogate as the pregnant woman forms the focus of the midwife's duty of care. The midwife's own personal beliefs and attitude towards surrogacy should not interfere with the care, support and service which Siân receives. Midwives may have a number of questions (based on their own beliefs and attitudes) which they would like to ask (but should avoid) such as:

'What made you decide to do this?'; 'How can you possibly carry the baby and then hand it over?'; 'Do you feel obliged or pressured into doing this?'

Siân's choice causes a dilemma for the midwife and service provision. What duty of care does the midwife have towards the commissioning couple? Who is going to provide preparation for parenthood? What postnatal care is required and where? How can the midwife ensure that the baby receives routine screening, vaccinations and other appropriate healthcare?

(continued)

Analysis

There are a number of issues surrounding surrogacy.

* attitudes to surrogacy – including Brazier Report, Warnock Report;
* who does surrogacy benefit?
* does the surrogate (Siân) really choose or is she 'coerced' or feels obliged to undertake this agreement?
* pressure from relatives (Mr and Mrs H);
* conflict – between Siân and her sister;
* rights – confidentiality, autonomy;
* accountability.

Legal perspective/issues

* commercialisation of surrogacy: 1985 Surrogacy Arrangements Act; COTS (2007) Childlessness Overcome Through Surrogacy;
* enforcement of the arrangement;
* legal status of the baby – adoption.

Case law

* Re *C* [1985] (payments) [2002] 1 FLR 909
* Re *A* [1987] (adoption, surrogacy) 2 All ER 826
* Re *P* [1987] (family) 2 FLR 421

What can be done?

* Midwives are required to provide a professional service to all childbearing women.
* The midwife must involve a supervisor of midwives.
* The midwife should take extra care to ensure that communication is appropriate and effective.
* The role and responsibilities of a midwife must be completed for mother, baby and the family.

Implications for practice

* RCM (1997) *Surrogacy: Defining Motherhood*. RCM, London;
* NMC (2008d) Code (confidentiality);
* handing over of baby/parental responsibility/parental orders;

- provision of postnatal care to the surrogate and her baby;
- consent for vitamin K and routine vaccinations.

Conclusion

Surrogacy challenges the maternity services to deliver safe, effective and high-quality care to all parties. Normal patterns of care will not be appropriate and the midwife will need to make adjustments. Logistically, the birth mother and baby may not be together for long and the midwife needs to support the birth mother's needs throughout.

Activity/reflection

- Identify if the NHS trust you are working for has a policy regarding surrogacy.
- Consider what antenatal preparation may be required by (a) the surrogate and (b) the commissioning individual.
- Suggest how a midwifery care plan may meet the needs of the surrogate.
- Identify the type of approach used to manage surrogacy arrangements.

Practice check

1. What safety or security measures does your trust have in place for babies?
2. With regard to baby identification labels, are you clear what name to use?
3. What should the midwife do when discharging the mother and the baby?

Useful websites

Surrogacy Services: www.surrogatefinder.com
Surrogacy in the Ukraine: http://mother-surrogate.com
UK Surrogacy Organisation: www.surrogacyuk.org

17 Professional malpractice, misconduct and negligence

Pre-requisites for this chapter

Please read Chapters 1–4 to ensure that you are comfortable with the terminology used in this chapter. You will also find definitions of the abbreviations used in the front of the book. The NHS Constitution underpins the key concepts of this chapter.

Introduction

Having a baby is the most common reason for admission to hospital in England and, in 2012, there were almost 700,000 live births. The number of births has increased by almost one-quarter in the last decade, placing increasing demands on NHS maternity services. Maternity care cost the NHS around £2.6 billion in 2012–2013. Maternity cases account for one-third of total clinical negligence payments and maternity clinical negligence claims have risen by 80 per cent over the last five years. Nearly one-fifth of trusts' spending on maternity services (some £480 million in total, equivalent to £700 per birth) is for clinical negligence cover. According to the NMC 0.6 per cent of nurses are reported to the regulatory body for alleged misconduct (NMC, 2014b).

This chapter will focus upon professional malpractice, misconduct and negligence. It is not possible to consider malpractice and negligence without recognising that management of organisations also impacts upon the provision of care. Organisational accountability is also considered in this chapter. Midwives do not go on duty to provide poor, substandard or negligent care. However, maintaining the high standards of care required to all childbearing women can be difficult, especially when expectations are high and the number of midwives is low. Midwives need to understand what things or practices can make them vulnerable to a negligence claim, the implications for professional practice and how to avoid providing care that falls short of the standards required.

Previous chapters have demonstrated that midwives cannot practise in ignorance of the law. Professional obligations come as part and parcel of being a professional and require midwives to undertake high-quality midwifery care. Midwives who fail to demonstrate those standards are accountable for not only their acts but also their omissions, or as Griffith *et al.* (2010) suggest: what you do and what you fail to do. Midwives are accountable to patients, the profession, employers and personally accountable to themselves. The legal frameworks are mainly civil and professional, but occasionally a criminal framework may be relevant (FGM, fraud, etc.).

The high standards of professional practice and the increasing expectations of women and their families regarding care during pregnancy and childbirth result in pressures in the delivery of all aspects of maternity care. Headlines in national, local and professional press frequently remind midwives of the risks involved in healthcare provision. Clinical governance, investigations into clinical incidents, report writing and action plans add to an already stretched and stressed workforce. Mistakes are costly not just in terms of finance, but morbidity, mortality, stress, anxiety and disappointment. This chapter focuses upon the perceived increase in negligence, legal framework and process. Midwives are accountable professionally, personally and contractually.

Midwifery healthcare ethics

The NHS Constitution (Department of Health, 2012b) identifies that the public have the right to expect that patients are at the heart of everything that we do. The provision of high-quality care should be safe, effective and focused upon the patient experience. Core values central to the NHS Constitution are respect and dignity, compassion, commitment to quality care, improving lives and maximising resources for the benefit of the whole community. With these values in mind, the midwife also has a specific role and responsibility regarding care during pregnancy and childbirth (NMC, 2010a). In addition to upholding basic human rights (Chapters 2 and 4) midwives also have duties to perform and skills to demonstrate (Chapter 5) in the upholding of ethical-based care (NMC, 2015). Midwives who fall short of the standards are personally accountable for their behaviours, acts or omissions. In Chapter 5 it was identified that the NMC is required to set out and maintain professional standards. The midwifery duty of care is found in the NMC Code (2015).

Trust

Midwives are required to be 'open and honest, act with integrity and uphold the reputation of your profession' (NMC, 2010a: 1). Midwives should act lawfully both in their professional and private lives. Student midwives during the course of their education and training gain insights and understanding as to how professional practice affects their personal lives. Social media are widely accessed and midwives need to be aware of the NMC (2010a) guidelines regarding its use. Lack of respect, judgemental comments, accusations and inappropriate language used in social media do not uphold the reputation of the profession. In addition, photographs or snapshots may be used as evidence of an individual being in a particular place at a particular time, which may not be where they are contractually bound. Women during pregnancy and childbirth need to be able to trust the midwife too.

Dignity and respect

These are central to the NHS Constitution and the NMC (2015) Code. Dignity is concerned with treating women and their families with kindness and consideration. Treating women as individuals has been fundamental to midwifery care and *Changing Childbirth* (Department of Health, Expert Maternity Group, 1993) focused upon choice, continuity and control for women accessing the maternity services. Other aspects of the ethical basis of dignity and respect are around confidentiality, consent, collaboration and clear professional boundaries. Midwives are required to provide screening programmes as recommended by the UK National Screening Committee.

Protect and promote health and wellbeing

In order to fulfil this standard of care midwives are required to share information with colleagues, work effectively as part of a team, delegate effectively and manage risk (NMC, 2010a). It is this part of the NMC Code that directly conflicts with the autonomy of the midwife.

High standard of midwifery practice

High standards of midwifery care are not only about using the best available evidence and keeping skills and knowledge up to date. To be able to demonstrate high standards of midwifery care midwives must also keep clear and accurate records (NMC, 2010a: 7). A key part of record-keeping is also to identify how effective interventions, medicines and care have been (see Chapter 7).

Uphold the reputation of your profession

Midwives are required to demonstrate personal and professional commitment to equality and diversity. An important aspect of this value is 'you must only cooperate with the media when you can confidently protect the confidential information and dignity of those in your care' (NMC, 2015: 9).

In short, midwives must be trustworthy and failing to comply with the NMC Code (2010a) can bring your fitness to practise into question, which can risk losing your registration. Midwives who fail to uphold the NMC Code or Midwives Rules and Standards risk having their fitness to practise investigated through the process of midwifery supervision (discussed in detail in Chapters 5 and 10).

What is professional malpractice?

Professional malpractice is when a midwife fails to uphold the Code of professional conduct, performance or ethics. The NMC fitness to practise directorate is responsible for the investigation, proceedings and reporting of allegations of malpractice and misconduct.

An allegation of impairment of fitness to practise on grounds of misconduct, lack of competence or ill health may be made by a member of the public, colleagues, employers or LSA. The investigations are thorough and if it is thought there is a case to answer the practitioner is referred to the NMC conduct committee. A number of sanctions may be applied.

The public and professionals can see the list of dates, names and nature of the NMC investigations. The findings (results) are recorded and published. All are located on the NMC website.

Each employer has a responsibility to check the NMC register on a regular basis and on any employment offered to ensure that the practitioner is registered.

The definition of what constitutes duty in professional practice is identified in the *Bolitho* v *City and Hackney Health Authority* [1997]. The *Bolitho* case requires that if a duty exists then the standard of care required is that of a reasonable man or in the case of maternity services what a reasonable body of midwives would do. Over-reliance on trust guidelines or policy is not tolerated by the courts; the midwife still has to demonstrate she has not blindly followed them. In a court all aspects of the policy will be scrutinised from the development, design writing and implementation of them! Policies must be evidence-based and up to date (see *Reynolds* v *North Tyneside Health Authority* [2002]).

Professional fitness to practise was questioned in the case of Paul Beland (NMC Hearing 2 November 2007). Paul conducted a home birth during an NHS trust suspended home birth service, without informing the supervisor of midwives (SoM). In 2004 Paul was suspended from practice by the LSA for failing to have vital equipment, leaving before care was completed during a home confinement and failing to document/complete care records.

Accountability and the NHS

The NHS Constitution (Department of Health, 2012b) identifies the rights to which patients, public and staff are entitled. The NHS 'belongs to us all' (Department of Health, 2012b: 2), which reinforces the notion that the common set of principles and values of the NHS bind together patients, staff, communities and the people it serves. The NHS Constitution (2012b) clearly identifies that there are seven principles which are the consensus or beliefs of the British public, NHS patients and staff. The seven principles are:

1. The NHS provides a comprehensive service, available to all.
2. Access to NHS services is based upon clinical need, not an individual's ability to pay.
3. The NHS aspires to the highest standards of excellence and professionalism.
4. The NHS aspires to put patients at the heart of everything it does.
5. The NHS works across organisational boundaries and in partnership with other organisations in the interest of patients, local communities and the wider population.
6. The NHS is committed to providing best value for taxpayers' money and the most effective, fair and sustainable use of finite resources.
7. The NHS is accountable to the public, communities and patients that it serves.

Ethical-based care is underpinned by values and beliefs about the way in which care is planned, provided and evaluated. The values of the NHS have been identified as: working together for patients, respect and dignity, commitment, compassion and improving lives; the NHS does not exclude, discriminate against or leave people behind regarding healthcare (Department of Health, 2013: 5). While these ethical values are important, patient rights enforce them. Patient rights are the way in which the NHS is accountable. Patients have the right to have any complaint about NHS services acknowledged within three working days and to have it properly investigated (NHS, 2013: 9). Maternity services are a good example of how patient rights are upheld. It is not uncommon for women who have accessed the NHS with their first pregnancy to return subsequently and identify that 'it was not like this, last time'. Improvements to the safety, effectiveness and experiences for childbearing women are ongoing and midwives are at the forefront in developing birth environments, care pathways and professional relationships to improve quality of care.

Governance

Governance is the collective term given to the 'systems and processes by which Trusts lead, direct and control their functions in order to achieve organisational objectives, safety, and quality services' (Department of Health, 2006: 11). Governance is applied to all aspects of maternity care, from education, research, clinical and risk management. Clinical governance is supported by a number of quality frameworks. Quality frameworks for the maternity services are provided from a number of sources – for example: RCOG, NPSA (surgical checklists), NICE (guidelines and clinical pathways), in addition to the policies and procedures of the local NHS trusts.

Clinical safety is paramount throughout the NHS. Safety in the maternity services is achieved by having clinical procedures, reduction of risks and high standards of care. Mothers and babies have the right to be looked after and cared for in as safe an environment as possible. The Clinical Negligence Scheme for Trusts (CNST) assesses maternity units on an annual basis against CNST standards and awards the unit a level between one and three. In 2010 the maternity service at Guys and St Thomas' became the first in the country to achieve a top accreditation of level three (*Practising Midwife*, 2010: 11).

Never events are defined as 'serious, largely preventable patient safety incidents that should not occur if the available preventable measures have been implemented by healthcare providers' (Department of Health, 2011b). The Department of Health publishes a list of these serious but avoidable patient safety incidents (Department of Health, 2011b). For the maternity services, never event number 25 concerns maternal death due to postpartum haemorrhage after elective Caesarean section. However, numbers 1 (wrong site surgery); 3 (retained foreign object post-operation); 8 (intravenous administration of epidural medication); 9 (maladministration of insulin); 15 (falls from unrestricted windows); 19 (misplaced naso- or oro-gastric tubes); 20 (wrong gas administered); 21 (failure to monitor and respond to oxygen saturation; 22 (air embolism); and 23 (misidentification of patients) are all relevant. These never events may be considered to be systems and human factor failures and as such are reported and investigated using clearly defined procedures and processes.

NHS hospitals are required to meet good standards of care at all times. Ethical standards around privacy and dignity, and legal standards around storage of records and confidentiality, are all measured. Often, when the NMC is investigating a complaint or alleged substandard care it emerges that the problem is not specific to an individual care worker. There may also be 'systems' failures whereby the organisation has wider issues that impact upon patient care.

Quality monitoring of maternity services

The Care Quality Commission (CQC) are charged with upholding standards of care delivery in England. The CQC is one part of the clinical governance that the government has over the NHS. In addition there are also the following quality monitoring aspects:

- Reporting of equipment faults go to the Medicines and Healthcare products Regulation Agency (MHRA).
- Serious Incidents (SIs) – not to be confused with statutory instruments! Serious incidents are identified and listed by the NHS trusts and are required by midwives to be reported.
- The NHS regulator (Monitor) also has a quality role in the maternity services. Monitor is an independent regulator of NHS foundation trusts. Its role is currently to assess applicant trusts and to regulate them. It is said to regulate the foundation trusts using a risk-based approach. The key aspects of this are 'timely, focused and proportionate' (Monitor, 2012). The Health and Social Care Act (2012) identified that Monitor is the new role as a 'sector regulator for England'. The primary function of this is to protect and promote patients' interests. It also demonstrates how proposed new legislation may change, strengthen and amend roles and responsibilities.

While Monitor regulates the NHS trusts, the NMC regulates midwives. Midwifery supervision is the quality mechanism used by the regulatory body. Annual inspections by the LSA identify areas of excellence and concern as part of their statutory functions. Sometimes it comes to the attention of the regulatory bodies that there are problems in provision of healthcare. In July 2011 the NMC undertook an unannounced extraordinary visit to University Hospitals Morecambe Bay NHS Foundation Trust (UHMBT) in conjunction with the Care Quality Commission (CQC). The maternity services are based in Furness General Hospital (labour ward, maternity wards) and Royal Lancaster Infirmary (neonatal unit). The review was a result of concerns relating to the quality of supervision of midwives and maternity care at the trust. The scope of the visit was confined to the provision of statutory supervision within UHMBT. In December 2011, the Quality Care Commission (QCC) revisited University Hospitals Morecambe Bay. The NMC updated the Hospitals Action Plan for the trust in March 2012:

> We are maintaining close monitoring of the safety and wellbeing of mothers and babies via our Local Supervising Authority reporting system. There is evidence that supervisors of midwives are providing leadership and driving the cultural changes necessary to ensure that the safety of women and their babies remain the focus of their activities.
>
> (NMC, 2012)

A return visit was undertaken in June 2012. This degree of scrutiny by the QCC and the NMC is expensive and time consuming. Following the Francis Report (2013) it is hoped that by identifying specific problems early, working with care providers and engaging with staff that quality standards will improve in the NHS. A more recent example has been the NMC report in Guernsey.

Public inquiries

The effect of numerous public inquiries, reports and reviews regarding health and social care have highlighted problems which a stretched and complex organisation such as the NHS has. The cost of inquiries, investigations and case reviews are not just financial. Stress and anxiety experienced by healthcare providers is increasingly seen. While recruitment of student midwives is buoyant, levels of attrition of student midwives have increased. Midwives leaving and unfilled midwifery posts are examples of how maternity services are struggling to cope. The RCM annual reports on the state of the maternity services highlight the numerical challenges in providing a maternity service (RCM, 2011, 2012b, 2013b).

Coroner Cases – Helen Rhyder (Banbury)

Midwives are providing maternity care for increasingly complex pregnancies. Whenever there is a maternal or baby death the case is referred to a Coroner. The Coroner's inquest is intended to identify any neglect, misconduct or criminal evidence which contributed to the mortality. In the case of Helen Ryder (NMC, 2011) failure to monitor a high risk patient and failure to provide basic care needed by a vulnerable patient resulted in Helen's dismissal from the NHS Trust and removal from the NMC register. A coroner in Coventry (Coventry Telegraph, 2012) identified that a maternal death was caused by a serious infection that was missed by hospital staff. The NHS Trust identified that lessons had been learnt and intensive sepsis training has been provided to enable staff to respond appropriately to the early signs and symptoms of infection.

What is negligence and is there any evidence of increased litigation?

Negligence is a civil wrong or tort. Negligence may be defined as 'a careless act' or 'an act or omission which causes damage'. When taken in the context of healthcare, clinical negligence usually refers to failure to act in a way that a reasonable person would act in the provision of healthcare. Clinical negligence has a long history and key case law such as the *Bolam* case [1957] have influenced the concern that healthcare providers have regarding compensation. Any person seeking compensation for personal injury or death must prove the following elements of negligence: duty of care, breach of duty of care, causation and harm.

Allegations of negligence may be defended in the following ways:

- denial of facts;
- a missing element;
- contributory negligence;
- willing assumption of risk (volenti non fit injuria);
- exemption of liability;
- limitation of time.

The final defence of limitation of time is not usually relevant to the maternity services as negligence in relation to birth injury or harm caused during birth to the baby may not be evident at the time. A delay or late diagnosis in children is not uncommon and birth injuries are not restricted in law to a time limitation.

Negligence claims are uncommon in maternity services, but when actions are taken they are upsetting and depressing for all concerned. The press and media use horrific headlines to create news reports, which ensure public attention and suggest that neglectful care and misconduct are prevalent. Headings like 'perineum hacking' provoke anxiety and stress for pregnant women who have yet to labour. The reality is that 694,241 women birth their babies in England each year (RCM, 2013b). The number of negligent cases is comparatively few. However, the national shortage of midwives coupled with the rising birth rates are not likely to see a reduction in negligence claims. The RCM (2012b) identifies that negligence claims are expensive to the NHS both in terms of time and money. Increasingly, whole departments have been created to provide legal advice services to NHS trusts. The situation is not helped by advertisements in local and national press regarding 'no win, no fee' and the blame culture which exists within our society. Symon (1998) identifies the views of midwives and obstetricians regarding litigation. Interestingly, Symon's research demonstrated that there is a strong perception that negligence litigation has increased and that as a result of this clinical practice has changed. Certainly, midwives currently working in the NHS are increasingly using risk assessment tools and reporting concerns (serious incident reporting).

The legal framework of negligence is one way of demonstrating liability regarding carelessness. In addition to the awarding of damages the midwife will be subjected to challenges regarding her care, registration and good character. Professional integrity will be subjected to scrutiny and may be found wanting. Expert witnesses have been used by the courts to provide specific medical and midwifery expertise to enable the courts to understand professional standards.

There are thought to be approximately 650,000 births across England and Wales every year (NRLS, 2014). The majority of births are safe and midwives and other healthcare professionals work hard to provide care and ensure that the data collection and information provision are carried out.

The NHS Litigation Authority (NHSLA) provides information and data regarding the number and type of claims it handles. All clinical claims since 1 April 1995 have been handled under the Clinical Negligence Scheme for Trusts (CNST). The CNST is a voluntary risk-pooling scheme for the NHS trusts, foundation trusts and primary care trusts. Any claims prior to April 1995 are handled under the Existing Liabilities Scheme (ELS), which is centrally funded by the Department of Health. Regional health authorities (abolished in 1996) have a smaller Ex RHA Scheme to cover negligence claims. In 2005/2006 the NHSLA reported receiving 5,697 claims (including potential claims) under its CNST scheme; in 2006/2007, 5,426 claims; and in 2007/2008, 5,470.

Symon (2006c) suggests that the apparent increase in medical negligence litigation is also blamed for a number of side-effects such as defensive practice, lowered recruitment and the need to set aside a proportion of the healthcare budget to pay damages and insurance premiums against further potential damage claims. In order for a successful negligence claim the following elements must be demonstrated: duty of care, breach of duty of care, causation and harm (damage) (Jones and Jenkins, 2004).

Duty of care

Any midwife providing care while employed in an NHS trust or privately for maternity services has a duty of care to women and their families. The duty of care is identified in the NHS Constitution (Department of Health, 2012b) and clearly requires midwives to fulfil these duties in the course of their employment. Duty of care consists of professional practice, clinical standards, evidence-based practice, compliance with care pathways and clinical judgement and decision making. While these duties are broad considerations that midwives must comply with, there is scope for demonstrating personalised care. The patient's right to safe, effective and respectful care underpin the duty of care. The NMC (2010a) Code identifies the professional standards regarding duty of care and this includes consent and information-giving and summoning medical help at an appropriate time. The duty of care also means that there is a legal obligation to ensure that the midwife always acts in such a way as to not cause harm (negligence).

Legal cases provide us with the detail with regard to duty of care. The key regarding duty of care is: what is reasonable? If it is reasonable to expect that somebody will be harmed by a midwife's action or inaction, then reasonable foreseeability demonstrates a duty of care is owed. For example in *Donaghue* v *Stevenson* (1932) the court established that a duty exists to those who are closely or directly affected (proximity) by an act or omission. Thus, a duty of care exists if the midwife could reasonably contemplate that an individual could be affected. An example would be a partner present at the birth of his baby – it would be reasonable to contemplate that his proximity means that the midwife has a duty of care towards him.

The extent of your duty of care is demonstrated in the case of *Sidaway* v *Bethlem Royal Hospital* [1985], whereby a professional is required to exercise skill and judgement in the improvement of the physical and mental wellbeing of a patient. Clearly, for a midwife the implications of the *Sidaway* case are that the duty of care encompasses the full role and responsibilities of the midwife identified in the NMC Code.

Choice cannot be provided unless the resources are available. The mother cannot insist upon having access to them. The law gives no legal right for the client to insist that services are available. Failure to provide (waiting) does not necessarily imply that there has been a breach of statutory duty. In the case of *Pearce* v *Bristol* [1998], it was found that the mother was not able to insist upon a Caesarean section.

Breach of duty of care

Assuming that a duty of care is demonstrated, in order for a negligence claim to be successful it must be demonstrated that there is a breach in the duty of care. Standards of care can vary from practitioner to practitioner and from time to time. The courts have provided clarification as to what standard of care is expected and that any findings must be made in keeping with the clinical practices of the time.

Low or poor standard of care is when the standard falls short of what is required by a reasonably competent midwife. The standard of 'reasonably competent' was identified in the case of *Bolam* v *Friern HMC* [1957]. The *Bolam* case led to the so-called 'Bolam test' which is applied by the courts to confirm if the standard of care provided was that of a practitioner who is reasonably competent in the opinion of his or her peers.

In the case of *Whitehouse* v *Jordan* (House of Lords) [1981] Jordan was found guilty in 1980 of negligence regarding a failed forceps delivery that occurred in 1970. In the appeal the court ruled that Jordan was not guilty of negligence as he should be judged by the standards of care at the time in question (1970), and not by the standards at the time of the trial (1980). In 1970 it was not uncommon to undertake a trial of forceps. This case has implications for all subsequent maternity cases as the court must be informed of standards of practice which were in place at the time of the allegation of negligence.

Failure to stick to an identified care pathway would not normally be subjected to a negligence claim as long as the midwife can demonstrate clinical reasoning. Griffith (2009a) identifies that where professional practice deviates from care pathways this is not considered negligent if variance can be demonstrated.

Causation and harm

In order for a negligence claim to be successful there must be a causal link between the duty and the harm (see *Wilsher* v *Essex Area Health Authority* [1986]). Mortality or any harm that a mother or her

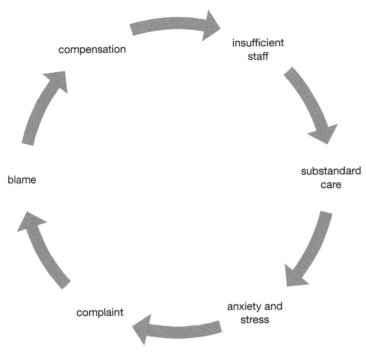

Figure 17.1 The cyclical nature of negligence and the NHS

baby suffers has to have resulted from the alleged negligent act. In negligence claims harm is usually considered to be personal injury, pain and suffering, although the loss of the ability to have children and post-traumatic stress disorder also are relevant here.

The ethical dilemma here is how you can measure the severity or impact of harm in order to be able to provide financial compensation. Realistically no amount of money can return a loved one.

Liability and compensation

Strict liability and vicarious liability are the two common types of liability. A midwife employed in the NHS automatically has indemnity provided by the employer. Changes to indemnity regulations have meant that midwives can no longer work independently of the NHS. If a negligence case is proven and liability is found, the NHS trust is required to pay compensation. The spiralling cost of litigation cases has caused many NHS trusts financial difficulties. Figure 17.1 illustrates the cyclical nature of negligence and malpractice. Throughout the cycle, staff numbers and behaviours have an impact.

Clinical risk

Given the nature of work in midwifery and obstetrics, it is important to ensure that all staff are able to meet policies and quality standards in the delivery of care. Most NHS trusts have a strategy for monitoring, managing and escalating risks encountered in clinical environments. Clinical management tools such as SBAR (Situation, Background, Assessment, Recommendation) are used to clearly identify if a case requires handover, escalation or transfer. Root cause analysis (RCA) considers compliance with relevant procedures and processes as well as human factors which impact upon dangers or risk to the woman and her family. Frequently, obstetric trigger lists identify those events which must be reported and investigated. Events are usually coded as serious, significant and untoward. Some NHS trusts use grades (red/orange/yellow/green). Managers (clinical risk) using standardised processes review these incidents and a report is prepared and presented to management group meetings. An RCA and action plan is identified for all serious incidents or events. The final part of the process is providing feedback to staff via email, newsletter and multidisciplinary team meetings. The function of the clinical risk team is to be proactive in monitoring, managing and escalating risks; investigate reported incidents; and foster a culture of support for risk management. Professor Brian Toft and Simon Reynolds (2005) identify that organisations that learn from mistakes and have taken steps towards active learning influence and promote a culture of safety.

Clinical Negligence Scheme for Trusts

The CNST is the way in which the government tries to exert control over the increasing number of negligence claims in the NHS. Maternity services in England account for a 'significant portion of the number and costs of claims reported to the NHSLA each year' (NHSLA, 2010). There are identified levels of risk for each trust. In order to identify the level of risk each trust is assessed against specific standards and an assessment made as to how they meet or do not meet the standards. This annual review is significant from a number of perspectives. A good review and achievement of clinical risk standards demonstrates excellence in patient care and management. Practitioners are also able to use the review to understand how 'safe' their working practices are. Managers are able to audit how compliant with procedures and best practice the service is. Clinical Risk Maternity Management Standards (NHSLA, 2010b) are organised into the following categories:

1. organisation
2. learning from experience
3. communication
4. critical care
5. induction, training and competence
6. health records
7. implementation of clinical risk management
8. staffing levels.

Each NHS trust is measured on the above categories and awarded a level of operational safety. Levels are level 0, 1, 2 and 3. Level 1 is associated with good performance in all categories across the entire maternity service and good risk management. Clinical risk management uses a number of tools to monitor and report clinical standards of care. Special terms are given to clinical situations, which can then be managed to enable the organisation to learn from any good practice or mistakes.

Never events (Department of Health, 2013) are 25 types of incident which are serious and preventable patient safety incidents. In 2009/2010 the National Patient Safety Agency (NPSA) identified a strategy (framework) for healthcare workers, clinicians, managers and Board members.

The NPSA is currently reviewing the safety issues surrounding the use of intravenous gentamicin to neonates and the safety for women with placenta previa following Caesarean section. In addition, the NPSA has adapted the WHO surgical safety checklist for the maternity services.

Prevented never events

This is the term given to anticipation or identification of the possibility of patient harm, whereby the midwife protects the woman before harm potentially occurs by being vigilant and actively preventing the event. Patient safety is like safeguarding – it requires all healthcare workers to engage in protecting the client from the risk of harm.

Fresh eyes approach

A fresh eyes approach has been used in relation to ECTGs (electrocardiotocographs or fetal monitors). As a management tool a 'fresh eyes approach' is useful as it enables a midwife who is not directly involved in providing care to take an independent look at the care provided. The author suggests that this approach be used for other aspects of maternity care and could be part of clinical supervision.

Defensive practice or 'just in case' obstetrics

A 'just in case' approach is where a practitioner advises or undertakes a treatment or intervention 'just in case', with a view to reducing the likelihood of litigation. The threat of litigation reduces practitioners to defensive practice such as elective Caesarean section, induction of labour or continuous electronic fetal monitoring. While these practices do not guarantee safety or reduce litigation, practitioners may feel that they are 'covering themselves' in that they have eliminated some risks associated with childbirth. From an ethical perspective defensive practice reduces women's rights, demonstrates paternalism and reinforces the notion that control is in the hands of the healthcare professional.

Chapter summary

The modern NHS is accountable for provision and delivery of high-quality healthcare. The system of governance is in place to ensure a safe and quality maternity service. All staff are required to demonstrate the six Cs (Department of Health, 2012a) and uphold the NHS Constitution (Department of Health, 2012b). Quality mechanisms and management tools enable midwives to identify priorities and meet healthcare needs. Poor midwifery practice is uncommon; if mistakes are made it is the woman's right to receive an explanation and apology. Midwives need to be able to recognise the trauma experienced and know how to avoid a similar mistake. Patient expectations are high and for the maternity services the demand and individual requirements of childbearing women are extensive. The financial cost of a negligence claim is extensive as legal fees, staff time and costs associated with harm and provision of healthcare may be for a lifetime. The emotional costs (for all concerned) are difficult to measure. There is no other NHS service where the nature, extent and costs are so keenly felt. Maternity services are the most demanding and the most rewarding of healthcare environments.

Case study: Sasha

Sasha, a 28-year-old primigravida, gives birth to a baby girl following a five-hour labour. Sasha has her husband as her birth partner, care during labour is provided by a midwife with 22 years' experience. Following the birth, the baby is placed skin-to-skin on Sasha's chest and the umbilical cord is clamped and cut by the midwife. During the cutting of the cord the midwife cut through the baby's finger at the same time.

Evaluation

In this unusual and rare emergency situation the harm caused to the baby must be managed and treatment provided. There are other issues of harm which also need consideration. In addition to managing the clinical situation the ethical basis for care must be considered. Sasha has already been through labour and her recovery will be impacted by the stress of the trauma to her daughter. The dilemma is that in order to provide the baby with appropriate care it is necessary to remove the baby from her mother.

Giving birth is a memorable experience, which is closely followed by a period of adjustment to being a new family. The experienced midwife is supporting the process of mother–baby attachment by placing the baby 'skin to skin'.

The midwife has requested medical aid to manage the emergency and will need to continue providing care for Sasha. A paediatrician will undertake the clinical management of the severed finger of the baby. Additional midwifery help is required to ensure that Sasha and her partner are cared for while the midwife is being cared for as well.

Analysis

Is the midwife fit for practice? Unless the midwife has identified that she is unwell or unable to work it is presumed that a midwife is fit for practice and will maintain the standard of care and uphold the NMC Code. The above incident would suggest that care has fallen short of what would normally be expected of a registered midwife and a report would need to be made. A supervisor of midwives (SoM) would be involved and would ensure that the midwife was supported, as she would undoubtedly be anxious, upset and traumatised by the situation.

Is the midwife negligent? It would be for the courts to decide. The NHS trust will conduct its own investigation, Clinical governance procedures will be followed. The midwife will also be investigated by the LSA and a full case review undertaken.

What can be done?

The first issue is that emergency care must be provided for the baby. Midwives providing care during labour must be able to call for medical and midwifery aid in an emergency. An NHS trust that does not have the correct workforce configuration is putting patients at risk.

The second issue is whether the midwife was negligent. While on initial consideration it would appear to be negligence, an investigation is necessary to establish the facts. In addition to the midwife manager's investigation, a supervisor of midwives will also investigate and the midwife will be required to make written statements (usually one for the manager and one for the investigating SoM). The midwife manager has a duty to provide support to the midwife at this time and allow the midwife time to write a statement.

Implications for practice

Cutting the umbilical cord is a routine practice following the birth of the baby. NHS trusts have guidelines in place for undertaking this procedure. Busy maternity hospitals provide midwives with equipment (delivery packs, cord clamps and cord cutters) to undertake clinical procedures. An incident involving equipment must be reported to the MHRA (MHRA, 2003).

Conclusion

This unusual case is a reminder of the responsibility and multiple aspects of the role of the midwife. All midwives (regardless of experience) must demonstrate fitness to practise and be fit for purpose while providing care. During the process of childbirth there are many risks both to mother and baby. It is essential that midwives are able to reduce and eliminate risks to a professional standard. What may be perceived as straightforward on initial consideration has the potential to become complex. What may be perceived as complex may become straightforward. Midwives must be familiar with the seven steps to patient safety and be self-aware regarding their own abilities and attributes. If a problem or incident occurs it must be reported, managed and the incident learned from. The NMC is responsible for protecting the public from substandard or poor care.

Case study: Sky

Sky (20 years of age) required suturing after an episiotomy during a vaginal birth. The midwife followed the procedure for the perineal repair. The midwife needs a clear view of the wound to be able to suture and places three swabs into the vagina to secure a clear view. The intention is to remove the swabs following completion of the procedure. Only two swabs were removed. Sky went home and the error was only brought to light when the swab fell out three days later.

Evaluation

The relevant ethical principle here is that of non-maleficence. The midwife has failed to remove all swabs and has placed Sky at risk of harm. In addition, it is vital that the correct procedure is followed once the incident is identified. The midwife has failed to remove the swab, failed to

(continued)

count the swabs at the end of the procedure, failed to document and fallen short of the standard required of a healthcare professional.

Analysis

The ethical principle relevant here is non-maleficence. The midwife should not harm patients and as a result of failing to remove a swab the midwife has increased the risk of harm to Sky from infection. In addition, the midwife has failed to uphold the standards of conduct and ethics required by the regulating body (NMC).

The midwife has not fulfilled the duty to provide a high standard of care or promoted the health and wellbeing of Sky. It is likely that the incident will be investigated, and as part of the investigation the midwife will be required to allow notes to be reviewed and a statement to be written. Clinical supervision of midwives is undertaken by the LSA and an SoM will be allocated to investigate and another to support the midwife.

Sky should formally complain to the NHS trust. The person who is informed of 'fallen out swab' must ensure that Sky is able to and is supported in making a complaint. Following receipt of the complaint, the NHS trust should uphold 'best practice' and reply promptly, informing Sky of what is being done and how the complaint is being managed. An apology should be issued at the earliest opportunity and the person being informed of the 'swab fall out' should be familiar with and able to follow the NHS trust's complaint procedure.

Sky will also require clinical follow-up and a care pathway should be identified to ensure that future care meets professional standards.

It is likely (given the current climate of blame) that Sky may wish to seek compensation for poor care. While litigation might not be first on her mind she may be persuaded by others to consider this option. Sky would be unlikely to be successful in a negligence claim, as she does not have all the elements for successful litigation (she is missing the element 'harm').

What can be done?

- The complaints procedure should be identified and explained to Sky.
- The midwife should be informed of the NHS trust's response of the complaint. The midwife should be given the opportunity to uphold the NMC (2010a) Code in showing concern and treating Sky respectfully. An opportunity for a personal apology should be considered.
- The NHS trust and the LSA will conduct an investigation simultaneously. An SoM will also support the midwife during the investigation process and in the writing of a statement.
- The NHS trust will review policy and procedures regarding suturing following vaginal birth and will ensure that the guidelines are based upon current standards and best practice.
- The midwife will be asked to supply all notes and documents to the manager, she would be advised to keep a copy of the documents.
- Confidentiality will be maintained and those with 'privileged' information connected with the case will be required to conduct themselves professionally.
- The midwife will reflect upon the clinical incident and will need to identify any actions or professional development.

Implications for practice

The failure to remove the swab meets the definition of a 'never event'. All swabs should have been counted at the start of the procedure and again at the end. The fact that Sky did not suffer any harm as a result of the swab being retained does not mean that 'all is well, that ends well'. The retained foreign object (never event 3) compromised patient safety and must be reported using the correct procedure. The never events policy framework (Department of Health, 2013: 5) identifies that failure to learn lessons from a single event (such as Sky) 'could be perceived as organizational failure', and Board leaders such as the Chief Executive and Nurse Directors are accountable.

Conclusion

This case study identifies that clinical errors made by a midwife are reported, investigated and dealt with by a number of processes (reporting, midwifery supervision, incident investigation, patient safety, never events and patient complaint). It is thought that never events are mainly system failures. However, the above case illustrates poor clinical practice by an individual midwife. Reporting serious incidents is a legal requirement of the Care Quality Commission (CQC) regulations: 'to err is human, to cover up is unforgivable, and to fail to learn is inexcusable' (Donaldson, in *Never Events Policy Framework*, Department of Health 2011b: 7).

Practice check

1. Check local trust policy/guidelines regarding episiotomy and repair. Is the policy evidence-based and up to date?
2. If the local trust policies were audited: are they regularly updated?
3. As a midwife can you demonstrate that you are working to the standard of a skilled professional?
4. Do you have the opportunity to attend maternity incident meetings?
5. Can you identify if your NHS trust learns from mistakes?
6. The NHS Constitution (Department of Health, 2012b) applies to all staff: how far are you able to go towards upholding the pledges?

Useful websites

Department of Health:
https://www.dh.gov.uk; www.gov.uk/government/publications/the-nhs-constitution-for-england
House of Commons Public Accounts Committee: www.publications.parliament.uk/pa
Monitor – the independent regulator of NHS foundation trusts: http://monitor-nhsft.gov.uk/home
National Health Litigation Authority: www.nhsla.com
National Patient Safety Agency (NPSA): www.npsa.org.uk
National Reporting and Learning Service (NRLS): www.nrls.uk

18 Whistleblowing and complaints

Pre-requisites for this chapter

You should be familiar with the NHS Constitution and with the key recommendations of the Francis Report and confidential enquiries into mortality, including the CIPOLD Report.

Introduction

Midwives are effective and efficient care providers to women and their families during childbirth. The NHS has benefited from high standards of professional care for childbearing women. However, if you scrutinise midwifery education and training, how much preparation is given to developing a midwife with attributes and virtues that support moral practice? What types of ethics are considered in the midwifery curriculum? How do students learn and understand that ethical principles are an integral part of everyday midwifery care and not just rhetoric around good communication skills? A virtue-based approach to midwifery does not focus upon midwifery practice (skills and knowledge) but focuses upon values and the ability of the midwife to provide high standards of care in challenging circumstances (high client expectations, numerous choices/demands and lack of appreciation by women and managers). Key findings of the Francis Report (2010, 2013) was that healthcare was not demonstrating compassionate care to a consistent standard, patients were not always the priority and entrants to the nursing profession should be assessed for their aptitude to deliver and lead proper care, and demonstrate an ability to commit themselves to the welfare of patients.

Customer care is an important aspect of business and service delivery. Most major businesses develop and provide staff training for customer care. They usually have complaints procedures and staff dedicated to responding to customer comments and concerns, as well as complaints. Establishing an efficient and user-friendly complaints system enables businesses to enhance their image, increase satisfaction and reduce staff stress. The NHS has in recent times recognised the importance of customer care and has begun to address complaints with a humanistic approach. Complaints procedures have been identified and formulated. The reason for this is that if a complaint is handled well the outcome for the business is usually less of a problem and less expensive than the mismanagement of a complaint. Complaints made by patients are thought to be increasing and the media have contributed to a blame culture. Stories that the NHS is failing patients, that staff are behaving badly and NHS trust data are inaccurate, is fuelling an environment in which staff feel undervalued and stressed. Patients and their families are increasingly aware that reporting healthcare experiences is important and that episodes of care should be satisfying and prompt. Patients know that some treatments and interventions are risky, but any problems and blame can be attached to the NHS and compensation is your right if harm is proven. To deconstruct the emergence of the blame culture is outside the scope of this text. However, it is important to note that when an NHS Trust provides compensation it effectively reduces the capital spent on staff.

Professional practice is fundamental to quality healthcare. Practitioners are accountable and must always be prepared to justify all decisions and actions. The NMC has raised the profile of midwifery supervision in an attempt to demonstrate robust regulation and control of midwifery professional practice. Midwives need to be able to articulate and demonstrate the role and responsibilities as identified in the Midwives Rules and Standards. Women and their families are able to access the Department of Health, NHS, local NHS trusts and NMC information on nature and extent of maternity services and midwifery care that is expected. Women and their families are able to contribute to and participate in choices and should be supported by professional practice that enables them to feel confident with the care and comfortable with the care providers.

Compensation for adverse events and outcomes is a valid and ethical outcome. Managers have to be able to interrupt the downward spiral associated with substandard care, negligence and professional malpractice and compensation pay-outs, rising staff costs and fewer staff. In the maternity services alone, shortages of midwives are challenging the ability to provide minimal postnatal care and threatening one-to-one care during labour. The Clinical Negligence Scheme for Trusts (CNST) was introduced to manage spiralling costs of litigation in the NHS. Implications for NHS trusts are that a CNST assessment is undertaken on an annual basis and NHS trusts can manage potential claims in an effective way. The maternity services also have the Local Supervising Authority (LSA) whose function is to protect the public.

Whistleblowing is the process of exposing illegality, misconduct or dishonesty in an organisation. A whistleblower is an individual who decides to expose the alleged dishonesty, etc. (usually to an outside organisation or the media). Famous whistleblowers such as Edward Snowdon, Julian Assange and Mark Klein exposed issues with security and IT. Barbara Allitt and Julie Bailey famously identified and reported poor standards of care and abuse of patients in Staffordshire.

The Francis Report identified that for the Mid Staffordshire NHS Trust the provision of healthcare was itself diseased. The illness (poor-quality healthcare leading to premature patient deaths) was undetected by managers due to the pre-occupation with cost cutting, targets and poor financial management. Whistleblowers such as Julie Bailey identified the illness (problems) and were themselves subjected to bullying and tactics intended to undermine personal credibility. Julie reported that NHS staff contributed to personal harassment, including the necessity to close her business for a time. The government's response to the Francis Report was for Jeremy Hunt (Secretary of State for Health) to identify that 'the health and care system must change' (NHS Confederation, 2013: 1). *Putting Patients First and Foremost* (the official government response) identified a new statutory duty of candour for providers, not individuals, pilot schemes for students seeking NHS funding for nursing degrees to first serve up to a year as a healthcare assistant and criminally negligent practice to be referred to the Health and Safety Executive. A key recommendation to improve the culture of care involves staff training and motivation using a new model of performance frameworks to be developed by Health Education England (HEE) and NHS employers. The ethical principle of compassion is at the heart of modern healthcare and all staff must have compassion as well as skills (NHS Confederation 2013: 2) The recommendation is that all student midwives (like other NHS-funded students) will be recruited using a values-based approach to selection.

In previous chapters ethical issues have been considered from a principles approach. Ethical issues have been addressed using the four ethical principles of autonomy, beneficence, non-maleficence and justice (Beauchamp and Childress, 1994). This chapter will undertake a virtue-based approach. Virtue ethics consider the morals of the individual practitioner or patient. Instead of concentrating upon the principles of ethical-based care, this chapter will address the values and character traits of individuals who are motivated to whistleblow or complain and the law addressing these behaviours.

Ethical issues

The expectations of all patients accessing the NHS have escalated, none more so than in maternity care, as successive reports (*Changing Childbirth* (Department of Health, Expert Maternity Group, 1993), *First Class Delivery* (Audit Commission, 1997), *Maternity Matters* (Department of Health, 2007), *Delivering High Quality Midwifery Care* (Department of Health, 2009), *Midwifery 2020: Delivering Expectations* (Department of Health, 2010c)) have identified that childbirth should be safe but also should be emotionally satisfying. Women have raised expectations around all aspects of childbirth regardless of the complexity of their pregnancy. New challenges and opportunities for midwives (Department of Health, 2010) require them to provide high-quality care and fulfil women's health and social care needs and expectations. It should also be noted here that midwives themselves have raised expectations by informing women of choices, providing continuity of care and including partners in all aspects of child-birth. The government agenda with regard to the maternity services has always been ambitious and the maternity services have been considered to be a yardstick on which other health services are measured. Midwives are the foundation of the maternity services; women and their families are the focus of our care, and collaborative working promotes quality care.

Complaints, escalating concerns and whistleblowing

It is widely recognised that the culture of a working environment plays an important part in terms of the behaviour of staff and the policy and practices used. A blame culture is an environment whereby blame or fault is apportioned to an individual while ignoring other aspects of poor, substandard or sloppy practice. A blame culture feeds from a bullying attitude and need to protect oneself. Where a blame culture exists, it is unlikely that patients, staff or reports which identify malpractice are likely to be heard, understood or acted upon. Complaints, raising concerns (reporting) and whistleblowing are all ways in which poor care, malpractice and systems failures can be identified.

Generally, patients are reluctant to complain for fear of being labelled 'difficult' or 'demanding'. Patients may also be afraid that in making a complaint subsequent care may be compromised, restricted or lost. The dilemma for the patient is: will I be treated less well if I have complained? From the midwife's perspective, it is necessary to ask oneself 'how do I feel and behave if a woman or her family challenge, complain or confront me?' In other words, how should midwives respond to complaints?

In maternity care the stakes are particularly high as the midwife has both mother and baby to consider. While a woman may behave in a way in which a baby may be compromised (drugs, smoking, alcohol consumption), the expectation is that the midwife has a duty to behave in a way that promotes fetal wellbeing, while being caring and compassionate towards the mother. The dilemma for the midwife is trying to strike a balance between the woman's rights and the need to promote the health and wellbeing of a baby yet to be born (no rights).

Raising and escalating concerns is the way in which midwives can suggest to managers difficulties in providing high standards of care. Raising and escalating concerns (NMC, 2013) is a professional requirement and managers need to be able to respond to midwives who are concerned about patient care. Understanding the nature and extent of the midwife's concern relies upon the service sharing the same values as the midwife. While high-quality maternity care has an ethical basis, so too does the provision of maternity services. Women expect excellence and equity in the NHS and as such require choices, services and continuity in a service which is flexible to meet their needs, efficient and effective, available and attractive, while provided on a limited budget and finite resources. Midwives are encouraged to escalate their concerns if struggling to provide care. Compliance and complacency (Mander, 2011) must be considered, as both can impact upon maternal mortality.

Audit is an important management tool for identifying problems or trends in midwifery practice. Personal audit of clinical care, midwifery audit of medicines management and audit of incident reporting all help in the identification of issues. Using the information obtained during audit may provide the midwife with an opportunity to identify and share concerns regarding care. Failing to act upon or ignoring evidence of poor care, audit and reports or mortality rates is unprofessional and in itself professional misconduct.

Confidentiality is always important. Midwives are privileged to information which would not normally be shared with other care providers or often a partner or husband. The midwife has a duty to protect confidentiality and to ensure that the woman has confidence that the information provided will not compromise her safety.

Legal issues

Legislation in the form of the Public Interest Disclosure Act 1998 identifies that responsible whistle-blowers require protection from employers, so that they do not lose their jobs as a result of escalating concerns or whistleblowing.

The provision of healthcare is complex and requires evidence-based practice and effective and efficient quality care. Increasingly, a business approach utilising metrics such as waiting times, time to treat and standardised information systems has been adopted. Since 1985 primary legislation in the form of the Hospital Complaints Procedure Act has ensured that patients have opportunities to make their concerns known to management.

In 2008 the European Court of Human Rights ruled that whistleblowing was protected as 'freedom of expression'.

Accountability is demonstrated in that where serious harm or death has resulted from a breach of the fundamental standards, criminal liability should follow. Gagging clauses and non-disparagement clauses are a way of silencing staff or limiting the ability of staff to disclose issues regarding patient safety and care.

Clinical governance is the legal framework for concerns regarding clinical care and quality. NHS trusts are also managed by a Board and the business model uses a customer-experience approach to monitoring the health service provided. A customer (NHS patient) has raised expectations of healthcare which includes much more than treatments and interventions. The modern NHS is measured on buildings, waiting times, comfort and atmosphere. Patient satisfaction with all aspects of the NHS are being measured and reported. Reducing complaints and the correct handling of complaints is important for staff as well.

Professional practice

All health and social care professionals have guidelines which identify specific roles and responsibilities. All guidelines also identify that health and social care professionals should work together to provide high standards of patient care.

Quality care

In 2010 the government's white paper (strategy) identified that to improve the NHS patients would be put at its heart through an information revolution and greater choice and control. Many of the attributes (shared decision making, access to information, choices about care and control over their own care records) were common in the maternity services. The new emphasis is on patient choice of any provider, choice of consultant-led team, choice of GP practice and choice of treatment. We will extend choice in maternity through new maternity networks.

The government strategy identified that patients would be able to rate hospitals and clinical departments according to the quality of care they receive, and we will require hospitals to be open about mistakes and always tell patients if something has gone wrong. Maternity services are not excluded from the rating system. 'Families and friends' tests are being used to rate all aspects of maternity services, from parent preparation classes, care in labour and postnatal levels of satisfaction. It is thought service user involvement in the design, delivery and evaluation of maternity services will benefit staff, students, women and their families. The Quality Care Commission is responsible for the monitoring of the services and experiences of women and their families (see also Healthwatch England, a patient-focused website that focuses on health and social services).

The system will focus on personalised care that reflects individuals' health and care needs, supports carers and encourages strong joint arrangements and local partnerships.

The key ethical approach of the modern NHS is that everyone, whatever their need or background, benefits from the 2010 strategy. Equity in the NHS extends to equity regarding involvement.

Complaints procedures

In Chapter 17 (on negligence) it can be seen that a complaint is often the first step or event in a possible negligence claim. It is important, then, that all complaints received are responded to and result in an appropriate response if healthcare workers are to avoid legal actions. A complaint does not always become a negligence claim, but if it is handled incorrectly can cause stress and anxiety to patients, staff and employers. In the past midwives may have been asked not to say 'I am sorry' for fear that in saying this they were admitting to errors, malpractice or guilt. Post-Francis Report, it is evident that patients and their relatives are even more unhappy when healthcare workers are not sorry for failings in care or system. Nurses are the largest professional group among healthcare workers worldwide (Parahoo, 1997). In the UK nurses, midwives and health visitors represent the largest workforce within the NHS and yet they are least likely to be informed about complaints and least likely to be trained as to how to manage them.

Legal status of student midwives

Pre-registration students are not professionally accountable for acts and omissions, but the nurse who is supervising is! The situation is different for the midwifery shortened course as students who are already on the NMC register are bound by the NMC Code (2008d).

All students (as adult learners) are expected to control their own learning experiences in so much as they do not undertake anything for which they have not been trained. Student midwives are required to identify needs with tutors and mentors. In addition, students have a responsibility to discuss when they are worried or see something they feel is wrong.

NHS Constitution

HEE identifies that 'even though the scale of what happened at Mid Staffordshire makes it stand out, there are pockets of poor culture, poor behaviour, lack of care and lack of compassion around the rest of the NHS' (Cumming, 2013). Following the Francis Report, NHS England has introduced the Family and Friends Test (FFT) to gather views in all NHS maternity units on three aspects of the maternity services (antenatal, labour and postnatal care). The FFT has been successfully used in A&E and other acute patient services. It is not possible here to debate the assumption that maternity services are similar to acute patient services. While other tools have been used to evaluate maternity services, the FFT is being promoted on the basis that every pregnant woman or new mother will have an opportunity to be heard. Results of the FFT and maternity services were published in January 2014.

Chapter summary

The blame culture, found in all aspects of social life, supports a thriving industry around litigation; healthcare litigation has also increased. Patient safety is paramount and staff safety is also a priority. Financial costs of errors both in the delivery and management of the maternity services are challenging. There are many dilemmas associated with maternity services and midwifery care. For many midwives there is urgency for more support regarding complex care, increasing birth rates and raised expectations. There is a dilemma for the NHS: while students and training are important and the NHS cannot operate without them, utilising unqualified or unregulated staff as main care providers is a risky business. Suitably qualified and regulated practitioners are also vulnerable and human errors; competency, skill and immorality may compromise care. Recruiting, selection and retaining midwives with the ability to provide ethical-based, evidence-based and effective care is challenging. Midwives and midwifery will always be judged on the last episode of care. Women's memories of childbirth last a lifetime and their experiences will impact upon their personal, family and friends' lives.

The maternity services are unlike any other NHS healthcare provision and consideration should be given to utilising a tool to evaluate the service which reflects the expectations of women, their families and midwives.

The ethical dilemma for the midwife is that in articulating concerns, stress or anxiety around maternity care of childbearing women they risk investigation of their own practice, alienation of colleagues, doubts regarding professional behaviour and fear of unemployment.

Staying positive, acquiring and maintaining clinical and communication skills will enable midwives to continue to provide the highest quality maternity care. Good leadership and management will enable the provision of maternity services which meet the high expectations of childbearing women and their families. A personal midwifery philosophy based upon customer focus, professional rigour and innovative midwifery is the future for the maternity services.

Case study: Sharon

Sharon is a labour ward coordinator of a busy NHS trust maternity unit. The trust delivers approximately 6,000 women per year and have a midwife:delivery ratio of 1:33.

Sharon is 'in charge' on a busy late shift and is combining the provision of midwifery care and coordinating the labour ward. Sharon is the named midwife for a lady (Charlotte) whose labour was induced on the early shift. Meanwhile, three other women go on to deliver their babies and Sharon is required to admit a lady with a twin pregnancy to the labour ward. An emergency LSCS for another lady is required and Sharon organises this event and ensures that staff are in theatre and the neonatal unit staff (appropriate grade and number) are attending. Charlotte has not seen Sharon for some time and her husband goes on the hunt for Sharon. Charlotte's husband is unhappy as he has been with Charlotte a long time and he is impatient because she has not had the baby. Charlotte is uncomfortable and tired. While her husband is looking for Sharon, Charlotte is on her own, becomes upset and cries because she feels unsupported and her labour is going on for a long time. Charlotte's husband cannot find Sharon so he asks another midwife to come to see his wife. The midwife provides his wife with pain relief and checks the fetal heart rate, which is within normal limits. The midwife returns to provide care for her 'caseload' for the shift.

Evaluation

The above case could be considered from an ethical principles approach. However, a moral-based approach will be utilised to enable the application of the six Cs to the clinical case. The author justifies this approach based upon the fact that maternity services not only requires skilled practitioners, but those with the values, beliefs and attitudes that prioritise women-focused care.

The moral responsibility of the midwife (Sharon) is not only a commitment to demonstrate and provide competent midwifery care, but to provide excellent midwifery care when faced with challenges such as shortage of staff, unrealistic workloads and lack of appreciation of the complexities of childbirth by the public. How Sharon approaches care and management during this episode of care is influenced by the NMC Code (2010a) and the NHS Constitution (2012b).

Analysis

From the above case it would seem that the midwife (Sharon) is an experienced midwife who is managing a labour ward in which workloads are frequently changing and client expectations are high. The maternity service aims to provide one-to-one care during labour and midwives are the most likely person to provide this in the UK. The RCM recommends a midwife-to-birth ratio of 1:28. In the maternity service in which Sharon is employed the ratio is stated as 1:33 (the national average). Frequently, prospective midwifery students identify that maternity care is 24 hours, 7 days per week and 365 days per year. The reality is that a midwife frequently works a variety of shift patterns, may be called in at short notice to provide support and may not be able to take breaks easily. All prospective students state that they understand the commitment required but most fail to realise the impact upon family life and lifestyle this responsibility entails. Sharon is working a late shift and ensuring that midwifery care is provided to all women on the delivery suite is her focus. In addition to providing care for Charlotte, Sharon also has a role in managing the department and supporting the midwifery team. There is a legal requirement to ensure that employment legislation and working directives are upheld. Sharon's role will also include ensuring that government guidelines with regard to maternity metrics are complied with (birth notifications, data entry, coding and records).

What can be done?

The moral virtues or characteristics that ensure that Sharon makes good choices in her clinical practice will have been developed throughout her experiences as a midwife. Sharon will be mindful of the need to treat Charlotte kindly and considerately. Sharon cannot afford to remain as the main care provider for Charlotte if she is to ensure that other women and midwives are supported. Sharon will need all the leadership and management skills she has acquired to ensure that women are not discriminated against.

Implications for practice

- Sharon must escalate her concerns regarding staffing levels.
- The labour ward team require support from other midwives.
- A supervisor of midwives must listen to Sharon and respond to her concerns.
- Management may need to close the maternity unit from any new admissions to ensure that adequate care can be provided to those women already in labour.

Practice check

1. Who is responsible for acknowledging complaints in your maternity service?
2. Have complaints increased in the last six months? If so, why?
3. What are the latest results in your NHS trust for the family and friends test?

Activity/reflection

1. A friend of yours has recently given birth at her local maternity unit. While visiting her and the new baby at home you notice that the baby has red marks on each side of the face. Your friend is

uncomfortable and finding it difficult to sit down. She is due to attend the postnatal clinic at six weeks. What ethical issues can you identify for: (a) the midwife; (b) the maternity service?

2. On the postnatal ward a first-time mother identifies that the midwife who looked after her during labour was rough and shouted at her. What actions do you think you should take?

Reflection

Using Driscoll's interrogative model of reflection consider complaints using the following headings:

- What are complaints?
- What do I do if I receive a complaint or hear about substandard care?
- What can I do to improve patient care in my clinical area?

Useful websites

Clinical negligence, see Department of Health: www.doh.gov.uk
Cure the NHS (campaign group): www.curethenhs.co.uk
Francis Report: www.midstaffspublicinquiry.com
Francis Report on Whistleblowing (Freedom to Speak up) at: https://freedomtospeakup.org.uk
Litigation, see National Health Service Litigation Authority (NHSLA): www.nhsla.com/Pages/Home.aspx
National Patient Safety Agency: www.npsa.org.uk

Appendices

Appendix 1: cases

Baby P (Peter Connelly)

Peter Connelly died in London after suffering over 50 injuries over an eight-month period.

Baby P was born 1 March 1 2006 and died 3 August 2007. Baby P's identity was revealed following expiration of a court anonymity order 10 August 2009.

On 11 November 2008 two men were found guilty of the murder of Baby P. The mother had already admitted allowing or causing Baby P's death. There was insufficient evidence for a murder charge.

Baby P's case was widely reported for four reasons. First, the magnitude of Peter's injuries; second, criminal proceedings including a potential murder charge; third, because Peter lived in the London Borough of Haringey, the same authority that was involved in the case of Victoria Climbié, whose death had led to a nationwide review of child protection services (Laming Report, 2000); fourth, there were a number of high-profile dismissals and resignations of staff. Senior government officials were involved and social media added to the publicity.

To view the timeline go to: http://news.sky.com/skynews/Home/UK-News/Baby-P-Timeline-Of-The-Toddlers-Tragic-Life-Haringey-Social-Services-Premature-Death/Article/200811215151356

The Baby P Report (2008) details mistakes made in the handling of the case. The full text will not be made public.

Laming (2009) published a progress report following the death of Baby P, which identifies that too many authorities have failed to adopt reforms identified in his previous review. This is significant as management of Child Services, in particular safeguarding procedures, continue to dominate professional concerns.

Daniel Pelka

Daniel Pelka was born on 15 July 2007 and died on 3 March 2012. The Serious Case Review (Coventry Safeguarding Children Board, 2013) identifies that the circumstances of Daniel's death suggested that he had been suffering abuse and neglect over a prolonged period of time. Daniel had an older and younger sibling (the latter born August 2011, also in the UK); he was the middle child of a family who had migrated from Poland in 2005. Home was not a safe place for the family; domestic abuse and violence, alongside excessive alcohol use by Daniel's mother and her partners, later led to the household being described as 'volatile' by the Serious Case Review (CSCB, 2013: 6). It identifies the abusive experiences of Daniel and his siblings. The ethical issues for Daniel were around the sustained inhuman treatment and torture; his abuse was of all types. The legal issue was abuse and murder. However, the abuse of his older sibling should also be remembered. Poor professional practice regarding communication, use of a sibling as an interpreter and reporter, as well as issues with record-keeping contribute to lessons that must be learned from Daniel's sad life. Daniel's mother and her partner were charged with Daniel's murder on 9 March 2012. They were convicted of Daniel's murder on 31 July 2013.

Daniel Pelka suffered and died as a result of a systematic failure of safeguarding strategy and the ability of his mother to hide his abuse, manufacture an illness (eating disorder) and isolate him from his family. This case is particularly worrying for midwives as Ms Luczak was able to present an image of being caring and concerned about her children while physically, psychologically and neglectfully abusing Daniel. The Serious Case Review identified 'confused and ineffective communication', 'inappropriate advice' and 'lack of referral' which prevented purposeful intervention which may have made a difference in assessing the family situation.

The police were called to the family home on many occasions and there were 27 reported incidents of domestic abuse. Daniel's mother (Ms Luczak) accessed the maternity service in February 2011 and Daniel's sibling was born in August 2011. While undertaking the discharge of Ms Luczak and the new baby, the midwife made contact with the Children, Learning and Young People (CLYP) directorate and spoke with a duty officer. The family were known to the social workers and Ms Luczak identified that she was happy to go home. In October 2011 a referral was made to the community paediatrician. In December 2011 a home visit was carried out by an education welfare officer (EWO). Between December and February Daniel was investigated for poor weight gain, excessive appetite (he was reported to be constantly hungry and thirsty). He was prescribed iron syrup, zinc tablets and vitamin drops. On 2 March 2012 Daniel was absent from school. On Saturday 3 March Daniel was admitted to hospital having suffered a cardiac arrest and could not be resuscitated. Daniel's siblings remained in the family home until they were taken into foster care on Monday 5 March following examination of Daniel, which revealed bruising to his head and the exact nature of his emaciation and neglect.

Robert Hercz (1986) case to European Court of Human Rights.

- Right to prevent partner from having an abortion.
- Project Genesis: a child's life is too precious to owe its survival to the decision of one person (woman).
- Partner Vivian Haandstad termination of pregnancy.
- Society for the Protection of the Unborn Child: Right to be Born Society was founded by Robert Hercz.

Paton Case

- *Paton v Trustees of British Pregnancy Advisory Service* [1978] 2 All ER 987.
- Mr Paton asked the courts to prevent his wife going ahead with a termination.

- The English courts ruled that Mr Paton had no *locus standi* provided that terms of the Abortion Act 1967 were fulfilled.
- Mr Paton took the case to the ECHR, citing a breach of Article 8 (right to respect for family life).
- The ECHR ruled that the rights of the mother were protected under para. 2 of Article 8.
- The ECHR ruled that the father has no right to be consulted regarding termination of pregnancy.
- The fetus does not have legal personality/rights until it is born (Congenital Disabilities Act).

Sidaway v *Bethlem Board of Governors [1985]*

Mrs Sidaway underwent an operation for recurring pain in her neck, right shoulder and arm. Performed by a senior neurosurgeon, there was a 1–2 per cent risk of damage to the nerve root and spinal column.

The plaintiff was left severely disabled. She brought an action in negligence, claiming that she had not been given adequate warning of the risks.

During the hearing it transpired that the surgeon had told her of the risks of damage to the nerve root but not the risks to her spinal column.

Did the surgeon act negligently? The surgeon was conforming to what in 1974 had been accepted as standard medical practice *by a responsible and skilled body of neurosurgeons*. Therefore, the House of Lords rejected the claim that the surgeon had acted negligently.

Gillick v *West Norfolk and Wisbech AHA and the DHSS [1985] 1 AC 112*

Doctors consulted at a family planning clinic by a girl under 16 years would not be acting unlawfully if they prescribed contraceptives, so long as in doing so they were acting in good faith to protect her against the harmful effects of sexual intercourse.

Victoria Gillick (five daughters) went to court to challenge the decision.

Cabrera case (2009)

Mayra Cabrera, 30, died shortly after giving birth to her son Zac at Great Western Hospital (GWH) Swindon, Wiltshire in May 2004. The baby survived.

The inquest revealed that following delivery, Bupivacaine, a potent anaesthetic, was wrongly fed into a vein in her hand (usually given into the spinal cord). The inquest jury said that gross negligence by Swindon and Marlborough NHS Trust, specifically substandard storage of drugs in the maternity unit, had led to the death.

Mr Arnel Cabrera (38) had been told immediately afterwards that his wife had died from an amniotic fluid embolism but later learned (after instructing a lawyer) that she died because Bupivacaine had been administered wrongly.

The Cabreras came to Britain from the Philippines after Mrs Cabrera got a job as a theatre nurse in 2002. Mr Cabrera (IT consultant) was granted leave to stay until 2009, provided his wife was working at the hospital. Mr Arnel Cabrera was deported to the Philippines.

This landmark case 'shared responsibility' for the cause of the drug error. The NHS trust was liable.

Sally Clark case

Sally Clark was convicted of the murder of her sons. Dr Meadow was involved as an expert witness against 80 women convicted of cot death. Sally Clark was released from prison after three years. Her release was secured when additional evidence found that the post mortems of her babies revealed microbiology results that had not been disclosed to the police. *Staphylococcus aureus* was found from eight sites of the baby's body (Harry, her second son), including the cerebral spinal fluid.

Katie Thorpe case

The case of Katie Thorpe, from Billericay, who is a wheelchair user, raised fundamental issues of medical care and patients' rights, even though it has not been tested in court.

- Katie's mother, Alison, had asked the hospital to remove the teenager's womb because she believed it would improve her daughter's quality of life.
- Ms Thorpe, who held discussions with a consultant gynaecologist at the hospital, said she wanted Katie to avoid the 'pain, discomfort and indignity' of menstruation.
- The decision by a hospital in Essex not to carry out a hysterectomy on a 15-year-old girl with cerebral palsy was welcomed by charities supporting people with disabilities (January 2008).

Diane Blood (1999)

- 1997: widow allowed dead husband's baby.
- The Court of Appeal made a historic judgment in favour of a widow being inseminated with her dead husband's sperm. The 1990 Human Fertilisation and Embryology Act banned Diane Blood, 32, from using her husband Stephen's sperm without his written consent.
- The court has ruled Mrs Blood's case is unique – sperm should not have been removed in the circumstances.
- The court said Mrs Blood should be allowed to seek fertility treatment within the European Community but not in the UK.
- The Court of Appeal has clarified the law by confirming the extraction and storage of sperm without written consent is unlawful.
- Doctors at the Free University's Centre for Reproductive Medicine in Brussels took nine months to agree to give Mrs Blood fertility treatment.
- Mrs Blood publicly announced her pregnancy on 27 June 1998.
- She gave birth to her son Liam – weighing 5 lb 13 oz – four weeks early on 11 December 1998 at Jessop's Hospital in Sheffield.
- On 17 July 2002 Mrs Blood gave birth to her second son – using her husband's frozen sperm – Joel Michael at the Royal Hallamshire Hospital in Sheffield.
- She claimed victory in her legal battle to have her late partner legally recognised as the father of her children in February 2003.

Natalie Evans (2005)

Natalie Evans, from Wiltshire, started IVF treatment with her then-partner Howard Johnston in 2001. However, the couple separated and Mr Johnston withdrew his consent for Ms Evans to use the embryos, which had been fertilised with his sperm.

The Court of Appeal ruled in June that Ms Evans could *not* use the embryos. She is asking the court to consider whether UK law, which now requires her six stored embryos to be destroyed, is a breach of her human rights.

Ms Evans underwent IVF treatment following a diagnosis of ovarian cancer. Six embryos were created and placed in storage.

Ms Evans applied to the High Court for permission to use the embryos in IVF treatment.

She argued that Mr Johnston, from Gloucester, had already consented to their creation, storage and use, and should not be allowed to change his mind.

However, her case was dismissed both by the High Court, and later by the Court of Appeal. The House of Lords decided it would not consider the case.

The current Human Fertilisation and Embryology Act – which governs IVF treatment – says that consent from both man and woman is vital at every stage of the process.

Muiris Lyons of solicitors Alexander Harris, who represented Ms Evans, said:

> Natalie has now been left with no choice other than to take her case to Europe. She feels very strongly that she should be allowed to use her stored embryos. She cannot understand that the law requires them to be destroyed when they represent her last chance to have a natural child of her own. If the UK law says that Howard can change his mind at any time, then Natalie feels that the law is unfair and breaches her human rights. It gives a man an absolute veto, which outside of the world of IVF and fertility treatment he would not enjoy.

The European Court of Human Rights ruled in a majority verdict that, even in such exceptional circumstances as Ms Evans', the right to a family life – enshrined in Article 8 of the European Convention on Human Rights – could not override Mr Johnston's withdrawal of consent.

A panel of seven judges made the ruling, which read: 'The Court, like the national courts, had great sympathy for the plight of the applicant who, if implantation did not take place, would be deprived of the ability to give birth to her own child.'

It also ruled unanimously that the embryos did not have an independent right to life.

Beth Warren (2014)

Beth won the right to stop her dead husband's sperm being destroyed by the Human Fertilisation and embryology Authority (HFEA). HEFA are the regulator and had taken a technical approach to sperm storage. Mrs Warren had the right to grieve for her husband before making a decision regarding use or destruction of the sperm.

P, C & S v The United Kingdom [2002] 2 FLR 631

- European Court of Human Rights. A complex case which concerned possible violations of Article 6 and 8 of the ECHR.

- Emergency removal of a child at birth (Emergency Protection Order).
- It concerned an American mother; the father was a social worker. This case related to her second baby, born in Rochdale. The mother had been convicted in California of an offence relating to care of her first child with her previous husband (administering laxatives inappropriately).
- The court recognised that Social Services had legitimate reasons for concern but did not support removal of the child (six hours old) from its mother and father.
- See Bainham (2005: 550).

Appendix 2: practitioner mal practice cases

Dr Harold Shipman

- When investigating deaths, coroners failed to identify links between Dr Shipman and a series of deaths.
- Dr Shipman (GP) was convicted at Preston Crown Court in January 2000.
- He was convicted of murder, having killed at least 250 of his patients over 23 years.
- He committed suicide in Wakefield prison on 13 January 2004.
- The Coroners and Justice Act 2009 makes provision regarding the need to undertake a post mortem and if an inquest is appropriate. If a death is not thought to be a natural death, coroners are also able to summon a jury to decide on the cause of death.
- The inquiry has published six reports. The first concluded that Shipman killed at least 215 patients. The second found that his last three victims could have been saved if the police had investigated other patients' deaths properly. The third report found that by issuing death certificates stating natural causes, the serial killer was able to evade investigation by coroners. The fourth report called for stringent controls on the use and stockpiling of controlled drugs such as diamorphine.

Dr Roy Meadow

- Coined the term 'Munchausen's syndrome by proxy' in 1977.
- Was an expert witness for shaken baby syndrome in child protection cases.
- Offered testimony in the 1993 Beverly Allitt case.
- Was an expert witness in 80 cases of sudden infant death.
- Said 'one cot death is tragic, two is suspicious and three is murder'. Was involved in the conviction of over 80 women convicted of cot death murders.
- In the Sally Clark case his research (stats) and expertise (one in 73 million chance) were called into question.
- Sally Clark was released from prison on the grounds that the conviction was unsafe. Sir Roy Meadow's expertise was questioned regarding his use of statistics and sudden infant death. It was the failure of another (Dr Williams) to disclose some bacteriological results that also helped secure the conviction in the first place.
- Struck off the GMC register; reinstated upon appeal.

Dr Rodney Ledward

- Gynaecologist (Southeast England) struck off by the GMC (guilty of negligence in 13 operations).
- The inquiry (Ritchie Report, 2000) found there had been a climate of fear and intimidation preventing nurses and junior doctors from telling tales in case they lost their jobs.
- Recommendation was that each trust develop a list of *untoward non-clinical events* that trigger an incident report/identification.
- Dr Ledward died in 2000 (59 women alleged that they were raped or sexually assaulted by him).
- The Public Interest Disclosure Act (1988) has been extended to protect the whistleblower from victimisation (Dimond 2013: 185).

Nurse Beverley Allitt

- Beverley Allitt was given 13 life sentences in 1993 for murdering four children, attempting to murder another three and causing grievous bodily harm with intent to a further six at Grantham and Kesteven hospital in Lincolnshire.
- The former nurse was diagnosed as suffering from Munchausen's syndrome by proxy when she carried out the attacks between 1991 and 1993.
- Now 46 years old, she is held at the Rampton high-security hospital in Nottingham.
- Allitt murdered the four children by injecting them with high doses of insulin.
- Clothier Report 1992 recommendations: changes to occupational health, disclosure and CRB.
- The Children Act 2004 provides the legal framework for reforming Children's Services. The main aim of this legislation is to ensure that children are healthy, safe and able to learn. It is thought that through effective safeguarding of children and cooperation between agencies and families that babies and children will be protected.

Dr Leonard Arthur

- Tried for the attempted murder of baby John Pearson.
- The case brought attention to the dilemmas facing doctors while treating severely disabled babies.
- Mr Justice Farquharson presided, November 1981.
- The outcome of the trial confirmed that 'nursing care only' is an acceptable form of treatment.
- The administration of a drug (pain relief) is not an offence, even if it accelerates death.
- Sir Thomas Hetherington (Director of Public Prosecutions) identified that the decision to prosecute Dr Arthur was the most difficult of his career.
- A good debate regarding this case can be found in de Cruz and McNaughton (1989).

Paul Beland (midwife)

Professional accountability is demonstrated in the case of Paul Beland (NMC Hearing 2 November 2007). In 2004 Paul was suspended from practice for failing to have vital equipment, leaving before care was completed during a home confinement and failing to document. Paul Beland conducted a home birth during an NHS trust suspended home birth service, without informing the supervisor of midwives. He did not take emergency equipment, left the patient before care was completed and failed to complete records. He was found guilty by the NMC.

Appendix 3: NMC principles of good record keeping (NMC, 2009a: 4–5)

1. Handwriting should be legible.
2. All entries to records should be signed. In the case of written records, the person's name and job title should be printed alongside the first entry.
3. In line with local policy, you should put the date and time on all records. This should be in real time and chronological order and be as close to the actual time as possible.
4. Your records should be accurate and recorded in such a way that the meaning is clear.
5. Records should be factual and not include jargon, meaningless phrases or irrelevance or speculation.
6. You should use your professional judgement to decide what is relevant and what should be recorded.
7. You should record details of any assessments and reviews undertaken and provide clear evidence of the arrangements you have made for future and ongoing care. This should also include details of information given about care and treatment.
8. Records should identify any risks or problems that have arisen and show the action taken to deal with them.
9. You have a duty to communicate fully and effectively with your colleagues, ensuring that they have all the information they need about the people in your care.
10. You must not alter or destroy any records without being authorised to do so.
11. In the unlikely event that you need to alter your own or another healthcare professional's records you must give your name and job title, and sign and date the original documentation. You should make sure that the alterations that you make, and the original record, are clear and auditable.
12. Where appropriate, the person in your care, or their carer, should be involved in the record-keeping process.
13. The language that you use should be easily understood by the people in your care.
14. Records should be readable when photocopied or scanned.
15. You should not use coded expressions of sarcasm or humorous abbreviations to describe the people in your care.
16. You should not falsify records.

Confidentiality

17. You need to be fully aware of the legal requirements regarding confidentiality and ensure your practice is in line with national and local policies.
18. You should be aware of the rules governing confidentiality in respect of the supply and use of data for secondary purposes.
19. You should follow local policy and guidelines when using records for research purposes.
20. You should not discuss the people in your care in places where you might be overheard. Nor should you leave records, either on paper or on computer screens, where they might be seen by unauthorised staff or members of the public.

21. You should not take or keep photographs of any person, or their family, that are not clinically relevant.

Access

22. People in your care should be told information on their health records may be seen by other people or agencies involved in their care.
23. People in your care have a right to ask to see their own health records. You should be aware of your local policy and be able to explain it to the person.
24. People in your care have the right to ask for their information to be withheld from you or other health professionals. You must respect that right unless withholding such information would cause serious harm to that person or others.
25. If you have any problems relating to access or record-keeping, such as missing records or problems accessing records, and you cannot sort out the problem yourself, you should report the matter to someone in authority. You should keep a record that you have done so.
26. You should not access the records of any person, or their family, to find out personal information that is not relevant to their care.

Disclosure

27. Information that can identify a person in your care must not be used or disclosed for purposes other than healthcare without the individual's explicit consent. However, you can release this information if the law requires it, or where there is a wider public interest.
28. Under common law, you are allowed to disclose information if it will help prevent, detect, investigate or punish serious crime or if it will prevent abuse or serious harm to others.

Information systems

29. You should be aware of, and know how to use, the information systems and tools that are available to you in your practice.
30. Smartcards or passwords to access information systems must not be shared. Similarly, do not leave systems open to access when you have finished using them.

Glossary

Abortion	The termination of pregnancy whereby the intention is to ensure that the fetus is not alive and before 24 weeks' gestation.
Accountability	Being answerable to someone for something one has done or not done.
Adverse drug event (ADE)	Wrong route drug error.
Advocate (1)	A person who pleads for another during legal proceedings. May be appointed and may or may not be paid.
Advocate (2)	From a healthcare point of view, a healthcare practitioner who presents the patient's point of view (especially when they are unable to do so themselves).
Affidavit	A statement given under oath, in the presence of a solicitor. A sworn statement.
Altruistic	Unselfish, to benefit somebody else while incurring a 'cost' to oneself.
Assault	A threat of unlawful contact.
Battery	Unlawful touching.
Bona fida midwife	Midwife who registered under the Midwives Act 1902.
Certified midwife	A midwife who holds a certificate from the CMB entitling her to practise.
Clitoral reconstruction	A term to describe the exploration for clitoral tissue, subsequent exposure and removal of scar tissue.
Clitoral rejuvenation	Attempts to locate and expose the glans clitoris.
Coroner	A person appointed to hold an inquest into an unexpected death (also a death in unusual circumstances).
Declaration of Geneva	An oath taken at the time of being admitted as a member of the medical profession.
Declaration of Helsinki	Statement of ethical principles to provide guidance regarding medical research involving human subjects. Considerations related to the wellbeing of the human participant take precedence over the interests of science and society.
Declaration of Tokyo (1975)	Guidelines for doctors concerning torture, cruel or inhuman or degrading treatment (imprisonment or detention).

Deinfibulation	Opening of the scar to expose the urethra and vagina.
Doula	A birth partner or supporter who is paid for supporting a woman during labour.
Ethical-based	A formal process of making logical decisions based upon ethical values.
Female genital mutilation	Cutting or female circumcision; a cultural practice of cutting of the female genitalia. Culturally known as female circumcision.
Health administrative body	Established under the Health and Social Care Act 2012.
Hippocratic oath	A sworn oath usually taken by doctors to do no harm.
Local Supervising Authority	Established under the Midwives Act for the purpose of supervision of midwives.
Midwife	A person registered with the Nursing and Midwifery Council to provide care for childbearing women.
Never events	Preventable patient safety incident.
Plaintiff	The old term for a claimant in a civil court case.
Professional misconduct	Unworthy conduct of a midwife.
Reinfibulation	Re-stitching of interoitus, mutilation of the female genitalia.
Surrogacy	Whereby one woman (or surrogate) becomes pregnant with the intention of handing over the baby to the commissioning individual or couple.
Termination of pregnancy	The deliberate induction of labour to terminate the pregnancy (regardless of gestation).
Tort	A civil wrongdoing, for example negligence, trespass to person, breach of statutory duty.
Torture	Deliberate, systematic or wanton infliction of physical or mental suffering by one or more persons acting alone or on the orders of any authority, to force another person to yield information, to make a confession or any other reason.
Ultra vires	Outside the powers given by the law.
Statutory bodies	Organisations created in legislation to regulate or control.
Vicarious liability	The liability of an employer for the wrongdoing by an employee committed in the course of employment.

Bibliography

Ackerman B (2012) Statutory framework for practice. In *Mayes' Midwifery* (14th edition). Baillière Tindall, Edinburgh.

Anderson M (2014) Autonomy: a midwifery revolution, editorial. *Essentially MIDIRS*, Volume 5, Number 6: 5.

Association of Radical Midwives (1993) Report of the spring national meeting, *Midwifery Matters*, Volume 57: 27–28.

Association of Radical Midwives (1995) *Super-Vision: Consensus Conference Proceedings*. ARM, Books for Midwives Press, Hale.

Audit Commission (1997) *First Class Delivery: Improving Maternity Services in England and Wales*. Audit Commission.

Avery G (2013) *Law and Ethics in Nursing and Healthcare: An Introduction*. Sage, London.

Bainbridge J (2005) Can midwives make a difference to women suffering domestic violence? *British Journal of Midwifery*, Volume 13, Number 11: 717.

Bainbridge J (2008) Abortion: sticking with the 24-week limit. *British Journal of Midwifery*, Volume 16, Number 7: 474.

Bainham A (2005) *Children: The Modern Law* (3rd edition). Family Law, Bristol.

Barker K (2012) Promoting supervision of midwifery to women. *British Journal of Midwifery*, Volume 20, Number 6: 454.

Barker K (2013) Reflections on the annual review. *British Journal of Midwifery*, Volume 21, Number 5: 310.

Barnett C (2005) Exploring midwives' attitudes to domestic violence screening. *British Journal of Midwifery*, Volume 13, Number 11: 702–705.

Beake S and Bick D (2007) Maternity services policy: does the rhetoric match the reality? *British Journal of Midwifery*, Volume 15, Number 2: 89–93.

Beauchamp TL and Childress JF (1994) *Principles of Biomedical Ethics* (4th edition). Oxford University Press, Oxford.

Beauchamp TL and Childress JF (2001) *Principles of Biomedical Ethics* (5th edition). Oxford University Press, Oxford.

Beauchamp TL and Childress JF (2009) *Principles of Biomedical Ethics* (6th edition). Oxford University Press, Oxford.

Beauchamp TL and Childress JF (2013) *Principles of Biomedical Ethics* (7th edition). Oxford University Press, Oxford.

Bent AE (1989) The education and practice of midwives in the 20th century. In *Myles Textbook for Midwives* (11th edition). Churchill Livingstone, Edinburgh.

Berg RC and Underland V (2013) The obstetric consequences of female genital mutilation/cutting: a systematic review and meta analysis. *Obstetrics and Gynacology International*, Special Issue.

Berggren V, Yagoub AE, Satti AM, Khalifa MA, Aziz FA and Bergstrom S (2006) Postpartum tightening operations on two delivery wards in Sudan. *British Journal of Midwifery*, Volume 14, Number 7: 407–410.

Bergstrom L, Roberts J, Skillman L and Seidel J (1992) 'You'll feel me touching you, sweetie': vaginal examinations during the second stage of labor. *Birth*, Volume 19: 19–20.

Bick D (2009) Postpartum management of the perineum. *British Journal of Midwifery*, Volume 17, Number 9: 571–577.

Bick D and MacArthur C (1995) Attendance, content and relevance of the six week postnatal examination. *Midwifery*, Volume 11, Number 62: 9–73.

Birth Place Study – National Perinatal Epidemology Unit (2011) *Birthplace in England Study*. Available at www.npeu.ox.ac.uk/birthplace.

Birthplace in England Collaborative Group (BECG) (2011) Perinatal and maternal outcomes by planned place of birth for healthy women with low risk pregnancies: the birthplace in England national prospective cohort study, *British Medical Journal* Volume 343: d7400. Available at www.bmj.com/content/343/bmj.d7400, accessed 29 June 2014.

Birthrights (2013) *Dignity in Childbirth. The Dignity Survey 2013: Women's and Midwives' Experiences of UK Maternity Care*. Available at http://tinyurl.com/o49fgez, accessed 29 June 2014.

Borton T (1970 [2001]) Models of critical reflection. In Rolf G, Freshwater D and Jasper M (eds) *Critical Reflection in Nursing and the Helping Professions*. Palgrave, Basingstoke.

Boyd C and Sellers L (1982) *The British Way of Birth*. Pan Books, London.

Brain M (1994) Foreword. In Dimond B, *Legal Aspects of Midwifery*. Books for Midwives Press, London.

Brazier M (2003) *Medicine, Patients and the Law* (3rd edition). Penguin, London.

Brazier M, Campbell A and Golombok S (1998) *Surrogacy: Review for Health Ministers of Current Arrangements for Payments and Regulation – Report of the Review Team*. Department of Health, London.

British Broadcasting Company (2012) Catholic midwives lose abortion 'conscientious objection' case. Available at www.bbc.co.uk/news/uk-scotland-glasgow-west-17203620, accessed 16 June 2014.

British Broadcasting Company (BBC) (2012) Abortion clinics checks costs million pounds. Available at www.bbc.co.uk/news/health-17620641, accessed 10 February 2015.

British Broadcasting Corporation (BBC) (2014) Surrogate jailed. Available at www.bbc.news/uk-england-devon-27868511, accessed 16 June 2014.

British Medical Association (2007) *The Law and Ethics of Abortion, BMA Views*. BMA. London.

British Medical Association (2011) *Female Genital Mutilation: Caring for Patients and Safeguarding Children*. British Medical Association, London.

British Pregnancy Advisory Service (2006) at www.bpas.org, accessed 16 June 2014.

Browne KD, Davies C and Stratton P (eds) (1988) *Early Prediction of Child Abuse*. Wiley & Sons. Chichester.

Browne KD (2002) *Early Prediction and Prevention of Child Abuse: A Handbook*. Wiley, Chichester.

Buka P (2008) *Patient's Rights, Law and Ethics for Nurses, A Practical Guide*. Hodder Arnold, London.

Caldwell K, Henshaw L and Taylor G (2005) Developing a framework for critiquing health research. *Journal of Health, Social and Environmental Issues*, Volume 6, Number 1: 45–53.

Cameron J and Rawlings-Anderson K (2001) Female circumcision and episiotomy: both mutilation? *British Journal of Midwifery*, Volume 9, Number 3: 137–142.

Campbell AV (1984 [2000]) Moral dilemmas in medicine. In Jones SR, *Ethics in Midwifery*. Moseby, London.

Capstick B (2004) The future of clinical negligence litigation? *British Medical Journal*, Volume 328: 457–459.

Cardale P (1990) Breaking away. *Nursing Times*, Volume 86, Number 28: 68–69.

Care Quality Commission (2011 [2014]) Investigation Report: Barking, Havering and Redbridge University Hospitals NHS Trust. Queens Hospital. Kind George Hospital. *BJM*, Volume 22, Number 1: 52.

Carr C (2012) *Unlocking Medical Law*. Routledge, Oxford.

Central Midwives Board (1965) *Report of the Work of the Central Midwives Board, Year End March 31st 1965*. CMB, London.

Central Midwives Board (1975) *Report of the Work of the Central Midwives Board Year End 31st March 1975*. CMB, London.

Central Midwives Board (1981) *Report of the Work of the Board*. CMB, London.

Central Midwives Board (1983) *Evolution to Devolution, 1902–1983*. CMB, London.

Centre for Maternal and Child Enquiries (2011) Saving mothers' lives: reviewing maternal deaths to make childhood safer: 2006–2008. The eighth report on confidential enquiries into maternal deaths in the United Kingdom. *British Journal of Obstetrics and Gynaecology*, Volume 118 (Supplement 1): 1–203.

Charity JL and Ord BA (2000) Ethical dilemmas in midwifery practice. In Fraser D (ed.) *Professional Studies for Midwifery Practice*. Churchill Livingstone, London.

Churchill H and Benbow A (2000) Informed choice in maternity services. *British Journal of Midwifery*, Volume 8, Number 1: 41

Clarke EJ (1993) The Children Act 1989: implications for midwifery. *British Journal of Midwifery*, Volume 1, Number 1: 26–30.

Clarke EJ (2009) Introduction of e-learning into the midwifery curriculum. *British Journal of Midwifery*, Volume 17, Number 7: 432–437.

Clarke EJ (2013) FGM: legal aspects. Presented at the British Journal of Midwives, study days in Cardiff, Leeds and Manchester.

Clarke EJ (2014) FGM underground: mind the gap. Presented at REPLACE 2 Conference.

Clarke R (2004) Midwifery autonomy and the code of professional conduct: an unethical combination? In Frith L and Draper H (eds) *Ethics and Midwifery*, Books for Midwives, Elsevier, London.

Clement S (1994) Unwanted vaginal examinations. *British Journal of Midwifery*, Volume 2, Number 8: 368–370.

Cluett ER and Bluff R (2000) *Principles and Practice of Research in Midwifery*. Harcourt, London.

Cluett ER and Burns E (2009) Immersion in water in labour and birth. *Cochrane Database of Systemic Reviews*, Volume 2: CD000111.

Confidential Enquiries into Maternal Death (CEMM) 1952–2003.

Confidential Enquiries into Stillbirth and Infant Deaths (CESDI) 1992–2003.

Confidential Enquiry into Maternal and Child Health (2004) Why mothers die (2000–2002) 6th Report.

Confidential Enquiry into Maternal and Child Health (2007) Why mothers die (2003–2005) 7th Report.

Confidential Enquiry into Maternal and Child Health (2007) Why mothers die (2006–2008) 8th Report.

Cooper IG (2000) Critical risk management. In Fraser D (ed) *Professional Studies for Midwifery Practice*. Churchill Livingstone, London.

Cooper TJ (2001) Informed consent is a primary requisite of quality care. *British Journal of Midwifery*, Volume 9, Number 11: 42–45.

Council for Healthcare Regulatory Excellence (2012) *Strategic Review of the Nursing and Midwifery Council*. CHRE, London. Interim Report.

Court Reporter (2011, 24 February) Midwife punished for lack of care to high-risk patient. *Banbury Guardian*: 1, 4.

Coventry Safeguarding Children Board (2013) Serious case review re Daniel Pelka. Coventry LSCB.

Coventry Telegraph (2012) Mum and Baby die days after birth. Coventry Telegraph Friday January 20th, 2012.

Coventry University (2004) Midwifery undergraduate curriculum. Coventry University.

Cronk M and Flint C (1989) *Community Midwifery: A Practical Guide*. Heinemann, London.

Crown Prosecution Service (2012) *Female Genital Mutilation Legal Guidance*. CPS, London.

Crown Prosecution Service (2014) *Strategy to Eliminate FGM*. CPS, London.

Cumming I (2013, 6 February) Health Education England statement on Francis Inquiry. Press statement.

Cummings J and Bennett V (2012) *Compassion in Practice, Six Cs*. Department of Health, London.

Cutner LP (1985) Female genital mutilation. *Obstetrical Gynaecological Survey*, Volume 40, Number 7: 437–443.

Dabrowski R (2012) Facing the future: what will the NHS look like under Hunt? *Midwives*, Volume 6: 38–41.

Dabrowski R (2013) Catholics appeal abortion decision. Available at www.rcm.org.uk/midiwves/news/catholics-appeal-abortion-decision, accessed 20 June 2014.

Dahlen H, Downe S, Duff M and Gyte G (2014) Vaginal examination during normal labour: routine examination or routine intervention? *International Journal of Childbirth*, Volume 3, Number 3: 142–152.

Daily Mail (2010) Midwife sliced off newborn baby's finger as she tried to cut the umbilical cord. Available at www.dailymail.co.uk/news/article-1280819, accessed 26 May 2010.

Davidson S and Raynor M (2012) Supervised practice: a midwife's reflective journey. *The Practising Midwife*, September: 34–36.

Davis J (2005) Doctors should be allowed to offer patients a simplified form of consent. *British Medical Journal*, Volume 331: 925.

de Cruz and McNaughton (1989) *By What Right? Studies in Medicine and the Law*. Penrhos Publications, Staffordshire.

Department of Constitutional Affairs (2007) *The Mental Capacity Act 2005: Code of Practice*. The Stationery Office, London.

Department of Health (1989) *Working for Patients*. HMSO, London.

Department of Health (1991) *Report on Confidential Enquiries into Maternal Deaths (1985–1987)*. HMSO, London.

Department of Health (1994) *Report on Confidential Enquiries into Maternal Deaths (1988–1990)*. HMSO, London.

Department of Health (1996) *Report on Confidential Enquiries into Maternal Deaths (1991–1993)*. HMSO, London.

Department of Health (1998) *Why Mothers Die: Report on Confidential Enquiries into Maternal Deaths in United Kingdom (1994–1996)*. HMSO, London.

Department of Health (2000) *No Secrets: Guidance on Developing and Implementing Multi-agency Policies and Procedures to Protect Vulnerable Adults from Abuse*. Department of Health, London.

Department of Health (2001a) *12 Key Points on Consent: The Law in England*. Department of Health, London.

Department of Health (2001b) *New Clinical Compensation Scheme for the NHS*. Department of Health, London.

Department of Health (2001c) *Modernising Regulation in the Health Professions*. Department of Health, London.

Department of Health (2001d) *Why Mothers Die: 5th Report on Confidential Enquiries into Maternal Deaths in United Kingdom (1997–1999)*. HMSO, London.

Department of Health (2002) *The Children Act Report 2001*. Department of Health, London.

Department of Health (2003a) *The Children Act Report 2002*. Department of Health, London.

Department of Health (2003b) *Consultation Document: DOH (2003) Making Amends: A Consultation Paper Setting Out Proposals for Reforming the Approach to Clinical Negligence in the NHS*. Department of Health, London. Available at www.doh.gov.uk/makingamends, accessed 30 May 2014.

Department of Health (2003c) *Reference Guide to Consent for Examination or Treatment* (2nd edition). Department of Health, London.

Department of Health (2004a) *The Children Act Report 2003*. Department of Health, London.

Department of Health (2004b) *The Chief Nursing Officer's Review of the Nursing, Midwifery and Health Visiting Contribution to Vulnerable Children and Young People*. Department of Health, London.

Department of Health (2004c) *Choosing Health: Making Healthy Choices Easier*. Department of Health, London.

Department of Health (2006) *Integrated Governance Handbook. A Handbook of Non-executives in Healthcare Organisations*. Department of Health, London. Available at http://webarchive.nationalarchives.gov.uk/+/www.dh.gov.uk/prod_consum_dh/groups/dh_digitalassets/@dh/@en/documents/digitalasset/dh_4129615.pdf, accessed 1 March 2015.

Department of Health (2007a) *Maternity Matters: Choice, Access and Continuity of Care in a Safe Service*. Department of Health, London.

Department of Health (2007b) *Trust Assurance and Safety: The Regulation of Health Professionals in the 21st Century*. Department of Health. London. Available at www.gov.uk/government/uploads/system/uploads/attachment_data/file/228847/7013.pdf

Department of Health (2009) *Delivering High Quality Midwifery Care: The Priorities, Opportunities and Challenges for Midwives*. Department of Health, London.

Department of Health (2010a) *Equity and Excellence: Liberating the NHS*. Department of Health, London.

Department of Health (2010b) *Guidelines for Consent*. Department of Health, London.

Department of Health (2010c) *Midwifery 2020: Delivering Expectations, Midwifery 2020 Programme*. Available at www.midiwfery2020.org, accessed 13 November 2013.

Department of Health (2010d) *The Munro Review of Child Protection: Part 1. A Systems Analysis*. Department of Health, London.

Department of Health (2010e) *What To Do if You are Worried a Child is Being Abused Based Upon Every Child Matters*. Available at www.dcsf.gov.uk/everychildmatters.

Department of Health (2011a) *Abortion Statistics in England and Wales*. Available at www.gov.uk/government/statistics/abortion-statistics-england-and-wales-2011, accessed 30 May 2014.

Department of Health (2011b) *The Never Events Policy Framework. An Update to the Never Events Policy*. Department of Health/Patient Safety, London.

Department of Health (2011c) *Enabling Excellence: Autonomy and Accountability for Healthcare Workers, Social Workers and Social Care Workers*. Department of Health, London. Available at www.gov.uk/government/uploads/system/uploads/attachment_data/file/216581/dh_124363.pdf.

Department of Health (2012a) *Compassion in Practice: Our Vision and Strategy*. Available at www.england.nhs.uk/nursingvision, accessed 30 May 2014.

Department of Health (2012b) *The NHS Constitution*. Department of Health, London.

Department of Health (2012c) Female Genital Mutilation CEM/CMO/2012/11, Gateway: 17675. Department of Health, London.

Department of Health (2012d) Abortion statistics, England & Wales: 2011. Press release. Available at www.gov.uk/government/news/abortion-statistics-england-wales-2011, accessed 16 February 2015.

Department of Health (2013) *The Never Events List; 2013/14 Update*. NHS England, Patient Safety Domain Team, London.

Department of Health (2014) *The Duty of Candour*. Department of Health, London.

Department of Health, Expert Maternity Group (1993) *Changing Childbirth*. HMSO, London.

Department of Health & Social Services (1984) *Report of the Committee of Inquiry into Human Fertilisation and Embryology (Warnock Report)*. HMSO, London.

Dimond B (1994) *Legal Aspects of Midwifery*. Books for Midwives Press, London.

Dimond B (2002) *Legal Aspects of Midwifery* (2nd edition) Books for Midwives Press, London.

Dimond B (2003) NHS redress scheme: clinical negligence compensation. *British Journal of Midwifery*, Volume 11, Number 9: 569–572

Dimond B (2004a) Law and the midwife. In Henderson C and Macdonald S (eds) *Mayes' Midwifery: A Textbook for Midwives*. Bailliere Tindall, London.

Dimond B (2004b) Abortion and the girl under 16 years old. *British Journal of Midwifery*, Volume 12, Number 8: 517.

Dimond B (2006a) *Legal Aspects of Midwifery* (3rd edition). Books for Midwives, London.

Dimond B (2006b) Termination of pregnancy. In *Legal Aspects of Midwifery* (3rd edition). Books for Midwives, London.

Dimond B (2008a) *Legal Aspects of Nursing* (3rd edition). Longman, Harlow.

Dimond B (2008b) *The Legal Aspects of Mental Capacity*. Blackwell Publishers, Oxford.

Dimond B (2013) *Legal Aspects of Midwifery* (4th edition). Longman, Harlow.

Donnison J (1977) *Midwives and Medical Men: A History of the Struggle for the Control of Childbirth*. Historic Publications, London.

Donnison J (1988) *Midwives and Medical Men* (2nd edition). Historical Publications Limited, London.

Dorkenoo E (1994) *Cutting the Rose, Female Genital Mutilation: The Practice and Its Prevention*. Minority rights Publications, London.

Dorkenoo E (1997) The wound that never heals. *Healthlines*, December–January: 26

Downe S (1994) Future midwifery supervision: midwifery supervision working party. *Midwifery Matters*, Volume 60: 25.

Driscoll J (1994) Reflective practice for practise. *Senior Nurse*, Volume 13, Number 7: 47–50.

Driscoll J (2000) *Practising Clinical Supervision*. Bailliere Tindall, Edinburgh.

Driscoll J (2007 [2010]) Practising clinical supervision: a reflective approach for healthcare professionals. In Howatson-Jones L (2010) *Reflective Practice in Nursing*. Learning Matters, London.

Duerden J (1995) Audit of midwifery supervision. In Association of Radical Midwives, *Super-Vision, Consensus Conference Proceedings*. ARM, Books for Midwives Press, Hale.

Duerden J (1996) An example of one audit and general issues concerning audit. In Kirkham M (ed) *Supervision of Midwives*, Books for Midwives Press, London.

Duerden J (2002) Supervision at the beginning of a new century. In Mander R and Fleming V (eds) *Failure to Progress*. Routledge, London.

Dyer O (1993) Gynaecologist struck off over female circumcision. *British Medical Journal*, Volume 307: 1441–1442.

Dyer O (2002) Gynaecologist is struck off for sterilising women without their consent. *British Medical Journal*, Volume 325: 1260.

Dyer C (2002) Paediatricians did not have duty of care to patient's mother. *British Medical Journal*, Volume 352: 1321

Edwards A (2008) Place of birth: can 'Maternity Matters' really deliver choice? *British Journal of Midwifery*, Volume 16, Number 12: 771–775.

Edwards N and Kirkham M (2013) Birth without midwife: a literature review. *MIDIRS Midwifery Digest*, Volume 23, Number 1: 7–16.

El Dareer AAR (1982) *Woman, Why do You Weep? Circumcision and its Consequences*. Zed Books, London.

El Dareer AAR (1983) Complications of female circumcision in the Sudan. *Tropical Doctor*, Volume 3: 131–133.

Enkin M, Keirse MJNC and Chalmers I (1989) *A Guide to Effective Care in Pregnancy and Childbirth*. Oxford medical publications, Oxford.

Ethics Research Center (2009) Definitions of values. www.ethics.org.

Ethics Research Center (2012) Definitions of values. Available at www.ethics.org/resource/definitions-values, accessed 14 February 2015.

European Economic Community (EEC) Midwives Directives 1980. European Union Directive 2005/36/EC/article 4.

European Institute for Gender Equality (2013) *Female Genital Mutilation in the European Union and Croatia Report*. EIGE, Belgium.

Farooqui O (1997) Female circumcision: a fair cut for women? *The British Journal of Family Planning*, Volume 23: 96–100.

Farrer M (1975) Midwife supervisor's role causes utter confusion. *Nursing Mirror*, 20 November: 35

Faulkner J (2005) RCM Ethics Advisory Committee: who are we and what do we do? *RCM Midwives*, Volume 8, Number 9: 364.

Female Genital Mutilation National Clinical Group (FGM NCG) (2012) Clinical standards for FGM services. Available at http://fgmnationalgroup.org, accessed 26 June 2013.

Ferguson P (1987) Midwives and conscientious objection. *Midwives*, Volume 110, Number 1310: 53–54.

Flemming Report (2013) *Confidential Inquiry into Premature Deaths of People with Learning Disabilities (CIPOLD)*. Department of Health, London.

Flint C (1986) *Sensitive Midwifery*. Heinemann, London.

Flint C (1991) Continuity of care provided by a team of midwives: the Know Your Midwife scheme. In Robinson S and Thompson A (eds) *Midwives, Research and Childbirth*, Volume II. Chapman and Hall, London.

Flint C (1993) Big sister is watching you. *Nursing Times*, Volume 89, Number 46: 66–67.

Floyd L (1993) Making home births safe for midwives. *Research and the Midwife Conference Proceedings*, 1993: 2–111.

Foundation for Women's Health Research and Development (FORWARD) (2004) North East London Doctor struck off GMC register. *FORWARD Newsletter*. www.forward.org.uk.

Frame S and North J (1996) Will history repeat itself? *ARM Midwifery Matters*, Volume 68: 3–4.

Francis Report (2010) *Independent Inquiry Report (2005–2009) into Mid Staffordshire NHS Foundation Trust*. Department of Health. Available at http://webarchive.nationalarchives.gov.uk/20130107105354/http:/www.dh.gov.uk/en/Publicationsandstatistics/Publications/PublicationsPolicyAndGuidance/DH_113018, accessed 19 February 2013.

Francis Report (2013) *Report of the Mid Staffordshire NHS Foundation Trust Public Inquiry*. Available at www.midstaffspublicinquiry.com, accessed 19 February 2013.

Fraser D (ed.) (2000) *Professional Studies for Midwifery Practice*. Churchill Livingstone. London.

Fraser D and Cooper MA (eds) (2003) *Myles Textbook for Midwives* (12th edition). Churchill Livingstone, London.

Fraser J (1997) *Child Protection, A Guide for Midwives*. Books for Midwives, Edinburgh.

Fraser J and Nolan M (2004) *Child Protection, a Guide for Midwives* (2nd edition). Books for Midwives, Edinburgh.

Frith L and Draper H (2004) *Ethics and Midwifery* (2nd edition). Books for Midwives, Edinburgh.

Garcia J, Garforth S and Ayres S (1985) Midwives confined? Labour wards policies and routines. Research and the Midwife Conference Proceedings, University of Manchester, 22 November 1985.

Gardner S (2012a) Informed decision making. *British Journal of Midwifery*, Volume 20, Number 5: 308.

Gardner S (2012b) Safeguarding against FGM: everyone's issue. *British Journal of Midwifery*, Volume 20, Number 6: 384.

Gardner S (2012c) Getting out there and making a difference. *British Journal of Midwifery*, Volume 20, Number 7: 460.

General Medical Council (2006) *Good Medical Practice*. GMC, London. Available at www.gmc-uk.org/guidance, accessed 29 March 2012.

General Medical Council (2008) *Consent: Patient's and Doctors Making Decisions Together*. GMC, London.

General Medical Council (2009) *Confidentiality*. GMC, London.

General Medical Council (2012) *Leadership and Management for All Doctors*. GMC, London.

General Medical Council (2013) *Intimate Examinations and Chaperones*. GMC, London.

Gibbs G (1988 [2001]) An educators framework for reflection. In Rolfe G, Freshwater D and Jasper M (eds) *Critical Reflection for Nursing*, Palgrave, Basingstoke.

Gillon R (1985) *Philosophical Medical Ethics*. Wiley, Chichester.

Gillon R (1994) The four principles revisited: a reappraisal. In Gillon R and Lloyd A, *Principles of Heathcare Ethics*. Wiley, Chichester.

Gillon R (2003) *Philosophical Medical Ethics* (2nd edition). Wiley, Chichester.

Gillon R and Lloyd A (1994) *Principles of Healthcare Ethics*. Wiley, Chichester.

Green C (2008) Pethidine use: the ethics. *The Practising Midwife*, Volume 11, Number 9: 14–17.

Griffith R (2009a) Maternity care pathways and the law. *British Journal of Midwifery*, Volume 17, Number 5: 324–325.

Griffith R (2009b) Medicines and the law – patient group directions. *British Journal of Midwifery*, Volume 17, Number 7: 460–461.

Griffith R (2012a) Protection and support for midwives who report poor practice threatened. *British Journal of Midwifery*, Volume 20, Number 2: 144–145.

Griffith R (2012b) Accountability in midwifery practice: answerable to society. *British Journal of Midwifery*, Volume 20, Number 7: 525–526.

Griffith R and Tengnah C (2008) *Law and Professional Issues in Nursing*. Learning Matters, Exeter.

Griffith R, Tengnah C and Patel C (2010) *Law and Professional Issues in Midwifery*. Learning Matters, Exeter.

Hamilton C and Nash L (2008) Legislation and the midwife. In Peate I and Hamilton C (eds) *Becoming a Midwife in the 21st Century*, Wiley, Chichester.

Harris J (1985) *Ethical Commandments in The Value of Life: An Introduction to Medical Ethics*. Routledge, London.

Harris J (1995) *The Value of Life: An Introduction to Medical Ethics*. Routlege, London.

Harris J (2005) Choose different types of consent. *British Medical Journal*, Volume 331: 925.

Health and Care Professions Council (2013) *Code of Conduct*. HCPC, London.

Health and Social Care Information Centre (2011) NHS maternity statistics April 2010–March 2011. Available at: http://www.hscic.gov.uk, accessed 26 May 2015.

Health and Social Care Information Centre (HSCIC) (2014a) Nearly 500 new cases identified. BBC News, 16 October. Available at www.bbc.co.uk/news/uk-29642997, accessed 22 October 2014.

Health and Social Care Information Centre (HSCIC) (2014b) Female Genital Mutilation Figures Published. Available at http://www.hscic.gov.uk/article/5147/FGM, accessed 7 November 2014.

Health Education England (2013, 6 February) Health Education England press statement on Francis Inquiry. Available at www.hee.nhs.uk, accessed 27 May 2014.

Health Professions Council (2008a) *Standards of Conduct, Performance and Ethics*. HPC, London.

Health Professions Council (2008b) *Standards of Proficiency*. HPC, London. Available at www.hpc-uk.org/publications/standards, accessed 17 May 2012.

Health Professions Council (2009) *Guidance on Conduct and Ethics for Students*. HPC, London.

Health Professions Council (2010) *Professional Conduct*. HPC, London.

Henderson C (1995) Why have a supplement on the statutory bodies? *British Journal of Midwifery*, Volume 3, Number 4: 201–202.

Henderson C and Macdonald S (eds) (2004) *Mayes' Midwifery* (13th edition). Stanley Thomas (Publishers) Ltd, London.

HM Government (2010) *Working Together to Safeguard Children: A Guide to Inter-agency Working to Safeguard and Promote the Welfare of Children*. Department of Health, London.

HM Government (2011) *Multi-agency Practice Guidelines: FGM*. HM Government, London.

HM Government (2014) *Female Genital Mutilation: The Case for a National Action Plan*. Secretary of State for the Home Department, London.

Hollins Martin, C (2007) How can we improve choice provision for childbearing women? *British Journal of Midwifery*, Volume 15, Number 8: 480–484.

Hope T, Savulescu J and Hendrick J (2008) *Medical Ethics and Law: The Core Curriculum* (2nd edition). Churchill Livingstone, China.

Inch S (1982) *Birthrights: A Parents' Guide to Modern Childbirth*. Hutchinson, London.

International Centre for Reproductive Health (IRCH) (2009) *Responding to FGM in Europe: Striking the Right Balance between Prosecution and Prevention*. IRCH, Ghent University, Belgium.

International Confederation of Midwives (1993) Code of midwifery ethics, identified in Vancouver. Updated, reviewed and adopted in Prague – ICM Council Meeting in 2014.

Jackson E (2006) *Surrogacy: Medical Law: Text, Cases and Materials*. Oxford University Press, Oxford.

Jackson S (2002) Reflective conversation pilot project. West Midlands Local Supervising Authority Consortium. *British Journal of Midwifery*, Volume 10, Number 3: 157.

Jenkins R (1995) *The Law and the Midwife*. Blackwell Scientific, Oxford.

Jessiman WC and Stuttaford M (2012) Supervisors of midwives as human rights defenders. *British Journal of Midwifery*, Volume 20, Number 6: 428–431.

JM Consulting (1998a) *The Regulation of Nurses, Midwives and Health Visitors: Invitation to Comment on Issues Raised by the Review of the Nurse, Midwives and Health Visitors Act 1997*. JM Consulting Ltd, Bristol.

JM Consulting (1998b) *Review of the Nurses, Midwives and Health Visitors Act 1997*. JM Consulting Ltd, Bristol.

Johnson AG and Johnson PRV (2007) *Making Sense of Medical Ethics, a Hands on Guide*. Hodder Arnold, London.

Jones SR (2000a) *Ethics in Midwifery* (2nd edition) Mosby, Edinburgh.

Jones SR (2000b) Assisted conception: a right or a dilemma? In Jones SR, *Ethics in Midwifery* (2nd edition). Mosby, Edinburgh.

Jones SR (2000c) Ethical dimensions of the midwife's role. In Jones SR, *Ethics in Midwifery* (2nd edition). Mosby, Edinburgh.

Jones SR (2004) Ethics and the midwife. In Henderson C and Macdonald C (eds) *Mayes' Midwifery: A Textbook for Midwives* (13th edition). Stanley Thomas (Publishers) Ltd, London.

Jones SR (2006) Surrogacy: the legal position and the midwife's duty of care. *British Journal of Midwifery*, Volume 14, Number 5: 256

Jones SR and Jenkins R (2004) *The Law and the Midwife* (2nd edition). Blackwell, Oxford.

Kant I (1949) Fundamental principles of the metaphysics of morals. In *Toward a Moral Horizon*, Pearson, Toronto.

Kant I (1964) Groundwork for the metaphysics of morals. In *Toward a Moral Horizon*. Pearson, Toronto.

Kempe RS and Kempe CH (1978) *Child Abuse: The Developing Child*. Fontana Press, Glasgow.

Kennedy Report (2001) *Bristol Royal Infirmary Inquiry, Chaired by Professor Ian Kennedy* (investigation into paediatric cardiac services 1984–1995). Available at www.bristol-inquiry.org.uk/final_report/report/index.htm.

Kennedy I (1988) *Treat Me Right: Essays in Medical Law and Ethics*. Clarendon Press, Cambridge.

Kennedy I and Grubb A (2000) *Medical Law* (3rd edition). Butterworths, London.

Kenyon C, Hills A, Winter C, Draycott T, Fox R and Siassakos D (2012) Women's perception of the term 'obstetrician'. *British Journal of Midwifery*, Volume 20, Number 7: 477–481.

Kightley R (2007) Delivering choice: where to birth? *British Journal of Midwifery*, Volume 15, Number 8: 475.

Kings Fund (2008) *Safe Births: Everybody's Business*. Kings Fund, London.

Kirby J (2002) 100 years of statutory supervision of midwives. *British Journal of Midwifery*, Volume 10, Number 3: 154–155.

Kirkham M (1989) Midwives and information giving during labour. In *Midwives, Research and Childbirth*, Volume 1. Chapman and Hall, London.

Kirkham (1995) The history of midwifery supervision. In *Super-Vision Consensus Conference Proceedings. Association of Radical Midwives (ARM)*. Books for Midwives Press, Hale.

Kirkham M (ed.) (1996) *Supervision of Midwives*. Books for Midwives Press, Hale.

Kirkham M (ed.) (2004) *Informed Choice in Maternity Care*, Basingstoke, Palgrave.

Kitzinger S and Walters R (1981) *Some Women's Experience of Episiotomy*. National Childbirth Trust, London.

Laming Report (2000) Confidential Inquiry into the Death of Victoria Climbié. Available at: http://webarchive.nationalarchives.gov.uk/20130401151715/http://www.education.gov.uk/publications/eOrderingDownload/CM-5730PDF.pdf

Lancet (2014) *Lancet Special Series on Midwifery: Women Should be in the Heart of Decision Making.* Launched 23 June 2014.

Lawrence C and Yearley C (2008) Regulating the midwifery profession: protecting women or the profession? In Peate I and Hamilton C (eds) *Becoming a Midwife in the 21st Century*, Wiley, Chichester.

Leap N and Hunter B (1993) *The Midwife's Tale.* Scarlett Press, London.

Ledward A (2011) Informed consent: ethical issues for midwifery research. *Evidence Based Midwifery*, Volume 9, Number 1. Available at: www.rcm.org.uk/ebm/ebm-2011/vol-9-issue1/infomed-consent-ethical-issues, accessed 7 March 2011.

Levy V (2004) Informed choice. In Kirkham M (ed) *Informed Choice in Maternity Care*. Palgrave, Basingstoke.

Lewin D, Fearon B, Hemmings V and Johnson G (2005) Informing women during vaginal examinations. *British Journal of Midwifery*, Volume 13, Number 1: 26–29.

Lewis G (ed.) (2004) *Confidential Enquiry into Maternal and Child Health: Why Mothers Die 2000–2002.* RCOG, London.

Lewis G (ed.) (2007) *The Confidential Enquiry into Maternal and Child Health (CEMACH), Saving Mothers' Lives: Reviewing Maternal Deaths to Make Motherhood Safer 2003–2005. The Seventh Report on Confidential Enquiries into Maternal Deaths in the United Kingdom.* CEMACH, London.

Lewison H (1996) Supervision as a public service. In Kirkham M (ed.) *Supervision of Midwives.* Books for Midwives Press, Hale.

Macdonald S and Magill-Cuerden J (2012) *Mayes' Midwifery* (14th edition). Bailliere Tindall, Edinburgh.

Mahran M (1981) Medical dangers of female circumcision. *IPPF Medical Bulletin*, Volume 15, Number 2: 1–3.

Malyon D (1998) Transfusion-free treatment of Jehovah's Witnesses: respecting the autonomous patient's rights. *Journal of Medical Ethics*, 24: 302–307.

Mander R (2011) Saving mothers' lives: the reality or the rhetoric? *MIDIRS Midwifery Digest*, Volume 21, Number 2: 254–258

Mander R and Fleming V (eds) (2009) *Becoming a Midwife*, Routledge, Oxford.

Mannion K (2008) Statutory supervision of midwives. In Peate I and Hamilton C (eds) *Becoming a Midwife in the 21st Century*. Wiley, Chichester.

Mason JK and Laurie GT (eds) (2006a) *Mason and McCall Smith's Law and Medical Ethics* (7th edition). Oxford University Press, Oxford.

Mason JK and Laurie GT (2006b) Termination of pregnancy. In Mason JK and Laurie GT (eds) *Mason and McCall Smith's Law & Medical Ethics*, (7th edition). Oxford University Press, Oxford.

Mazur DJ (2003) Influence of the law on risk and informed consent. *British Medical Journal*, Volume 327: 731–734.

McHale J and Tindle J (2001) *Law and Nursing* (2nd edition). Butterworth Heinemann, Oxford.

McHale J and Tindle J (2007) *Law and Nursing* (3rd edition). Butterworth Heinemann, Oxford.

McHugh N, Edwards N and Leap N (2013) A tale of two supervisors. *Essentially MIDIRS*, Volume 4, Number 5: 40–45.

Medicines and Healthcare products Regulatory Agency (2003) *Supplementary Prescribing*. MHRA, London.

Mellor J (2013) *Parliamentary and Health Service Ombudsman: Midwifery and Supervision Regulation: Recommendations for Change*. PHSO, London.

Mepham B (2005) *Bioethics, an Introduction for the Biosciences*. Oxford University Press, Oxford.

Meyer JHF and Land R (2004) Threshold concepts and troublesome knowledge (2): epistemological considerations and a conceptual framework for teaching and learning. *Higher Education*, Special Issue.

Middle JV and Wee MYK (2009) Informed consent for epidural analgesia in labour: a survey of UK practice. *MIDIRS Midwifery Digest*, Volume 19, Number 3: 375.

Momoh C (ed.) (2005) *Female Genital Mutilation*. Radcliffe, Oxford.

Monitor (2012) Available at www.gov.uk/government/organisations/monitor, accessed 3 March 2012.

Montgomery J (2003) *Health Care Law* (2nd Edition). Oxford University Press, Oxford.

Nakash A and Herdiman J (2007) Surrogacy. *Journal of Obstetrics & Gynaecology*, Volume 27, Number 3: 246–251.

National Commission of Inquiry into the Prevention of Abuse (1996) *Childhood Matters Volume 1*. HMSO, London.

National Health Service (1994) *The Patients Charter: Maternity Services*. Leaflet, Department of Health.

National Health Service (2013) *Putting Patients First and Foremost: The Initial Government's Response to Mid Staffordshire*

NHS Foundation Trust Public Inquiry. Available at: www.gov.uk/government/uploads/system/uploads/attachment_data/file/170701/Patients_First_and_Foremost.pdf, accessed 19 November 2013.

National Health Service Confederation (2013) *Summary of Government's Response to Francis Report.* NHSC, London. Available at www.nhsconfed.org, accessed 9 October 2013.

National Health Service England (2013) *Putting Patients first and foremost.* Department of Health. London.

National Health Service England (2014) *Standardise, Educate, Harmonise: Commissioning the Conditions for Safer Surgery. Report of the NHS England Never Events Taskforce.* Department of Health, London.

National Health Service Executive (2000) *Modernising Regulation: The New Nursing and Midwifery Council.* Department of Health, London.

National Health Service Litigation Authority (2010a) *Fact Sheet.* NHS Litigation Authority.

National Health Service Litigation Authority (2010b) *Clinical Negligence Scheme For Trusts: Maternity.* NHS Litigation Authority, London.

National Health Service Litigation Authority (2011) *Clinical Negligence Scheme for Trusts. Maternity. Clinical Risks Standards. Version 12012/13.* NHS Litigation Authority, London.

National Health Service Litigation Authority (2012) *Ten Years of Maternity Claims.* NHS Litigation Authority, London.

National Health Service Litigation Authority (2012–2013) NHSLA Fact sheet 5: trusts and health authority claims data. NHS Litigation Authority.

National Institute for Health and Clinical Excellence (2007) *Intra Partum Care: Management and Delivery of Care to Women in Labour.* NICE, London.

National Institute for Health and Clinical Excellence (2014) *Antenatal Care.* NICE, London.

National Patient Safety Agency (2010a) *National Framework for Reporting and Learning from Serious Incidents Requiring Investigation.* NPSA, London.

National Patient Safety Agency (2010b) *Seven Steps to Patient Safety, 2004–2009.* NPSA, London.

National Prescribing Centre (2004) *Patient Group Directions: A Practical Guide and Framework of Competencies for all Professionals Using Patient Group Directions.* NPC, London.

Nursing and Midwifery Council (2004) *Midwives Rules and Standards.* NMC, London.

Nursing and Midwifery Council (2005) *Guidelines for Records and Record Keeping.* NMC, London.

Nursing and Midwifery Council (2006a) *A–Z Advice Sheet: Consent.* NMC, London.

Nursing and Midwifery Council (2006b) *Standards for the Preparation and Practice of Supervisors of Midwives.* NMC, London.

Nursing and Midwifery Council (2006c) *Standards of Proficiency for Nurse and Midwife Prescribers.* NMC, London.

Nursing and Midwifery Council (2007a) *NMC Advice Sheet on Record Keeping.* NMC, London.

Nursing and Midwifery Council (2007b) *Overseas Midwives Programme: Standards for Adaption to Midwifery in the UK.* NMC, London.

Nursing and Midwifery Council (2007c) *Standards for the Supervised Practice of Midwives.* NMC, London .

Nursing and Midwifery Council (2008a) *Modern Supervision in Action: A Practical Guide for Midwives.* NMC. London.

Nursing and Midwifery Council (2008b) *Standards to Support Learning and Assessment in Practice.* NMC, London.

Nursing and Midwifery Council (2008c) *Supervision, Support and Safety: Analysis of the 2007–2008 Local Supervising Authority Annual Reports to the Nursing and Midwifery Council.* NMC, London.

Nursing and Midwifery Council (2008d) *The Code: Standards of Conduct, Performance and Ethics for Nurses and Midwives.* NMC, London.

Nursing and Midwifery Council (2008e) *Standards for Medicines Management,* NMC, London.

Nursing and Midwifery Council (2008f) *The PREP Handbook.* NMC, London.

Nursing and Midwifery Council (2009a) *Record Keeping: Guidance for Nurses and Midwives.* NMC, London.

Nursing and Midwifery Council (2009b) *Standards for Pre-registration Midwifery Education.* NMC, London.

Nursing and Midwifery Council (2009c) *Supervision, Support and Safety: Analysis of the 2008–2009 Local Supervising Authorities' Annual Reports to the NMC.* NMC, London.

Nursing and Midwifery Council (2010a) *Midwives Rules and Standards.* NMC, London.

Nursing and Midwifery Council (2010b) *Raising and Escalating Concerns: Guidance for Nurses and Midwives.* NMC, London.

Nursing and Midwifery Council (2010c) *Standards for Competence for Registered Midwives*. NMC, London.

Nursing and Midwifery Council (2010d) *Standards for Medicines Management*. NMC, London.

Nursing and Midwifery Council (2010e) *Supervision, Support and Safety: Analysis of the 2009–2010 LSA Annual Reports to the NMC*. NMC, London.

Nursing and Midwifery Council (2010f) *Supervisors of Midwives: How They Can Help You*. NMC, London.

Nursing and Midwifery Council (2011a) Changes to midwives exemptions. Nursing and Midwifery Council Circular 07/2011, available at www.nmc-uk.org/documents/circulars/2011circulars/nmccircular07-2011-midwives-exemptions.pdf, accessed 17 May 2014.

Nursing and Midwifery Council (2011b) *Supervision, Support and Safety: NMC Quality Assurance of the LSAs 2010–2011*. NMC. London.

Nursing and Midwifery Council (2011c) *The PREP Handbook*. NMC, London.

Nursing and Midwifery Council (2012a) *Midwives Rules and Standards*. NMC, London.

Nursing and Midwifery Council (2012b) Prescribing in pregnancy: the role of independent and supplementary nurse prescribers. Midwifery Council Advice.

Nursing and Midwifery Council (2012c) *Supervision, Support, Safety: Report of the Quality Assurance of the Local Supervising Authorities (LSAs) 2011–2012*. NMC, London.

Nursing and Midwifery Council (2012d) *Supervisors of Midwives: How They Can Help You*. NMC, London. Available at www.nmc-uk.org.

Nursing and Midwifery Council (2012e) *Conscientious Objection by Nurses and Midwives*. Available at http://Tinyurl.com/cp3n2ks, accessed 20 June 2014.

Nursing and Midwifery Council (2013) *Standards for the Supervised Practice of Midwives*. NMC, London.

Nursing and Midwifery Council (2014a) *Hearings*. Available at www.nmc-uk.org/hearings, accessed 13 June 2014.

Nursing and Midwifery Council (2014b) *Immediate Review of Midwifery Regulation*. NMC, London. Available at www.nmc-uk.org/media/Latest-news/Review-of-midwifery-regulation, accessed 13 March 2014.

Nursing and Midwifery Council (2014c) *Standards for the Preparation and Practice of Supervisors of Midwives*. NMC, London. Available at www.nmc-uk.org/Educators/Standards-for-the-education/Standards-for-the-preparation-for-the-supervision-of-midwives, accessed 20 June 2014.

Nursing and Midwifery Council (2014d) *Better Legislation for Better Regulation: The Case for Legislative Reform*. NMC, London.

Nursing and Midwifery Council (2015) *The Code: Standards of Conduct, Performance and Ethics for Nurses and Midwives*. NMC, London.

Parahoo K (1997) *Nursing Research: Principles and Process and Issues*. Macmillan, Basingstoke.

Parliamentary and Health Service Ombudsman (2013) *Midwifery and Supervision Regulation: Recommendations for Change*. PHSO, London.

Pattinson SD (2006) *Medical Law and Ethics*. Sweet and Maxwell, London.

Peat, Marwick, McLintock (1989) *Review of the UKCC and the Four National Boards for Nursing, Midwifery and Health Visiting*. Management Consultants, London.

Perinatal Institute (2012) *Birth Notes, Maternity Notes*. Available at www.pi.nhs.uk, accessed 20 June 2013.

Phipps, J (2012) Statutory supervision: achieving the balance. *British Journal of Midwifery*, Volume 20, Number 10: 736–739.

Popay S (2012) Another questionable procedure for maternity services? The policy of any qualified provider. *RCM Midwives*, Volume 15, Number 2: 42–43.

Powell C (2011) *Safeguarding Children and Young People: A Guide for Nurses and Midwives*, Open University Press, Maidenhead.

Practising Midwife (2010) Editorial, Volume 13, Number 11.

Pringle MK (1978) The needs of children. In *Child Abuse: A Reader and a Sourcebook*. Open University Press, Milton Keynes.

Public Accounts Committee (2014) *Maternity Services in England, Fortieth Report*. Parliament. Available at http://tinyurl.com/ml4bahn, accessed 21 March 2014.

Raynor M, Marshall J and Jackson K (2012) *Midwifery Practice: Critical Illness, Complications and Emergencies Case Book*. McGraw Hill, Maidenhead.

Renfrew M (1983) *Practical Guidance for Midwives Facing Ethical or Moral Dilemmas*. RCM, London.

REPLACE (2012) *FGM Toolkit for Working with Communities*. Available from: www.replacefgm.eu/toolkit, accessed 25 June 2014.

Report on the Committee on Nursing (1972) *Briggs Report*. HMSO, London.

Robinson J (1998) The demand for Caesareans: fact or fiction. *British Journal of Midwifery*, Volume 7, Number 5: 306.

Robinson J (2001a) Consent for emergency Caesareans. *British Journal of Midwifery*, Volume 9, Number 7: 452.

Robinson J (2001b) Intimate examinations: the complexities of consent. *British Journal of Midwifery*, Volume 9, Number 11: 4708–4709.

Rogers C and Yearley C (2013) National survey of supervision of midwives: time for reflection? *British Journal of Midwifery*, Volume 21: 356–363.

Rolfe G, Freshwater D and Jasper M (2001) *Critical Reflection for Nursing and the Helping Professions: A User's Guide*. Basingstoke, Palgrave.

Rosser J (1998) Breaking the rules. *The Practising Midwife*, Volume 1, Number 1: 4.

Rosser J (1999) Struck off: the midwife who obeyed doctor's orders (editorial). *The Practising Midwife*, Volume 2, Number 4: 5.

Roughley G (2007) Professional accountability for student midwives. *British Journal of Midwifery*, Volume 15, Number 7: 43.

Royal College of Anaesthetists (2010) *Best Practice in the Management of Epidural Analgesia in the Hospital Setting*. RCOA, London.

Royal College of Anaesthetists, Royal College of Midwives, Royal College of Obstetricians and Gynaecologists and Royal College of Paediticans and Child (2007) *Safer Childbirth: Minimum Standards for the Organization and Delivery of Care in Labour*. RCOG, London.

Royal College of Midwives (1983) *Practical Guidance for Midwives Facing Ethical or Moral Dilemmas*. RCM, London.

Royal College of Midwives (1987) *Towards a Healthy Nation: A Charter for the Maternity Services*. Policy document.

Royal College of Midwives (1997) *Position Paper No 18: Surrogacy: Defining Motherhood*. RCM, London. Available at www.rcm.org.uk/college/standards-and-practice/positionpapers, accessed 19 October 2008.

Royal College of Midwives (1998) *Position Paper No 21: Female Genital Mutilation*. RCM Welsh Board, Cardiff.

Royal College of Midwives (2011) *State of the Maternity Services Report* 2011. Available at: www.rcm.org.uk/sites/default/files/State%20of%20Maternity%20Services%20report%202011_0.pdf.

Royal College of Midwives (2012a) *Female Genital Mutilation: Report of a Survey on Midwives' Views and Knowledge*. RCM, London. Available at www.rcm.org.uk/sites/default/files/FGM%20Survey%20FINAL_0.pdf, accessed 13 June 2013.

Royal College of Midwives (2012b) *State of Maternity Services Report 2012*. Available at: www.rcm.org.uk/sites/default/files/State%20of%20Maternity%20Services%20report%202012_0.PDF.

Royal College of Midwives (2013a) *Headline News*. *Midwives Issue 6 Nursing and Midwifery Council (2008) The Code: Standards of Conduct, Performance and Ethics for Nurses and Midwives*. NMC, London.

Royal College of Midwives (2013b) *State of Maternity Services Report 2013*. Available at: www.rcm.org.uk/sites/default/files/State%20of%20Maternity%20Services%20report%202013_0.pdf.

Royal College of Midwives (2014) *RCM Support for Statutory Supervision of Midwives*. RCM, London.

Royal College of Midwives, Royal College of Obstetricians and Gynaecologists (2006) *Joint Position Statement Number 1: Immersion in Water during Labour and Birth*. RCM/RCOG, London.

Royal College of Midwives, Royal College of Nursing, Royal College of Obstetricians and Gynaecologists, Equality Now and UNITE (2013) *Tackling FGM in the UK: Intercollegiate Recommendations for Identifying, Recording and Reporting*. Royal College of Midwives, London.

Royal College of Nursing (1994) *Female Genital Mutilation*. RCN, London.

Royal College of Nursing (2006) *FGM: An RCN Educational Resource for Nursing and Midwifery Staff*. RCN, London.

Royal College of Nursing (2015) *Female Genital Mutilation: An RCN Resource for Nursing and Midwifery Practice* (2nd edition). RCN, London.

Royal College of Obstetricians and Gynaecologists (1994) *Legal and Ethical Issues of Court Ordered LSCS*. RCOG, London.

Royal College of Obstetricians and Gynaecologists (1997) *Intimate Examinations: Report of a Working Party*. RCOG, London.

Royal College of Obstetricians and Gynaecologists (2004) *The Care of Women Requesting Induced Abortion: Evidence Based Clinical Guideline Number 7*. RCOG, London.

Royal College of Obstetricians and Gynaecologists (2007) *Safer Childbirth: Minimum Standards for Service Provision and Care in Labour*. RCOG, RCM, RCPCH, RCA (replaces RCM/RCOG *Safer Childbirth*, 1999).

Royal College of Obstetricians and Gynaecologists (2008) *Maternity Dashboards Clinical Performance and Governance Score Card (Good Practice No. 7)*. RCOG, London.

Royal College of Obstetricians and Gynaecologists (2009a) *Female Genital Mutilation and its Management. Green Top Guideline No 53*. RCOG, London.

Royal College of Obstetricians and Gynaecologists (2009b) *Consent Advice No 7: Caesarean Section*. RCOG, London.

Royal College of Obstetricians and Gynaecologists (2010) *Termination of Pregnancy for Fetal Abnormaility in England, Scotland and Wales*. RCOG, London.

Royal College of Obstetricians and Gynaecologists (2015) *Obtaining Valid Consent. Clinical Governance Advice No 6*. RCOG, London.

Rushwan H (1980) Etiologic factors in pelvic inflammatory disease in Sudanese women. *American Journal of Obstetrics and Gynaecology*. 1 December: 877–879.

Schenker JG and Eisenburg VH (1997) Ethical issues relating to reproduction control and women's health. *International Journal of Gynaecology and Obstetrics*, Volume 58: 167–176.

Schneider GW and Snell L (2000) CARE: an approach for teaching ethics in medicine. *Social Science and Medicine* 51:1563–1567. Available at: http://www.UKCEN.net, accessed 28 May 2015.

Schroeder E, Petrou S, Patel N *et al.* (2012) Cost effectiveness of alternative planned places of birth in women at low risk of complications: evidence from the Birthplace in England national prospective cohort study. *British Medical Journal*, Volume 344, Number 7854: 18. Available at http://tinyurl.com/bobl34s, accessed 11 November 2014.

Shandall AA (1967) Circumcision and infibulation of females. *Sudan Medical Journal*, Volume 5, Number 4: 178–212.

Shaw E (1985) Female circumcision. *American Journal of Nursing*, Volume 86, Number 6: 684–687.

Silverton L (2014) RCM headlines: lack of voice in regulation. *Midwives*, Volume 3: 13

Skipworth A (1996) Audit of supervisors in the West Midlands. In Kirkham M (ed.) *Supervision of Midwives*. Books for Midwives Press, Hale.

Sleep J (1983) The West Berkshire Episiotomy Trial. Research and the Midwife Conference Proceedings, University of Manchester, November: 81 (out of print).

Sleep JM, Grant A, Garcia J, Elbourne D, Spencer J and Chalmers I (1984) West Berkshire perineal management trial. *British Medical Journal*, Volume 289: 587–590.

Stake RE (1995) *The Art of Case Study Research*. Sage, London.

Stapleton H, Duerden J and Kirkham M (1998) *Evaluation of the Impact of the Supervision of Midwives on Professional Practice and the Quality of Midwifery Care*. English National Board, London.

Stevenson O (ed.) (1989) *Child Abuse, Public Policy and Professional Practice*, Harvester Wheatsheaf, London.

Stevenson O and Smith J (1983 [1989]) Report on the implementation of section 56 of the Children Act, 1975. In Stevenson O (ed.) *Child Abuse, Public Policy and Professional Practice*, Harvester Wheatsheaf, London

Stewart S (2006) Internet research in midwifery: practical considerations and challenges. *British Journal of Midwifery*, Volume 14, Number 9: 527–529.

Storch JL, Rodney P and Starzomski R (2004) Toward a moral horizon, nursing ethics for leadership and practice. Prentice Hall, Toronto.

Sweet B (1982) *Mayes' Midwifery* (10th edition). Bailliere Tindall, London.

Sweet B (1988) *Mayes' Midwifery* (11th edition). Bailliere Tindall, London.

Sweet B and Tiran D (1997) *Mayes' Midwifery* (12th edition). Bailliere Tindall, London.

Symon A (1997) Consent and choice: the rights of the patients. *British Journal of Midwifery*, Volume 5, Number 5: 256–258.

Symon A (1998) *Litigation, the Views of Midwives and Obstetricians*. Hochland and Hochland, Cheshire.

Symon A (ed.) (2006a) *Risk and Choice in Maternity Care: An International Perspective*. Churchill Livingstone, Philadelphia.

Symon A (2006b) Are we facing a complaints and litigation crisis in the health service? *British Journal of Midwifery*, Volume 14, Number 3: 164.

Symon A (2006c) Midwives must not allow publicity to push then into defensive practice. *British Journal of Midwifery*, Volume 14, Number 9: 542.

Symon A (2006d) Institutional racism and discrimination: are they endemic in the NHS? *British Journal of Midwifery*, Volume 14, Number 6: 366.

Symon A (2009) A critical two minutes. *British Journal of Midwifery*, Volume 17, Number 6: 395.

Symon A (2010) Legal challenges to the NMC's Fitness to Practise decisions. *British Journal of Midwifery*, Volume 18, Number 6: 390–391.

Symon A (2011) Law carry the consensus of people. *British Journal of Midwifery*, Volume 19, Number 3: 193–194.

Symon A (2013) The Nursing and Midwifery Council faces more legal challenges. *British Journal of Midwifery*, Volume 21, Number 6: 449–450.

Tew M (1990) *Safer Childbirth: A Critical History of Maternity Care*. Chapman and Hall, London.

Thomas M and Mayes G (1996) The ENB perspective: preparation of supervisors of midwives for their role. In Kirkham M (ed.) *Supervision of Midwives*. Books for Midwives Press, Hale.

Thompson A (1994) Towards a code of ethics. *Modern Midwife*, January: 27.

Thompson FE (2004) *Mothers and Midwives: The Ethical Journey*. Books for Midwives Press, Edinburgh.

Thompson H (2012) Caesarean section at maternal request: an update. *British Journal of Midwifery*, Volume 20, Number 2: 98–103.

Thompson JB (2004) A human rights framework for midwifery care. *Journal of Midwifery and Women's Health*, Volume 49, Number 3: 175–181.

Thorlby R, Smith J, Williams S and Dayan M (2014) *The Francis Report: One Year On, Response of Acute Trusts in England*. Nuffield Trust, London.

Tingle J and Cribb A (ed.) (2002) *Nursing Law and Ethics* (2nd edition). Blackwell Publishing, Oxford.

Tinsley (2002) Record keeping for dummies: abstracts from 100 years of statutory supervision. *British Journal of Midwifery*, Volume 10, Number 3: 158

Tiran D (1997) The statutory framework and control of practice of midwives in the UK. In *Mayes' Midwifery* (12th edition). Bailliere Tindall, London.

Toft B and Reynolds S (2005) *Learning from Disasters, a Management Approach* (3rd edition). Palgrave, Basingstoke.

Towler J and Bramall J (1986) *Midwives in History and Society*. Croom Helm, London.

UKCC (1983) *Handbook of Midwives Rules* (1st edition). UKKC, London.

UKCC (1986) *Midwives Rules*. UKCC, London.

UKCC (1992) *Parts of the UKCC Register*. UKCC CJR/MW/JK/KC, London.

UKCC (1998) *Midwives Rules and Code of Practice*. UKCC, London.

UKCC (1999) *The Continuing Professional Development Standard*. UKCC, London.

UKCC (2000) *The Practice Standard*. UKCC, London.

UNICEF (1992) *Baby Friendly Initiative, UNICEF*. Available at: www.unicef.org.uk/babyfriendly, accessed 17 May 2012.

UNICEF (2008) UN to sign up to the Interagency statement on the elimination of FGM. Available at: www.unicef.org.uk/fgm, accessed on 17 September 2009.

United Nations (1966) International Covenant on Social, Economic and Cultural Rights. Article 12 at www.ohchr.org/EN/ProfessionalInterest/Pages/CESCR.aspx.

United Nations Convention on the Elimination of all forms of discrimination Against Women (UNEDW) (1981). Available at www.ohchr.org/en/hrbodies/cedaw/pages/cedawindex.aspx, accessed 25 June 2014.

United Nations Convention on the Elimination of all Forms of Discrimination Against Women (UNEDW) (1990). Available at www.ohchr.org/en/hrbodies/cedaw/pages/cedawindex.aspx, accessed 25 June 2014.

United Nations International Convention on Rights of Child (CRC). Available at www.ohchr.org/en/professionalinterest/pages/crc.aspx, accessed 25 June 2014.

Verrals S (1980) *Anatomy and Physiology Applied to Obstetrics* (2nd edition). Pitman Medical, Tunbridge Wells.

Verzin JA (1975) Sequelae of female circumcision. *Tropical Doctor*, Volume 5: 163–169.

Walker RJ (1980) *The English Legal System* (5th edition). Butterworths, London.

Walsh D (2012) *Evidence and Skills for Normal Labour and Birth* (2nd edition). Routledge, Abingdon.

Walton I (1995) Conflicts in supervision of midwives. In Association of Radical Midwives, *Super-vision, Consensus Conference Proceedings*, ARM, Books for Midwives Press, Hale.

Warwick C (2014a) NMC fee rise, members raise concern. *Midwives Magazine*, Volume 5: 17.

Warwick, C (2014b) Wake up call for government. *Midwives Magazine*, Volume 2: 10.

Warwick C (2014c) RCM response to the Mellor report. *Midwives Magazine*, Volume 2: 10.

Wheeler H (2012) *Law, Ethics and Professional Issues for Nursing*. Routledge, London.

White Ribbon Alliance (2012, 2014) Respectful Maternity Care Charter. Available at www.whiteribbonalliance.org/respectfulcare, accessed 16 June 2014.

Whyte A (1989) An act of love, not cruelty. *Community Care*, 7 September: 15–16.

Wilday RJ (1989) Ethics in midwifery. *Midwives Chronicle & Nursing Notes*, June: 176–182.

Williams C (2009) Whistleblowing or escalating concerns? *NMC News*, November: 16–19.

Witz A (1992) *Professions and Patriarchy*. Routledge, London.

Woolf, Lord (1996) *Access to Justice, Final Report*. HMSO, London.

World Health Organization (1981) International code of marketing of breast milk substitutes. Available at: www.who.int/nutrition/publications/code_english.pdf, accessed 12 March 2014.

World Health Organization (1995) Appropriate technology for birth. *Lancet*, Volume 2, Number 8452: 436–437.

World Health Organization (1996) *Female Genital Mutilation. Report of WHO Technical Working Group*. WHO, Geneva.

World Health Organization (1997, 2008) Female genital mutilation definition. Available at www.who.int/reproductivehealth/topics/fgm/overview/en, accessed 29 June 2014.

World Health Organization (2006) Study group on female genital mutilation and obstetric outcome: FGM and obstetric outcome. WHO collaborative prospective study in six African countries. *Lancet*, Volume 367, Number 9525: 1835–1841.

World Health Organization (2008a) Classification of female genital mutilation. Available at: www.who.int/reproductivehealth/topics/fgm/overview/en, accessed 12 March 2014.

World Health Organization (2008b) *Eliminating FGM: An Interagency Statement*. WHO, Switzerland. Available at: http://whqlibdoc.who.int/publications/2008/9789241596442_eng.pdf?ua=1, accessed 29 June 2014.

World Medical Association (1975, 2005, 2006) Declaration of Tokyo, WMA. Available at www.wma.net/en/20activities/10ethics/20tokyo, accessed 29 June 2014.

Worth, J (2006) Back street abortions. *MIDIRS Midwifery Digest*, Volume 16, Number 3: 337–338.

Maternity services relevant reports

The author selects relevant reports for your information (in chronological order).

Ministry of Health (1949) *Report of the Working Party on Midwives*. HMSO, London.

Department of Health and Social Security (1970) *Domiciliary Midwifery and Maternity Bed Needs (Peel Report)*. HMSO, London.

Report on the Committee on Nursing (1972) *Statutory Structure (Briggs Report)*. HMSO, London.

Maternity Services Advisory Committee (1982, 1984, 1985) *Maternity Care in Action, Part 1,2,3*. HMSO, London.

Department of Health (1989) *Working for Patients, Education and Training*. Working Paper 10.

Department of Health (1991) *Patients Charter*. HMSO, London.

House of Commons Health Committee (1992) *Second Report of Maternity Services (Winterton Report)*, Volume 1. Maternity Services House of Commons, London. (Author's note: precursor to the *Changing Childbirth* document.)

RCOG, RCM, and RCGP (1992) *A Framework for Maternity Care: Maternity Care in the New NHS – A Joint Approach*. RCOG, London.

Department of Health (1993) *Changing Childbirth Report Part 1: Report of the Expert Maternity Group (Cumberledge Report)*. Department of Health, London.

Department of Health (1998) *Midwifery: Delivering our Future. Report of the Standing Nursing and Midwifery Advisory Committee (SNMAC)*. Department of Health, London.

Audit Commission (1998) *First Class Delivery: A National Survey of Women's Views of Maternity Care*. NPEU, London.

Kennedy Report (2001) *Bristol Royal Infirmary Inquiry, Chaired by Professor Ian Kennedy* (investigation into paediatric cardiac services 1984–1995). Available at www.bristol-inquiry.org.uk/final_report/report/index.htm.

HM Government (2003) *Every Child Matters*. Green Paper.

CEMACH (2004) *Confidential Enquiry into Maternal and Child Health: Why Mothers Die 2000–2002*. CEMACH, London.

Department of Health (2004) *National Service Framework for Children, Young People and Maternity Services (NSF), Standard 11*. Department of Health, London.

Department of Health (2007) *Maternity Matters: Choice, Access and Continuity of Care in a Safe Service*. Department of Health, London.

Department of Health (2007) *Trust, Assurance and Safety: The Regulation of Health Professionals in the 21st Century*. White Paper.

Department of Health (2008) *High Quality Care for All: NHS Next Stage Review – Final Report (Darzi Report)*. Department of Health, London.

Department of Health (2009) *Delivering High Quality Midwifery Care: The Priorities, Opportunities and Challenges for Midwives*. Department of Health, London.

Department of Health (2010) *Midwifery 2020: Delivering Expectations*. Department of Health, London.

UK Government (2010) *Midwifery 2020: Delivering Expectations, Midwifery 2020 Programme*, London. Available at www.gov.uk/government/uploads/system.

Department of Health (2010) *Getting it Right for Children and Young People, Overcoming Cultural Barriers in the NHS so as to Meet their Needs (Kennedy Report)*. Department of Health, London.

Francis Report (2010) *Independent Inquiry Report (2005–2009) into Mid Staffordshire NHS Foundation Trust*. Department of Health. Available at http://webarchive.nationalarchives.gov.uk/20130107105354/http:/www.dh.gov.uk/en/Publicationsandstatistics/Publications/PublicationsPolicyAndGuidance/DH_113018.

Department of Education (2010) *The Munro Review of Child Protection: Part 1. Systems Analysis (Munro Report)*. Department of Education, London.

Kings Fund (2010) *Safe Births: Everybody's Business. An Independent Inquiry into the Safety of Maternity Services in England*. Kings Fund, Hobbs Ltd, England.

Department of Health (2012) *The Never Events Policy Framework, an Update to the Never Events Policy*. Department of Health, London.

Department of Health (2012) *Compassion in Practice, Nursing, Midwifery and Care Staff: Our Vision and Strategy*. Department of Health, London.

Scottish Executive (2012) *Keeping Childbirth Natural and Dynamic*. Scottish Executive, Edinburgh. Available at www.scotland.gov.uk/topics/health/NHS-Scotland/nursing/naturalchildbirth.

Berwick Report (2013) *A Promise to Learn: A Commitment to Act*. National Advisory Group (NAG) on the Safety of Patients in England. Available at www.gov.uk/government/uploads/system/uploads/attachment_data/file/226703/Berwick_Report.pdf.

Care Quality Commission (2013) *National Findings from the 2013 Survey of Women's Experiences of Maternity Care*. CQC, London. Available at www.cqc.org.uk.

CIPOLD (2013) *Confidential Inquiry into Premature Deaths of People with Learning Disabilities*. Available at www.bris.ac.uk/cipold/reports/executivesummaryeasyread.pdf, accessed 29 June 2014.

NHS England (2013) *The Never Events List; 2013/14 Update*. NHS England, London.

NHS England (2013) *Quality Care For All*, NHS England, London.

Francis Report (2013) *Report of the Mid Staffordshire NHS Foundation Trust Public Inquiry*, Robert Frances. Available at www.midstaffspublicinquiry.com.

Department of Health (2013) *Review into the Quality of Care and Treatment Provided by 14 Hospital Trusts in England (Keogh Report)*. Department of Health, London.

National Audit Office (2013) *Maternity Services in England*. NAO, London.

NHS England (2013) *Putting Patients First (NHS Business Plan)*. NHS England, London.

Royal College of Midwives (2013) *State of Maternity Services Report 2013*. RCM, London.

HM Government (2014) *Independent Review of Healthcare and Social Work in NHS Care Settings (Cavendish Report)*. Department of Health, London.

Cheyne H, Skar S, Paterson A, *et al.* (2014) *Having a Baby in Scotland 2013: Women's Experiences of Maternity Care, Volume 1: National Results*. Available at http://scotland.gov.uk/Publications/2014/01/8489.

House of Commons Public Accounts Committee (2014) *Maternity Services in England, Fortieth Report*. HCPAC, London. Available at http://tinyurl.com/ml4bahn.

Index

Please note that page numbers in italics relate to Tables

of 46, 48; law and healthcare 45; in maternity
care 45–9; and midwifery care 43–52; patients
121; supervisors of midwives as defenders of 48;
universal rights of childbearing women 46; *see also*
Human Rights Act 1998
human rights, cases: *Gillick v West Norfolk & Wisbech
Area Health Authority* (1986) 49–50, 90, 237; *R
(Axon) v Secretary of State for Health* 2006 50; *R v
HFEA (ex parte Blood)* 1999 50, 238; *R v HFEA
(ex parte Evans)* 2005 50; *Warren v HFEA (ex parte
Warren)* 2014 50–1
Human Rights Act 1998: birth environment 145–6;
child protection 123, 127; consent 83; effects
34–5; and European Convention on Human Rights
49; as example of primary legislation 33–5; legal
force 34; midwifery care 49; safeguarding 123;
significance 34; *see also* human rights
Human Rights in Childbirth 27
Hunt, Jeremy 227
Hunter, B 56

implicit consent 78
Inch, S 48, 55
independent and supplementary nurse prescribers
(INP) 113
infant formula manufacturers 18
infants: rights of 143; safeguarding 119–20; *see also*
childbirth; children; fetus
information giving 80, 81–2; antenatal period
89; degree of information to give 91; systems
243; *see also* patient information leaflets (PILs);
record-keeping
informed consent doctrine 81, 87
intention to practise (ItP) 40, 68, 71
International Centre for Reproductive Health (IRCH)
188
International Day of Zero Tolerance for Female
Genital Mutilation 178
inter-professional working 119, 126, 127
intimate care/examinations: capacity to consent 90–1;
vaginal examination every four hours 90–1, 92

Jackson, S 68
Jackson reforms 39
Jessiman, WC 48, 122
JM Consulting Ltd 61, 64
Johnson, AG 23, 24
Johnson, PRV 23, 24
judicial review 32
justice 21, 22

Kant, Immanuel 20
Keirse, MJNC 189
Kempe, CH 119
Kempe, RS 119
Kennedy Report (2001) 44, 261

Kings College London, Gordon museum of pathology
44
Kings Fund 72, 137
Kirby, J 68
Kirkham, M 27, 130, 134
Kitzinger, S 190
Klein, Mark 227

labour: capacity to consent compromised 88–9;
intimate care/examinations, consent for 90–1;
pain relief in 28, 108–9; record-keeping 98; *see
also* birth; childbirth; childbirth rights; delivery;
delivery suite
labour ward coordinator 51–2
Laming Report 2000 122
Lancet 77
Laurie, GT 53, 159
law: case law 36–8, 85, 86; complexity of 32; of
consent 77–8; division into civil and criminal
proceedings 37, 38; enforcement 37; and
healthcare, legal framework 45; *see also* consent;
courts; English legal system; legislative framework
for midwifery; primary legislation; secondary
legislation and statutory instruments
Law Commission 137
Leap, N 56, 130
Ledward, A 25
Ledward, Rodney (doctor) 240–1
legal documents 97
legislative framework for midwifery 40–1, 53–73;
consent to treatment 83–5; control and regulation
of midwives 66–7; Directives 61, 112; effects
of legislation 66; intention to practise 40, 68,
71; misconduct and fitness to practise 68–9;
primary legislation 55–61; primary purpose
of midwifery legislation 53, 54; professional
accountability 68–9; secondary legislation and
statutory instruments (Orders and Regulations)
62–5; *see also* English legal system; law; primary
legislation; secondary legislation and statutory
instruments
legislative framework for midwifery, and specific
statutes: Health Act 1999 61; Henry VIII's Act of
1512 54; Midwives Act 1902, 1918, 1926, 1936
and 1951 33, 40, 56–8; National Health Service
Reorganisation Act 1973 71–2; Nurses, Midwives
and Health Visitors Act 1979, 1992 and 1997 33,
40–1, 58–61
Lewin, D 90
Lewison, H 138
liability and compensation 219
life: beginning of human life 155; right to 145, 239;
sanctity of life principle 155, 157
LIFE (charity organisation) 157
Local Safeguarding Boards (LSBs) 84
Local Safeguarding Children Board (LSCB) 122, 124

9 780415 675253